EVERYDAY EXPOSURE

Sarah Marie Wiebe

EVERYDAY EXPOSURE

Indigenous Mobilization and Environmental Justice in Canada's Chemical Valley

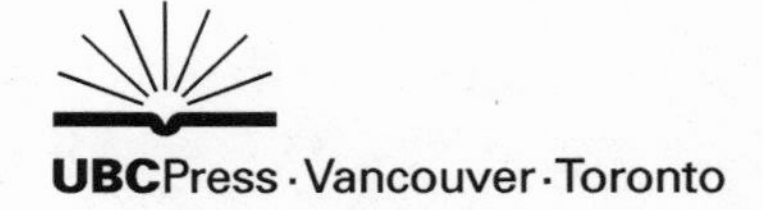

25 24 23 22 21 20 19 18 17 1   5 4 3 2 1

Printed in Canada on FSC-certified ancient-forest-free paper (100% post-consumer recycled) that is processed chlorine- and acid-free.

Library and Archives Canada Cataloguing in Publication

Wiebe, Sarah Marie, author
Everyday exposure : indigenous mobilization and environmental justice in Canada's chemical valley / Sarah Marie Wiebe.

Includes bibliographical references and index.
Issued in print and electronic formats.
ISBN 978-0-7748-3263-2 (hardback). – ISBN 978-0-7748-3264-9 (pbk.). –
ISBN 978-0-7748-3265-6 (pdf). – ISBN 978-0-7748-3266-3 (epub).

1. Aamjiwnaang First Nation. 2. Ojibwa Indians – Health and hygiene – Ontario – Sarnia. 3. Pollution – Political aspects – Ontario – Sarnia. 4. Pollution – Social aspects – Ontario – Sarnia. 5. Human ecology – Ontario – Sarnia. 6. Environmental justice – Ontario – Sarnia. 7. Sarnia (Ont.) – Environmental conditions. I. Title.

GE240.C3W53 2016   304.2089'97333071327   C2016-904117-4
C2016-904118-2

Canada

UBC Press gratefully acknowledges the financial support for our publishing program of the Government of Canada (through the Canada Book Fund), the Canada Council for the Arts, and the British Columbia Arts Council.

This book has been published with the help of a grant from the Canadian Federation for the Humanities and Social Sciences, through the Awards to Scholarly Publications Program, using funds provided by the Social Sciences and Humanities Research Council of Canada.

Printed and bound in Canada by Friesens
Set in Myriad SemiCondensed and Minion by Artegraphica Design Co. Ltd.
Copy editor: Robert Lewis
Proofreader: Helen Godolphin
Cover designer: StepUp Communications
Cover image: Laurence Butet-Roch, *An Eastern Cottonwood, Rooted in Chemical Valley*

UBC Press
The University of British Columbia
2029 West Mall
Vancouver, BC V6T 1Z2
www.ubcpress.ca

To Tashmoo Avenue –
a place of friendship, inspiration, laughter, and light

Miigwetch

Prologue: Lungs of the Earth

Silently sleeping
Smothered in smoke
Shattered scenery
Suffering from smog
Choking lungs
From the dark mist
Swallow the air
Creeping death
Lurks in the background
Unseen to the eyes
Hanging my head
Low to the earth
Cries from the heart
to breathe
to breathe
Ribs ache
Tired and weary
Reaching for the sun
a sun that's faded into clouds
Those clouds surround me
Covered in emptiness and ashes
Snowy tears fall around me
Drowning me in the thick puffs of smoke

Poem by Mckay Swanson,
Aamjiwnaang First Nation,
December 2014

Figure 1
Lungs of the Earth, by Aaron Vincent Elkaim

Contents

Figures and Tables

Figures

Tables

Foreword
A Canadian Tragedy

JAMES TULLY

Every once in a while, an outstanding work of scholarship comes along that transforms the way a seemingly intractable injustice is seen and, in so doing, also transforms the way it should be approached and addressed by all concerned. Such a work is *Everyday Exposure: Indigenous Mobilization and Environmental Justice in Canada's Chemical Valley* by Sarah Marie Wiebe. The injustice is the systemic social and ecological suffering of Indigenous peoples and their communities within the jurisdictions and policies of the Canadian federation. She shows how this unjust system persists and deepens despite well-meaning attempts to address it in what is perhaps the worst case: the horrendous "slow violence" of health and ecological suffering of the Aamjiwnaang First Nation surrounded by Chemical Valley. In meticulous detail, she delineates the complex system or assemblage of private and public law, power relations, different types of knowledge, ambiguous jurisdictions, history of treaty making, geopolitical interests, consultations, deliberations, partnerships, protests, reviews, and differentially situated actors in which policies are developed and applied. With this multilayered policy assemblage in clear view, she shows precisely how it repeatedly fails to generate and enact policies that effectively address either the unregulated production of petrochemical and polymer toxins and pollutants that devastate the lives and homeland of Aamjiwnaang citizens or the ongoing intergenerational human harms and ecological devastation to Aamjiwnaang citizens and their home.

Sarah Marie Wiebe developed a unique method to carry out this research. She draws on the best critical literature in a wide range of fields: policy studies,

Indigenous scholarship, political theory and science, ecology, health studies, feminism, intersectionality, governmentality, decolonization, reproductive justice, and most important, in-depth interviewing and engagement. She brings the useful insights of these diverse approaches together in a comprehensive method and fashions them to fit this specific case. However, her objective is not only to bring to light this made-in-Canada tragedy and to provide a method for studying it in other cases; her objective is also to show us that there is a way to transform this unjust system into a just one.

Through her "creative engagement" with the Aamjiwnaang people, Sarah Marie Wiebe learned that a way of transformation already exists here and now in the daily lived experience of Aamjiwnaang citizens taking care of themselves and their home. At the heart of this alternative, place-based, relational, and embodied way of being in the world with human and more-than-human relatives is the practical knowledge that humans acquire primarily through their sensuous and perceptual participation with the living earth they inhabit – that is, knowledge of the anthropogenic ecosystems in which humans and the earth's ecosystems co-evolve. And the basic mode of participation is gift-gratitude-reciprocity relationships of interdependency and mutual responsibility with the living earth. The animate earth takes care of us, and we in reciprocity take care of "it" – "all our relatives."

This Indigenous (Anishinaabe/Anishinabek) way of being is learned through practice and stories. It is mobilized in the ecological citizenship practices through which Aamjiwnaang citizens attempt to take care of their contaminated bodies and home. Yet it is misunderstood, discredited, and marginalized or co-opted from the perspective of the dominant nonrelational forms of being and knowing of the policy assemblage. From this perspective, as Sarah Marie Wiebe documents, what happens within Chemical Valley is said to be unrelated to what happens without. There are no "offsite impacts." Scientific research has not shown a verifiable causal relation between health and environment, and the Aamjiwnaang methods of gathering data are said to be unreliable. If there are unusual health problems in Aamjiwnaang, they are said to be due to "lifestyle choices," and biomedical knowledge treats the diseased bodies in isolation from the environment. In this atomistic world, no one has responsibilities that derive reciprocally from relationships of interdependency and interbeing because no such relationships exist. Even if some responsibility is shown to be due, given the structure of corporate law and the ambiguity of jurisdictions in Canadian federalism, it is almost always possible to shift the responsibility to someone else or, if this fails, to shelve the report, commission another study, or prolong the response indefinitely. And so on, time after time. It is a vicious social system that generates and rewards an ethos of irresponsibility.

The most important and challenging argument of *Everyday Exposure* is that this tragedy can be overcome. The key is to base policy on Aamjiwnaang interdependent ways of being and knowing in the first instance – that is, on the perceptual relationship of the senses and nervous system of the human body with the living earth and on the epistemology and practices of reciprocal responsibilities that follow from it. This is what she calls "sensing policy." This would involve a radical decolonization and transformation not only of policy but also of the whole policy assemblage of Canadian federalism. Indigenous people cannot achieve this outcome on their own, as this case study shows. It requires the mutual aid of non-Indigenous policy communities and partners throughout the assemblage. Securing this aid is not impossible. As Sarah Marie Wiebe points out, the embodied, place-based, relational, and responsible way of Aamjiwnaang citizens resonates with recent approaches in holistic health studies, deep ecology, eco-phenomenology and eco-feminism, ethnobotany, the Gaia hypothesis in the life sciences, ecological citizenship, scientific responses to global pollution, climate change and the Anthropocene, the shift from linear to cyclical cradle-to-cradle economics, and community-based lifeways. These place-based forms of research, participation, and engaged policy making are slowly finding their way into the ways that local communities around the world self-organize and coordinate with policy communities, universities, and governments.

As difficult and challenging as this transformation appears, the point is surely that there is no alternative. The policy assemblage that is devastating the Aamjiwnaang people and their ecosystems is part of the Canadian federal policy assemblages that are devastating other Indigenous communities and, more slowly yet just as inexorably, non-Indigenous communities. No one is offsite or not responsible. The choice is change or self-destruction. This is the deep truth of the relational view that Sarah Marie Wiebe learned from Aamjiwnaang citizens she worked with and that she explains so clearly in this remarkable book. The rest is up to us.

Preface

Fighting for life, a large eastern cottonwood digs its roots deep into the earth. Branches outstretched, arms spread wide, trunk standing tall. Anchored. Confident. Resilient. Day and night, it breathes. Soaking in sunlight, giving back to the atmosphere. Dark reactions take place. Assimilating carbon into organic compounds, the tree exhales. Humans inhale. A reciprocal human–more-than-human dance ensues. Come spring, its veins sprout hope, transporting water and nutrients throughout the core of its being and into the air.

Located a stone's throw from the Aamjiwnaaang First Nation's band office, the steadfast tree holds its ground. Adjacent to the community baseball field – a periodic source of pleasure and play – the tree stands alone. It rests metres away from the densest concentration of pollution in the country and quite possibly the world. Only a barbed wire fence separates it from the noxious neighbours across the street. Vast bulbous plumes of chemical effluent burst into the air, over the highway, and onto the community, engulfing the tree. This image is an acute reminder of how life becomes compromised. Like the eastern cottonwood, citizens living here survive. Struggling to thrive, they fight back while defending their land, their culture, and their home.

Like this tree, stories have roots. As numerous Anishinabek scholars emphasize, stories are rooted in "both the origins and the imaginings of what it means to be a participant in an ever-changing and vibrant culture in humanity" (J. Borrows 2013, xii; Doerfler, Sinclair, and Stark 2013; L. Simpson 2011). Stories provide a methodological and theoretical approach to Anishinabek scholarship. They embody "ideas and systems that form the basis for law, values and community"; thus they are "rich and complex creations that allow for the growth and vitality of diverse and disparate ways of understanding the world" (J. Borrows 2013, xii). Stories haunt and heal. As Lindsay Borrows (n.d., 4) states, "when governments make decisions without stories, people suffer." This book tells the story of a community fighting for justice in an environmentally compromised setting, which impacts residents' entire way of life. From my vantage point as a privileged academic who is committed to creative, intersectional policy and to decolonizing scholarship, I tell this story through images, poetry, voices, and documents, and I express my gratitude with the greatest respect to those who generously shared their knowledge with me. As a collection of stories that travel through time, this book aims to engage diverse knowledges, incite critical thought, and inspire reflection. Creating space for dialogue about the tough matter of environmental and reproductive injustice in Canada's Chemical Valley is an ongoing concern. Indeed, this story is not over yet. Looking backward helps us to understand where we've come from so that we may better understand just how far we have yet to go.

A benzene leak at the neighbouring industrial facility Novacor sparked a partial evacuation of the Aamjiwnaang First Nation Reserve during the summer of 1992. It included Tashmoo Avenue, home to the reserve band office, adjacent to the Chippewa Day Care Centre. Police and firefighters remained on standby as local officials issued an advisory and rerouted a school bus full of children headed for home. Neither plant officials nor the Ontario Ministry of Environment called the community daycare. Novacor spokesman Frank Barber noted that the "monitors located on the property line didn't detect benzene vapors leaving the site" (Mathewson 1992). In other words, there was "no offsite impact" beyond Novacor's fence line. Only after daycare workers noticed heavy, stinking, steaming air spewing toward their community were seventeen resting children whisked away to another location on the reserve. With financial support from industry, the daycare has since been relocated, although the band office, resource centre, and recreational facilities remain in place. Living with the potential for emergency has become a permanent feature of this community's daily landscape.

Citizens in Aamjiwnaang live in a perpetual state of alert. The following year, in 1993, a Suncor toluene release highlighted communication breakdown between industry, citizens, and government officials. That year, lightning struck a neighbouring chemical holding tank, simultaneously striking fear in the minds of local residents about their vitality. At 4:00 a.m. the local St. Clair High School became a safe haven for some evacuated residents, whereas others had been mistakenly sent home early, prior to an "all-clear" declaration

(McCaffery 1993). Chief Phil Maness demanded answers as Sarnia's mayor, Mike Bradley, expressed concern about the apparent communication gap between the plants, emergency planners, radio, and Aamjiwnaang residents (ibid.). In response, Police Chief Murray McMaster claimed that "uncoordinated good intentions created confusion during the Suncor emergency evacuation" (Bowen 1994). The police report called for better emergency management and cooperation between stakeholders in the Chemical Valley area. Sarnia's emergency planning coordinator, Bruce Middleton, acknowledged his concern about the delay in reaching the radio stations and said that it was likely due to overcommitted personnel (ibid.). As a release that extended beyond plant boundaries, this Code 6 incident generated calls for better offsite planning.[1]

Public safety response beyond the fence line falls heavily upon the shoulders of Aamjiwnaang citizens. Police Chief McMaster has argued that, as part of a municipal primary control group comprising police, fire, and civic officials, a point person must be designated by the band to direct the community whenever an emergency affects the reserve (Bowen 1994). He recommends that residents must act responsibly to spread the word according to established protocols in the event of evacuation (ibid.). During Suncor's release, the siren system failed to alert residents due to a malfunction caused by a dead battery. Mayor Bradley's response reiterated the importance of regular siren testing (ibid.). Now, each Monday at 12:30 p.m., sirens wail in Chemical Valley as Aamjiwnaang citizens safeguard their land and life.

Fast-forward to over a decade later when children, staff, and supporters of the Aamjiwnaang Binoojiinyag Kino Maagewgamgoons Day Care Centre took to the streets on Wednesday, January 16, 2013, to claim their right to a cleaner environment.[2] At an Idle No More demonstration,[3] concerned citizens demanded better communication between industry officials and local residents. The previous Friday, a mercaptan leak from an adjacent Shell refinery had caused a stink, resulting in road closures, renewed rerouting of school busses, and a shelter-in-place warning. Alert sirens, which enframe the reserve, had once again failed to sound. Reports of nausea, headaches, sore throats, and swollen eyes had surfaced over the weekend. On Wednesday citizens marched from the daycare toward the band cemetery along the St. Clair Parkway at the reserve's northwestern perimeter. Whether or not this community can find shelter in this place is a matter of continued dispute.[4] The normalization of scenarios like these deeply affects the community, heavily impacting human and more-than-human life.

Acknowledgments

While writing this book, the spiral of my life took me back and forth between Coast Salish, Algonquin, and Anishinabek territories. In June 2015, as I finalized my reflections, at least for the time being, Canada's Truth and Reconciliation Commission released its final report. Thinking about Indigenous-Canadian relationships, mutual respect, and reconciliation has led me to reflect upon the places and people that informed and inspired my intellectual growth as a scholar. Many fuelled the pages to follow: family, friends, my academic mentors, the Aamjiwnaang Environment and Education Departments, Green Teens, and the Kiijig Collective. I could not have asked for more engaging and academically rigorous mentors than Michael Orsini, Dayna Scott, and Martin Papillon. Kathryn Trevenen and Andrew Biros's voracious engagement with this manuscript also significantly enhanced these pages as they went to press. It was a pleasure to learn about the world of bio-monitoring and environmental science from Nil Basu and his research team. Furthermore, I am especially grateful to Ottawa- and Lambton County–based archivists Jason Bennett, Dana Thorne, and Luke Stempien. Their assistance from a distance significantly contributed to the book's historical depth.

This project would not have been possible without the continuous support of the Aamjiwnaang Environment Department. I appreciate Sharilyn Johnston's ongoing confidence in me as well as in this project. Each encounter with Christine Rogers – colleague, advisor, and friend – brought memories, laughs, and adventures. Thank you to community advisors Mike Plain, Wilson

Plain Sr., and Christine Rogers for keeping me accountable to the community. The energies, passions, and insights of Ron Plain, Ada Lockridge, Mckay Swanson, and Bonnie Plain, in artistic collaborations, controversies, and conversations, guided me through the contested terrain of environmental justice.

An evolving sense of "home" enabled me to press forward during the years of research for this book. Thank you to my family for tolerating my desire to push personal and intellectual boundaries of thought and for listening to me, supporting me, and laughing along with me even when they did not understand where I was or what I was doing. The presence of Jonathan – my brother – during the early stages of this pursuit provided much needed comfort as I found my bearings in an unfamiliar place. He is both a star and a rock in my life. To the Grays – Vanessa, Lindsay, and Arlene – thank you for warmly welcoming me.

Conversations that began on Canada's West Coast spawned this project's evolution on Ontario's West Coast, bordering Lake Huron, instilling in me a philosopher-surfer ethic. I eternally appreciate provocations that began during Jim Tully's graduate seminar on imperialism and political theory at the University of Victoria. During that time, preceding his current position as chief of the Tsilhqot'in First Nation, Russell Myers's persuasive prompting encouraged me to reflexively take up questions about settler colonialism. Those pivotal discussions significantly informed my engagement with the themes covered in this book. Particular thanks to the UVic crew: Jen and Carly Bagelman, Rhea Wilson, Megan Purcell, Jen Vermilyea, David Newberry, Delacey Tedesco, Charles Horn, Can Mutlu, Noah Ross, Jarrad Reddekop, Bjorn Ekeberg, and Sagi Cohen. This text was reviewed and made much stronger by Jen Bagelman, Laurence Butet-Roch, and Gabriel Genest Blouin.

The presence in my life of Stefan Currie-Roberts throughout all of this time meant the world to me. Of many friends, Laurence Butet-Roch stands apart as my "Roch" and intellectual coadventurer, whose artistic eye helped me to focus as I began this research and as I concluded this book. The hospitality and friendship of Sophia Muller and Helaina Gaspard kept me connected to the Ottawa intellectual community. I am grateful to Arlene Gray, Nicole Knowles, and the late Noelle Paquette for their joyful spirits and for getting me up and running; to the Boreal Collective and the Kiijig Collective for laughs and lessons learned and for the honour of sharing the creative process with them; to Ian Alexander, a ray of sunshine in Sarnia's sea of gray, who inspired the fledgling filmmaker in me as we saw this project take flight; to Jonathan Taggart for orienting me to place; and to Jordan Manley for walking me through place. To Marie-Chantal

Locas, merci pour ton amitié et ton accompagnement à travers cette aventure académique. Rita Dhamoon, Heidi Kiiwetinepinesiik Stark, and Simon Glezos each offered incisive remarks to hone this text. Conversations with faculty and students during the Indigenous Studies Workshop series at the University of Victoria further enriched the pages to follow. It was also a true pleasure to share this work within the wonderful intellectual community at the University of Wyoming. Caskey Russell's and Teena Gabrielson's warmth and hospitality nurtured this manuscript in its final stages.

Generous support from several invaluable sources made the research required for this book possible, including the Institute for Studies and Innovation in Community University Engagement (ISICUE) at the University of Victoria, a Joseph-Armand Bombardier CGS Doctoral Fellowship from the Social Sciences and Humanities Research Council of Canada, an Ontario Graduate Scholarship, and a Population Health Improvement Research Network Award. ISICUE provided an ideal enabling and reflective space to craft this manuscript. I am indebted to the team who make this place so dynamic: our fearless leader, biker-chick and director Leslie Brown, as well as Budd Hall, Maeve Lydon, Beata Jirkova, Martin Taylor, and Crystal Tremblay. I am also thrilled to have shared ideas with and learned from brilliant interns and students who engaged with us in this space, notably Kelly Aguirre, Greg Atkinson, Amy Becker, Mallory Colletta, Alison DuBois, Bruno de Oliveira Jayme, Robyn Spilker, and Cate White. I am incredibly grateful to my editor Randy Schmidt at UBC Press for his guidance and insight and to my reviewers for pushing me to finesse this project as it entered the publication process.

Images depicted in this text by Laurence Butet-Roch stem from her ongoing project *Our Grandfathers Were Chiefs*, which began in 2010. They are provided here with her consent and that of those photographed. Project details and additional images are available online at http://www.lbrphoto.ca/photos/Our-Grandfathers-Were-Chiefs/1. Both Laurence Butet-Roch and Aaron Vincent Elkaim independently shot breathtaking photographs of a pollution-engulfed eastern cottonwood tree, taken on the reserve near the band office in 2011. Laurence's image graces the book cover. In my view, this image captures the haunting aesthetic of Chemical Valley's local impact. With careful composition, the image of the cottonwood tree brings to life Aamjiwnaang's affective landscape – at once beautiful, harrowing, visceral, and threatening. Two members of the Aamjiwnaang First Nation, Mckay Swanson and Mike Plain, wrote compelling poetry inspired by these images; their words eloquently bookend the manuscript. Both Laurence and Aaron are members of the Boreal Collective and inspire me in ways beyond words. It is an honour to call them collaborators and friends. It is an even greater honour to not only witness but also share a sense of vision with them as we collaboratively bring this story to light and into sight. For more about the Boreal Collective, see http://wwwborealcollective.com.

EVERYDAY EXPOSURE

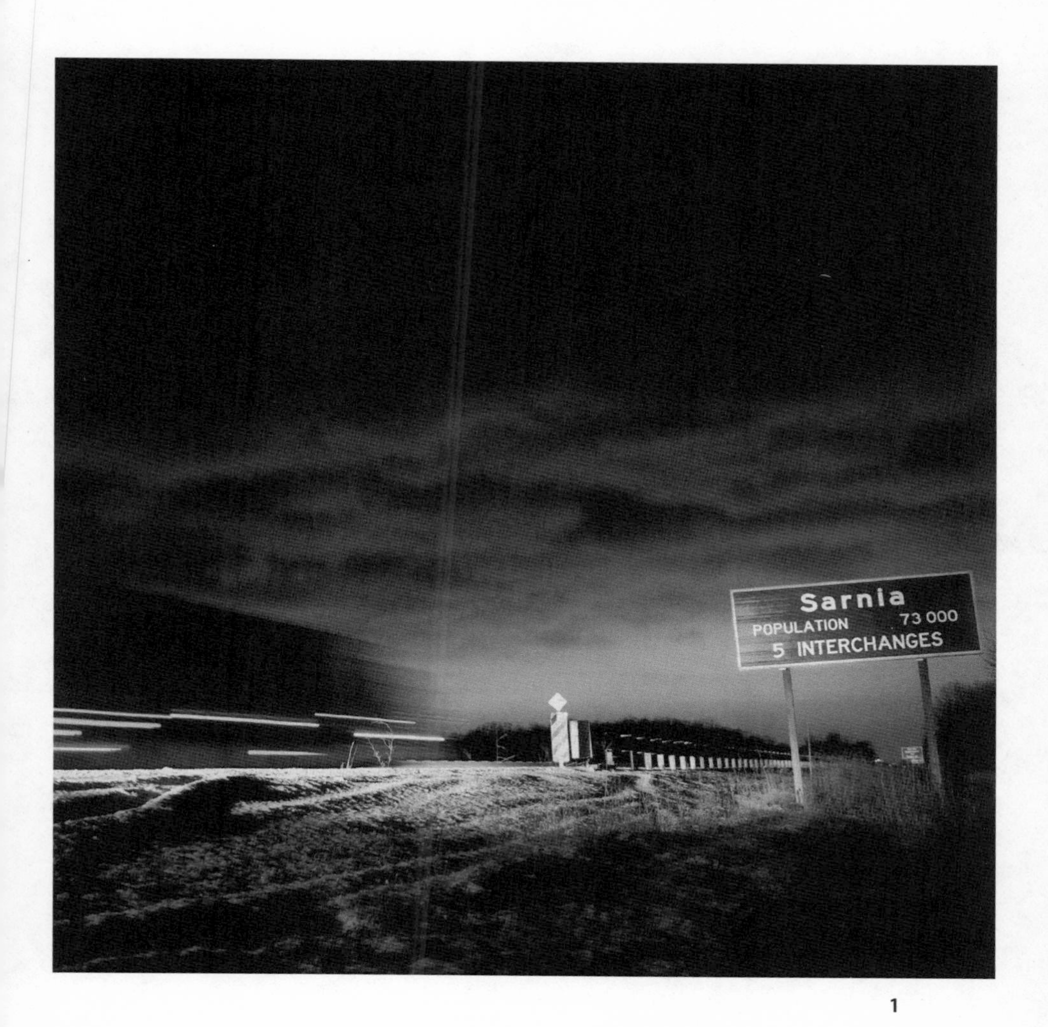

1

2

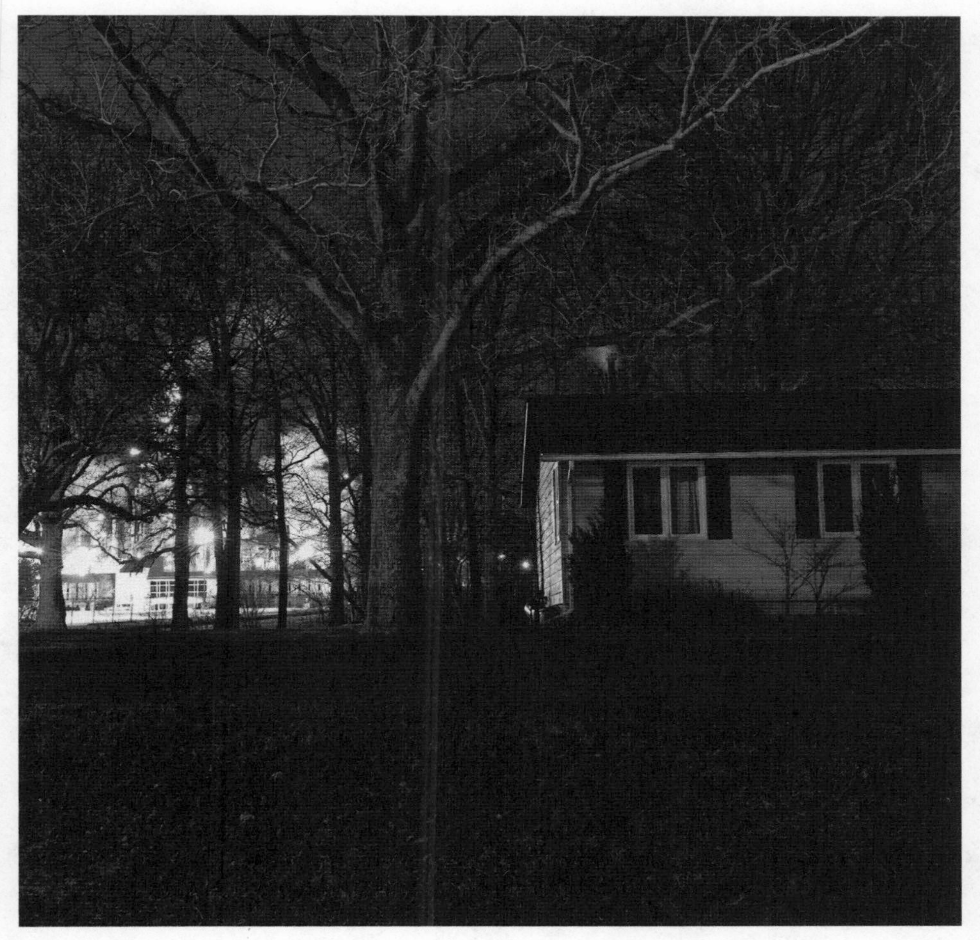

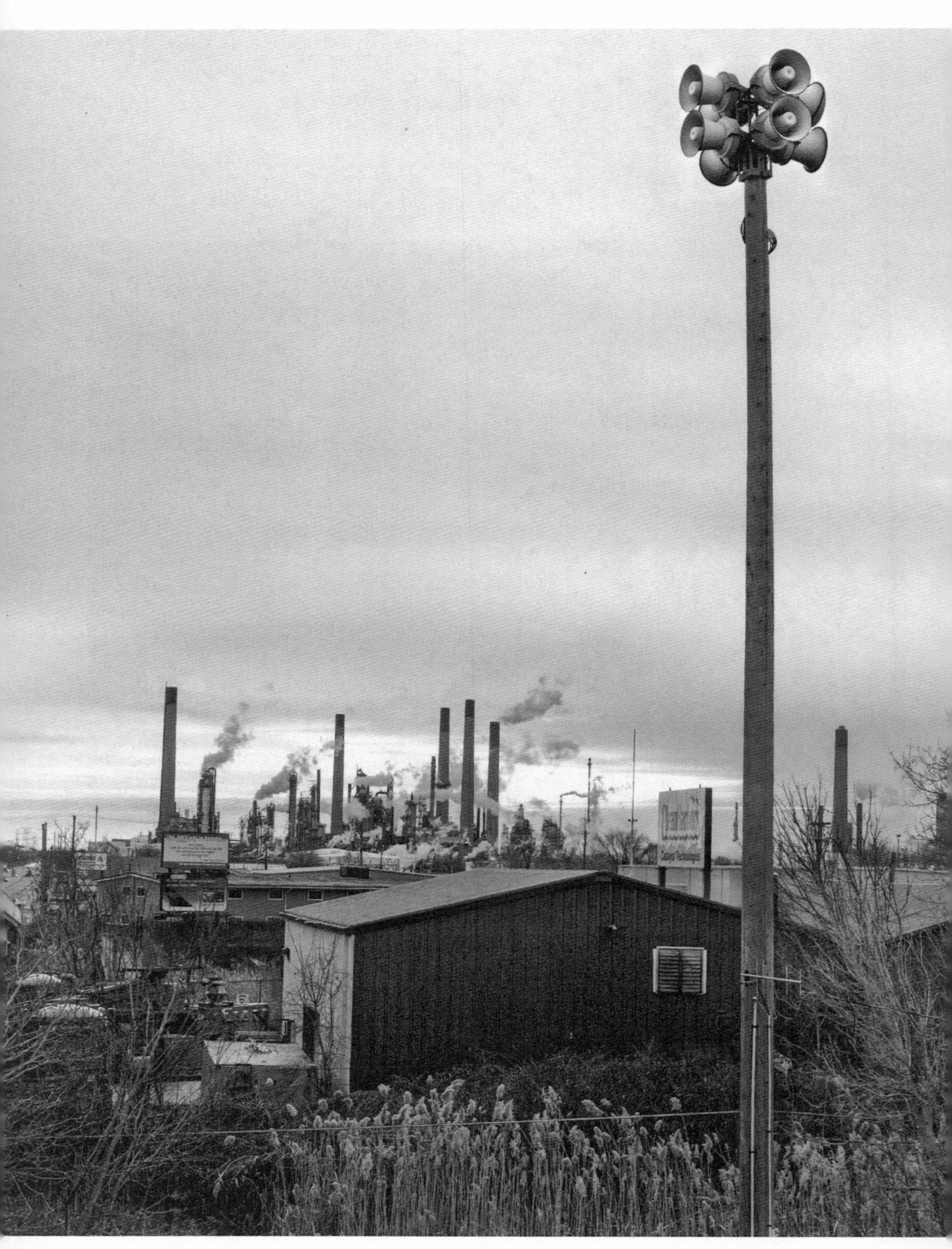

4

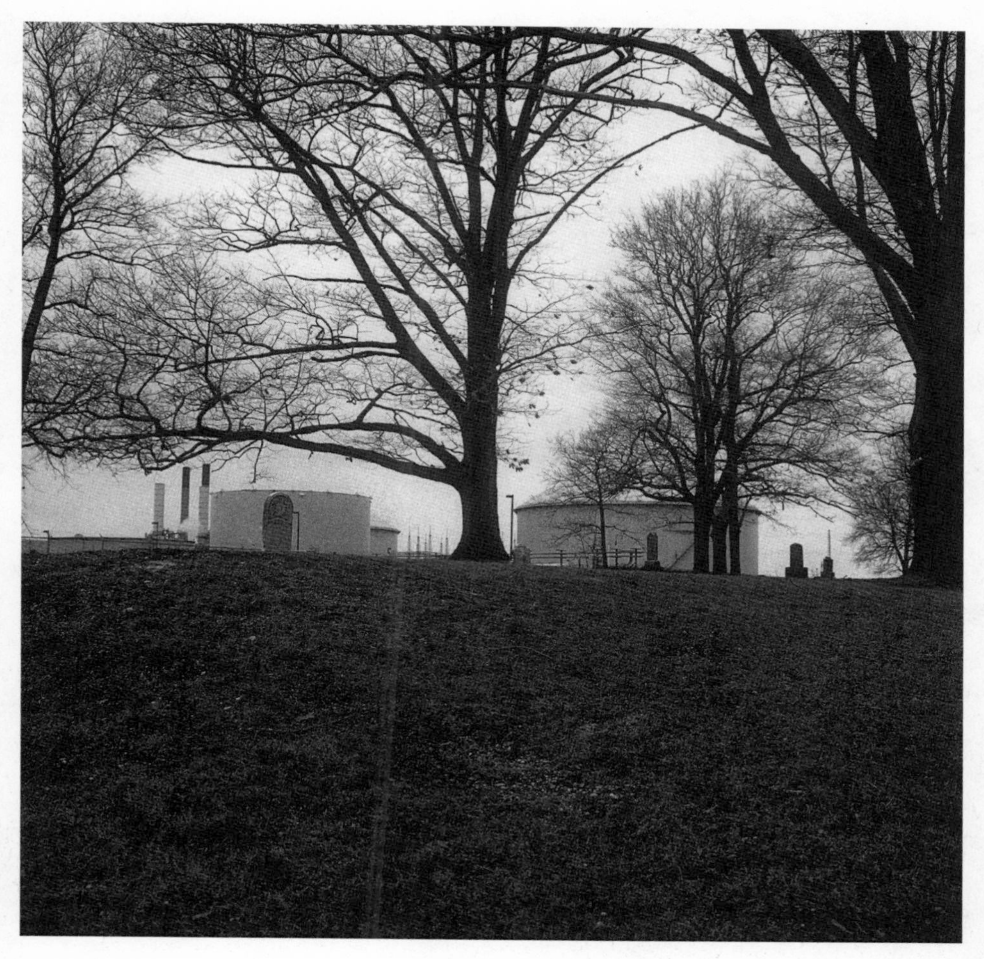

Atmosphere

Home, bittersweet home

Arriving in Sarnia at night, you are greeted by an orange glow that extends its embrace. It hovers permanently over the city. Visible from miles away, it guides you forward like the Northern Star. As you approach, it spreads beyond the pines, beyond the fields, over the road. You gaze upward, wondering when you will see its edge. It feels like you are entering a twilight zone. You are then met with a bouquet of strange scents: rotten eggs, decaying onions, burning gasoline, and many more that don't compare to anything you've ever smelled before.

Such a grisly welcome would turn away most visitors. But, in the heart of Canada's Chemical Valley – an industrial complex housing the country's densest concentration of petrochemical plants – rests a home and a haven for over 850 Anishinabek people who inhabit a patch of land measuring 12.57 square kilometres where trees still reign tall and where the occasional deer or wild turkey still roams freely in the bush. By continuously safeguarding this territory, the Aamjiwnaang First Nation prevents it from suffering a dismal fate, one where its value would rest in the money that can be made from its exploitation rather than in the lives it spawns.

Although a refuge, their surroundings also act as a constant reminder of what they've lost, of the atrocities perpetrated against Indigenous communities in the country, and of the enduring injustices they come up against. Behind each towering smokestack is a legacy of scorn; each wailing siren acts as an omen, warning us all that we continue to disfigure and destroy the beautiful yet haunting landscape that Aamjiwnaang residents call both prison and home.

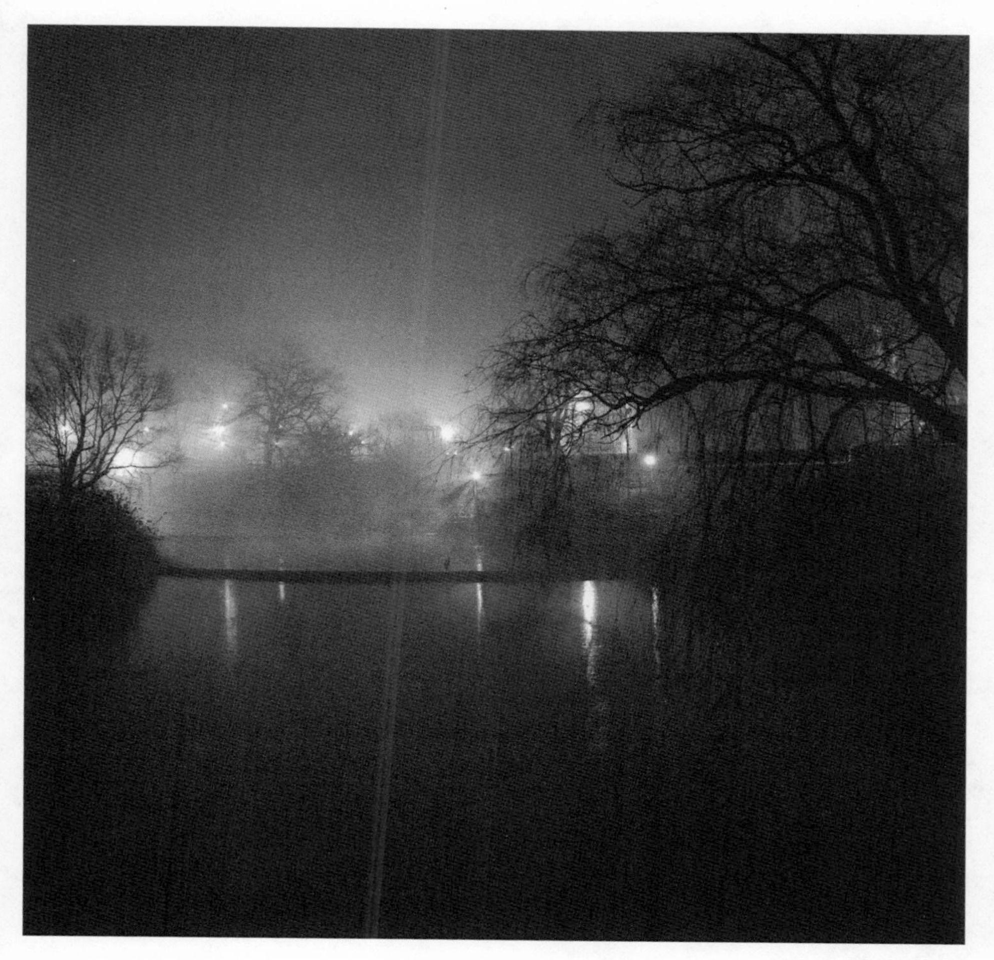

6

CAPTIONS

1 Located at the confluence of the St. Clair River and the Great Lakes along the St. Lawrence Seaway, Sarnia quickly became an industrial hub. Every major multinational petrochemical company impresses itself upon the landscape with a facility in the area. Their activities are responsible for the orange glow that can be seen from afar, welcoming you to Chemical Valley. December 2010.

2 Approximately 60 percent of releases of air pollutants by the industries located in Sarnia happen within five kilometres of Aamjiwnaang First Nation. Ineos Nova and Lanxess, respectively specializing in polystyrene and polymer products, are located across the road from the band office, the playground, and a community resource centre. January 2012.

3 On the Canadian side of the Canada-US border, more than forty large industrial and petrochemical facilities surround Aamjiwnaang. They spew out more greenhouse gases than the province of British Columbia and more toxic air pollutants than Manitoba, New Brunswick, or Saskatchewan. The nighttime light is courtesy of Suncor. December 2010.

4 The sirens around Chemical Valley remind people that the release of unwanted and dangerous chemicals into the air, water, or ground could occur at any given time. However, many locals consider this system less than reliable since it provides little information as to how one should react. December 2010.

5 There is no place to rest in peace in Aamjiwnaang. Even its cemetery lies in the shadow of Suncor's facilities. Constant mechanical humming is heard in the background. Every Monday at 12:30 p.m., the test sirens wail. Given its location on the other side of a mere chain-link fence, it further infiltrates this place of meditation. January 2012.

6 Talfourd Creek runs through the Aamjiwnaang First Nation Reserve and alongside the Suncor facilities until it reaches the St. Clair River. PCB, nickel, cadmium, arsenic, and lead contamination render it dangerous for humans and wildlife alike. What was once a source of pleasure – bathing, food, fishing – is now a source of constant worry. January 2015.

Photos and text by Laurence Butet-Roch

1

Skeletons in the Closet
Citizen Wounding and the Biopolitics of Injustice

Home is both refuge and prison for citizens of Canada's Chemical Valley. There, human and more-than-human residents dwell on a threshold between a state of normalcy and emergency. Chemical Valley is a heavy industrial zone, located in southwestern Ontario and responsible for approximately 40 percent of Canada's chemical manufacturing, with sixty-two plants on both sides of the Canada-US border. It is Ontario's worst air pollution hotspot (Ecojustice 2007a; Scott 2008). Chemicals from Aamjiwnaang's industrial neighbours include benzene, hydrogen sulfide, and sulphur dioxide. In Chemical Valley, individuals must be prepared for hazardous incidents at any given time. In general, alerts occur in the case of a chemical spill, fire, explosion, nuclear emergency, extreme weather event, or transportation accident. In Aamjiwnaang, such occurrences have become the norm.

Because warnings can be heard over loudspeakers, megaphones, and sirens, Chemical Valley is an audible place, which deeply affects those who live there. Noise pollution bears upon those living in this "sacrifice zone" (Lerner 2010). Each Monday at 12:30 p.m., the test sirens sound. These relics of the Second World War remind citizens of the constant invasion of their air by the neighbouring chemical facilities. Alongside wailing sirens, bodies clench as individuals jump for their radios, phones, and televisions to see whether there is any imminent threat. For some, this is little more than the everyday scene, which has destroyed the previous serenity of this place; they barely flinch. In such a seemingly post-apocalyptic environment, sounds mask the silence with which invisible chemicals penetrate bodies.

On June 8, 2011, community members gathered and laid yet another cancer-stricken loved one to rest in their cemetery. The graveyard – whose perimeter is surrounded on all sides by a chain-link fence, smokestacks, junkyards, somewhat clandestine surveillance cameras, and conciliatory cedar trees – looks like an island, displaced from the remaining reserve territory. During the ceremony, as is customary, members gathered around to sing, dance, and drum. That day, the neighbouring industrial vibrations accompanied the beat of the drum as the corpse was lowered beneath the earth's surface, drowning out the audibility of ceremonial song. Although one might expect that being laid to rest is a peaceful procedure, here it is anything but, as industrial flaring overbears ceremonial reverberations. Not only is Chemical Valley heard, but it is also a stunning aesthetic masterpiece. Sirens, stacks, and steeples dominate the airspace and ensconce the Aamjiwnaang First Nation.

According to Anishinabek beliefs, the world we live in is not "the real" world.[1] It is a mirror, reflecting what is to come in the spirit world. As bodies enter the spirit world in Aamjiwnaang, the earth perpetually vibrates in response to what is felt above and below the ground. Elders state that the spirits are trapped; they haunt this place, unable to reach the world they are destined for. The greatest grievance here is that not only do Indigenous peoples in Canada experience the ongoing effects of the tragedies of colonization and the legacy of the residential schools, but now their spirits also remain captured between past and future, which affects the ability of Indigenous peoples to survive and thrive in the present. As the Royal Commission on Aboriginal Peoples (RCAP 1996) has emphasized, many wish to keep such secrets – "ghosts of the past" – hidden. The haunting semblance of these ghosts lingers today. Although all is not lost, the residential schools were but one nail in the coffin marking what has been lost in this community. With colonization came warfare, epidemics, and the reduction of a vast population to the mere "sample size" remaining today. The Aamjiwnaang First Nation graveyard is the ultimate symbol of Canadian entrapment, a living trace of our collective history and reflective of all that we would like to store away beyond immediate vision and out of mind: our skeletons in the closet.

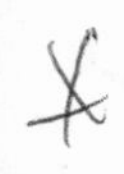

Sensing Policy

To breathe life into Canadian policy, a site-specific, experiential, and place-based account of everyday struggles for environmental reproductive justice is needed. According to the US Environmental Protection Agency (2011), environmental justice "is the fair treatment and meaningful involvement of all people regardless of race, color, national origin, or income with respect to the development, implementation, and enforcement of environmental laws, regulations and policies." With origins in the US African-American, Hispanic, and Indigenous communities, the environmental justice movement in the United States is well documented (Bryant 1995; Bullard 1993; Soja 1996, 2010). Much of this movement is grounded within individual and community experiences in particular places as they seek environmental justice. Although there have been some studies in Canada, the discourse of "environmental justice" and substantive policy making has been minimal. Nevertheless, some academics are actively engaged with research on environmental justice (Clarke and Agyeman 2011; Agyeman et al. 2009; Haluza-DeLay 2007; McGregor 2009; Scott 2005, 2008). Moreover, *environmental reproductive justice* – the inextricable connection between physical and cultural survival – is less prominent than environmental justice in research and practice (Hoover et al. 2012). This is especially the case within the Canadian context.

In 2005 members of the Aamjiwnaang First Nation teamed up with health researchers to conduct community-based participatory research. One key finding rocked the community: a stark decline in the number of male births (Mackenzie, Lockridge, and Keith 2005; see Appendix 1). As discussed in Wiebe and Konsmo (2014), the term "reproductive justice" originated within US organizations to promote the rights of women of colour and Indigenous women and to link "reproductive rights" with "social justice." That discussion evaluates struggles for reproductive justice in Canada to make crucial connections between the reproductive body, social justice, and place. Configured historically, geographically, and experientially, this approach considers bodies to be "contextually specific" (Parr 2010, 1). In this respect, the affected, feeling, *sensing* body is a conduit for knowledge. Parr (ibid., 9) focuses on the robust materialities of everyday encounters as "directly and fleshly as possible." This emphasis on "flesh" underscores the significance of the body and embodied ways of knowing. Reframing environmental justice to account for reproductive justice helps us to examine how citizens in Aamjiwnaang employ and mobilize experiential knowledge.[2] This approach draws into focus the following components of analysis: *multilayered analysis, lived experience, geopolitical location,* and how *situated bodies of knowledge* make the living sense of policy both more visible and sensible. These four features are crucial to making policies that account for diverse experiences and ways of knowing and that are ultimately more democratic and just.

In telling the story of ongoing struggles for environmental reproductive justice, it is crucial that place and cultural knowledge be made central to citizen claims. Cues from Indigenous scholarship, gleaned both from relevant literature and from narratives presented to me in conversations with local carriers of that knowledge, are integral to this project (Alfred and Corntassel 2005; J. Borrows 2002, 2010, 2013; Coulthard 2014; Doerfler, Sinclair, and Stark 2013; L. Simpson 2011). Counter to a discursive framing that separates individuals from their environment and aligned with Alfred and Corntassel's (2005, 597) argument that some expressions of Indigeneity offer a radically different kind of "being," or place-based subjectivity, I situate bodies in place to document citizen struggles for environmental reproductive justice. To examine ongoing citizen struggles for knowledge in Aamjiwnaang, a biopolitical and interpretive analysis inspired by the works of "postmodern" theorists Michel Foucault, Gilles Deleuze, and Félix Guattari demonstrates how all knowledge is power-laden and thus political.

At the core here is a concern with the individual, neoliberal, biopolitical subjectivity assumed and offered by much of official and unofficial public health discourse and policy. In addition to framing what we can or cannot say, discourse can be understood as "actions, sites of production, practices, embodiments and images that support or resist a particular way of thinking and talking about a subject" (Rutherford 2011, xxiii). Discourse is ultimately about the construction and enactment of power through repressive and productive means. It entails an ensemble of institutional, linguistic, practical, visual, and embodied sign systems. To examine the ensemble, or *assemblage*, of Indigenous environmental justice, both a textual analysis of Canadian public policies and a discursive analysis of concerns raised by citizens of the Aamjiwnaang First Nation are employed in answering the following questions: How do environmental and reproductive injustices impact Aamjiwnaang citizens, and how do they respond?[3] Moreover, what do citizen struggles in Chemical Valley tell us about the meaning and expression of citizenship in Canada and beyond? What are the implications for our understanding of citizenship if we take seriously the practices and discourses of Aamjiwnaang community members articulated in their own terms?

To address these questions, Chapter 3 contextualizes citizens' *multilayered* struggles over knowledge by discussing the relationship between biopower and the *policy assemblage* for Indigenous environmental justice, encompassing Canadian jurisdiction for on-reserve environmental health. Biopower involves twin biopolitical poles: population management and individual practices of citizen responsibility for self-care and rule. Subsequently, Chapter 4 documents local citizens' corporeal concerns and practices to account for *lived experience*. Chapters 5 and 6 examine the Aamjiwnaang First Nation's activities on the ground as they cope with their health and habitat to make sense of how they should respond to their slow-moving pollution problem. Whereas Chapter 4 documents citizens' stories presented in their own terms, Chapter 5 examines *geopolitical location* and discusses how Aamjiwnaang came to be situated in the middle of Chemical Valley. Chapter 6 then assesses *situated bodies of knowledge* based upon in-depth interviews with residents and policy makers. In doing so, it examines struggles over knowledge and scientific expertise in the context of a local health study as the community seeks recognition of the impacts of these exposures on their reproductive health. This focus on knowledge illuminates the contested nature of what constitutes data, science, expertise, and ultimately "truth."

The term "biopower" refers to the ways that biological processes of daily life become infused with politics in disciplinary and productive ways. As much biopolitical scholarship reveals, in addition to being a concept about how the "vital or productive processes of human existence" become implicated in new forms of power through the "capacities of bodies and conduct of individuals," biopower is a form of both repressive and productive power (Braun 2007, 8; Dean 2010; Rose 2007). As the following chapters demonstrate in visceral detail, disciplinary techniques include the maximization of bodily forces through efficient systems of population management; at the same time, biopolitics takes the nation as an object and makes it legible through various knowledge systems. Moreover, examining bodily interrelations and interactions with policy offers a *multilayered* approach to policy analysis that extends from the community to the provincial and federal governments. Such an account takes into consideration how ongoing struggles have developed over a century of settlement, industrialization, and cultural dislocation. The components of *multilayered analysis, lived experience, geopolitical location,* and *situated bodies of knowledge* are crucial to the enhancement of scholarship on environmental reproductive justice in Canada.

We must bear in mind that this situation of injustice is not a matter of historical accident. As Brown (1995) contends, due in large part to the institutional configurations of state rule, citizens live within "states of injury." The apparent "policy void" that has resulted in the lack of environmental reproductive justice in Canada can be attributed to the same systemic problem. How, then, can we make sense of citizen concerns in a climate of state withdrawal, and how can situated stories speak back to decision makers in order to inform better policy making in Canada? Turning to community members' concerns highlights the ways that their experiences and voices interact with and confront the policy assemblage for Indigenous environmental justice. Such a textured approach sheds light on the prismatic ways that biopower operates today. It also provides some visibility to the ongoing injustices, with the ultimate aim of contributing to how this situation can be seen, lived, and felt to be otherwise in order to enable escape from the ensnarement of this "biopolitical trap" (Rancière 2004, 301).

Introducing Wounded Citizens

On October 29, 2010, Ecojustice – a national charitable legal firm dedicated to defending the right of Canadians to a healthy environment – launched constitutional litigation against the Province of Ontario's Ministry of Environment (MOE) and Suncor Energy Products Incorporated on behalf of two members of the Aamjiwnaang First Nation: Ron Plain and Ada Lockridge. The case challenges the "deficient manner in which the Ministry of Environment regulates pollution in the area around Ada and Ron's community of Aamjiwnaang" (Duncan, field notes, Queen's Park, Ontario, November 1, 2010). Following close to a decade of local and global environmental activism in a battle against the province's environmental legislation, the litigants articulated frustration with the ministry's continued approval of permits to allow the advancement, expansion, and encroachment of pollutants on their land, in their homes, and on their bodies: "I felt as if my family's health and well-being was being sacrificed, at a cost" (Plain, field notes, Queen's Park, Ontario, November 1, 2010). Fatigued by the lack of attention to the cumulative impacts of the pollutants and to the consequential health effects, members of this First Nation took action to speak out against the provincial government and industry. A ministry approval to allow Suncor, a petroleum and ethanol refinery, to expand its chemical refining production in an oversaturated industrial area within a few kilometres of their reserve was the coup de grâce for these individuals. They contend that the approval constitutes a violation of their basic human rights under the Canadian Charter of Rights and Freedoms, particularly Section 7 on the right to life, liberty, and security of the person and Section 15 on the right to equality for all Canadians.

Citizen bodies in Aamjiwnaang are continuously exposed to creeping contamination. This exposure causes alarm: "I was taught growing up that it was a good thing when the flares are going, 'cause it's more dangerous down on the ground, and not to burn off, but I never thought about what was burning and how it can affect our health" (Lockridge, field notes, Queen's Park, Ontario, November 1, 2010). Flaring – the act of disposing of gas that cannot be processed or sold by burning it off and releasing it into the atmosphere – is meant only to

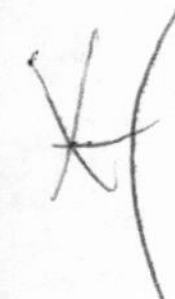

be an emergency practice for when gases build up. In Chemical Valley citizens live with this practice in a perpetual state of emergency, resonant of what Nixon (2011) refers to as "slow violence."[4] Such chronic violence takes place over time and is often state-sanctioned, invisible, and not considered to be violence at all. Shedding light on the policy assemblage of Indigenous environmental justice brings into focus the operation and inner workings of uneven power relations in Canada's colonial present.

To examine these asymmetrical relations and the ways that they establish a certain kind of political order, we can understand the policy assemblage of Indigenous environmental justice as a deeply political social technology. This assemblage of *institutional configurations, discursive fields,* and *citizen practices* thus presents structural and discursive ways of thinking about power relations that enable a particular kind of slow violence, injury, and ongoing wounding (Jain 2006, xi, 2–3; Nixon 2011).[5] These relations reveal that the contemporary manifestations of colonial biopower in Canada, from universal state policies to intimate sites and lived experiences, are distributed through policies across scales from the Canadian Constitution to the individual citizen. Injury and wounding in Chemical Valley thus emerge as incidental features of Canadian politics with direct consequences for the meaning and practice of citizenship. Although this injurious culture appears to be fixed to the Canadian policy landscape, writing about power relations in this way requires nuance and respect for the agency of those resisting on the ground. As assemblages are fluid, there exists the possibility that this landscape can be thought of, felt, lived, and experienced otherwise. A turn to the visceral weight of policy in Chemical Valley brings to life the everyday impact on citizens.

The Ministry of Environment grants approval to facilities that seek to emit certain substances in Ontario. Pursuant to the province's 1993 Environmental Bill of Rights, all approvals appear on the Environmental Registry's website, which contains "public notices" about environmental matters proposed for a thirty-day period of public consultation. The conventional process for obtaining a certificate of approval (COA) outlined in Section 9 of the Environmental Protection Act (EPA) depicts how industries must estimate maximum emissions to air, soil, and water based on standards for specific pollutants established by the Act's regulations. These criteria are commonly referred to as "point of impingement" (POI) standards.[6] They set a limit on the concentration of a pollutant that can be present at any POI, often defined as the fence line, or property line, of an industrial facility (Ecojustice 2010, 7). Under the EPA, the minister has the discretion to consider cumulative effects beyond the fence line. In contrast to the COA procedure, under Sections 18, 157, and 196 of the EPA, the ministry has the authority to permit companies to operate outside the POI standards (ibid., 9). The ministry allowed Suncor to enhance its production through amendment of one such control order, a discretionary, industry-government negotiated process that did not require public consultation.

This particular incident allowed a 25 percent increase in chemical production – up to 180 tonnes of sulphur a day – at the Sarnia refinery, a facility that produces transportation and heating fuels, liquefied petroleum gases, residential fuel oil, asphalt, feedstock, and petrochemicals (Ecojustice 2010, 9, 13). Approximately 75 percent of the crude oil at Suncor's petroleum refinery in Sarnia is synthetic crude supplied from Suncor's tar sands operations, which contain high levels of sulphur. In its productions, it emits sulphur dioxide, hydrogen sulphide, oxides of nitrogen, carbon monoxide, particulate matter, and benzene (ibid., 10). Each entails corollary adverse health effects; yet some of these chemicals, such as benzene, remain unregulated under the EPA rubric. Benzene is sweet and colourless. It evaporates quickly in air and dissolves slightly in water. It is highly flammable, can cause bone marrow not to produce enough red blood cells, and has been known to cause anemia and leukemia (MOE 2005). Others, such as hydrogen sulphide, are known neurotoxins that are frequently released in the flaring process. Several adjacent neighbouring facilities produce similar chemicals. However, the cumulative effects of such a high conglomeration of facilities continue to be unregulated by the existing legislative framework. The applicants became aware of the specifics of this amendment only through a formal request under the Freedom of Information and Protection of Privacy Act, shifting the burden of responsibility for monitoring Suncor's production from the government to this community. Suncor is but one facility among sixty-two located on both sides of the Canada-US border (Ecojustice 2007a; Scott 2008).

Suncor's presence affects every angle of the reserve's perimeter. Not only does this facility encircle the traditional burial ground, dislocating it from the reserve, but the stacks also pierce the sky at such a height that they are visible from nearly every residential home on the Aamjiwnaang First Nation Reserve. Resting easy in death is no simple feat, as noise and vibrations are some of the sensations felt when citizens of this community lay loved ones to rest. Children play in their yards amid a landscape bearing sounds akin to jets blasting for takeoff. Residents and their children express fear of entering the streams and creeks, perceived to be a toxic stockpile. Against the backdrop of sirens, smells, and soot, as rates of cardiovascular and respiratory illness rise, individuals look at their surroundings with distress.

Members of this community experience and articulate numerous physical and psychological health harms. In addition to respiratory, cardiovascular, reproductive, and skin diseases, fear is an everyday reality (Ecojustice 2007a). Knowing neither the contents of what is spewing into the air, soil, and water nor their impact on individual bodies is a cause of discomfort. Individuals become susceptible to these unknown substances; yet bearing the burden of proof for bodily harm remains onerous. Over the years, Aamjiwnaang residents became frustrated with hearing that their "lifestyle choices" were to blame for adverse health effects. A leading community advocate stated, "Don't tell me that nowhere else in the world people don't smoke, don't drink, they don't use drugs, they don't use makeup, they don't have carpets in their house. I always thought, like many others have, that the government was taking care of us. But now I believe that's not true" (Lockridge, field notes, Queen's Park, Ontario, November 1, 2010). Many Aamjiwnaang citizens wish to live a healthy and productive life; however, they have lost some of their personal autonomy with respect to health outcomes, and they bear a disproportionate responsibility for proving toxic exposure and adverse health effects. Some residents have moved away and have never turned back. This forced mobility follows a long history of cultural dislocation and socio-economic disadvantage for First Nations peoples within Canadian society at large and Aamjiwnaang in particular.

Subsequent to nearly a decade of responsible neighbourly activities, which included documenting spills, odours, noises, and vibrations, calling the ministry's Spills Actions Centre, "bucket brigades," biomonitoring, body-mapping, shutting vents and windows, and sheltering-in-place, this community became weary.[7] When communities mobilize to gain expertise, the interactions between community members and the makers of public policy are charged with political meaning and laden with asymmetrical power relations. Communities facing environmental injustices frequently bear a disproportionate burden of environmental risk exposure as well as the costs associated with gaining expertise and knowledge about this exposure. Thus the polluted become "powerless" when faced with pollution (Scott 2008, 335). As communities embark upon resistance strategies, from biomonitoring to bucket brigades, they seek to make inroads and change environmental monitoring and regulation. Although bucket brigade activities in Aamjiwnaang served as a precursor to getting an air monitor on the reserve, the burden of "proof" and responsibility for environmental management continues to fall upon the shoulders of Aamjiwnaang's citizens at a distance from governmental regulation. As Scott (ibid., 338) discusses, citizens transition from "victims" to "agents of change." They are simultaneously co-opted and empowered by this kind of agency.

Aamjiwnaang: A *Place* Where Spirits Live in the Water

Despite the alarming landscape, this place is *home*. The Aamjiwnaang First Nation Reserve, or Sarnia Reserve 45, is home to approximately 850 Anishinabek people, also known as the Chippewas of Sarnia. Located just across the Canada–US border from Port Huron, Michigan, the reserve is at the southernmost tip of Lake Huron, approximately seven kilometres south of Sarnia's core. For nearly half a century, Aamjiwnaang's land has been almost completely surrounded by one of Canada's largest concentrations of petrochemical manufacturing. Much of the original reserve, founded by Treaties 27½ and 29 in 1825 and 1827, has dwindled over the years due to various surrenders, the peak of which occurred through controversial land deals in the 1950s and 1960s when development companies sought to purchase the entire reserve. This attempt was enabled through the federal government's fiduciary responsibilities, in line with the Indian Act. The land base has since been compressed as a partial consequence of land sales and surrenders, highway expansion, and municipal annexations. According to one local historian, the Anishinabek people effectively became "prisoners in their own home" (Plain 2007). Pipelines, factories, and petroleum storage tanks occupy today's territory and encircle the reserve.

In September 2011 the World Health Organization (WHO) surveyed 1,100 cities in ninety-one countries and declared Sarnia to have the worst air quality in the country (Jeffrey 2011). Canada ranked third in the world when it came to air quality; yet the airshed above Sarnia was found to have the highest concentration of particulate matter per cubic metre in all of Canada, on par with a population-dense city like New York. According to Dean Edwardson, general manager of the industry-funded Sarnia-Lambton Environmental Association, housed at Suncor's Sustainability Centre, "60% of what's measured comes from the U.S." (ibid.). Pointing to coal-fired plants across the river, he considered the WHO's findings to markedly differ from local monitoring statistics. This discrepancy raises the question of who is responsible for providing accurate information to citizens of Sarnia about the contaminants in their environment.

The Sarnia area, including the city of Sarnia and the township of St. Clair, can be further characterized by a dense concentration of industrial facilities. A MOE (2005) report identified chemical plants, natural gas sites, petroleum refineries, plastics recyclers, fertilizer plants, electric generation stations, a wastewater treatment plant, and a landfill site. This report did not include inactive sites, which also house and store waste products and litter the landscape in this area (see Figure 2 below). It hosts Canada's largest hazardous waste dump

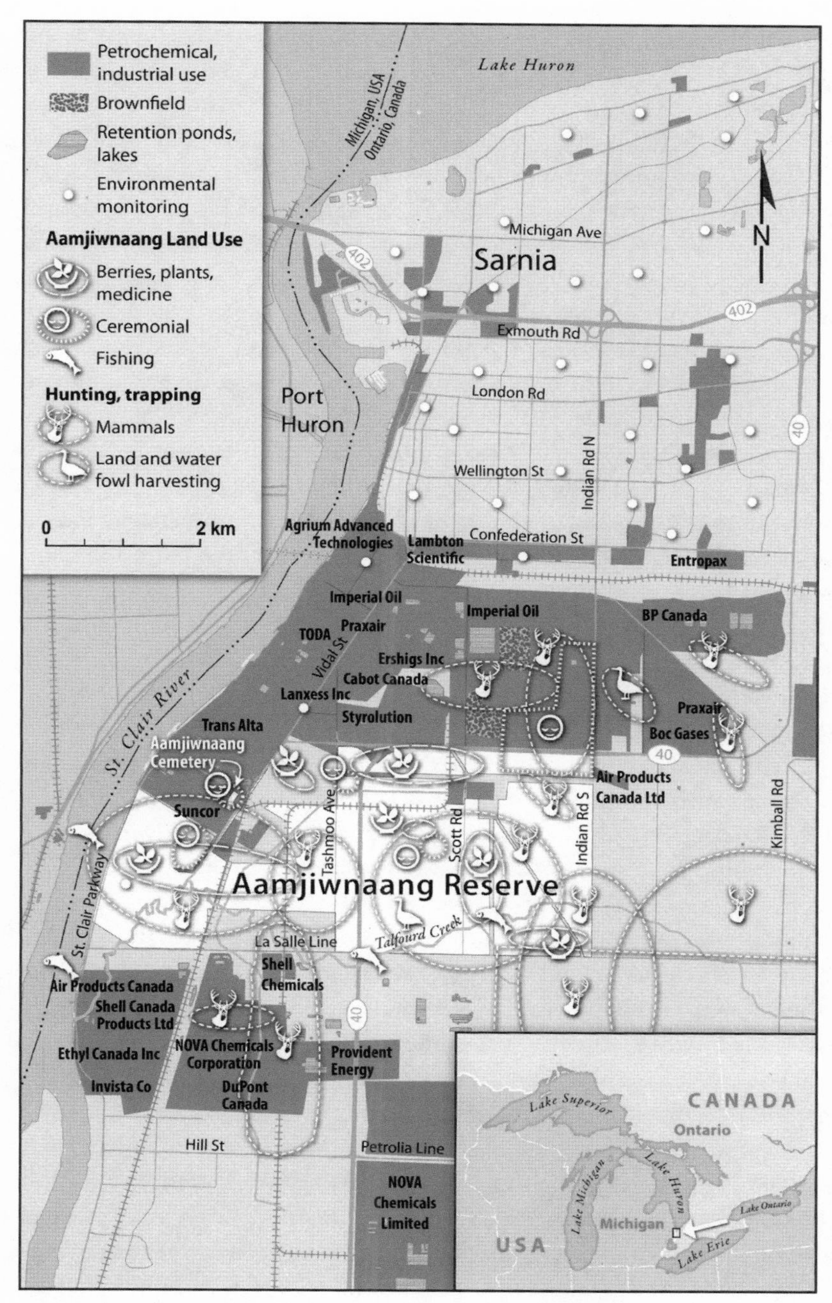

Figure 2 Map of Aamjiwnaang traditional land use and industrial sites. Cartography by Ken Josephson.

and is a hub for the production of synthetic rubber, polyvinyl chloride, and plastics.

According to this report, a common risk of petroleum refining is exposure to hydrogen sulfide, which contains a rotten egg smell. However, "concentrations above 150 ppm may overwhelm the olfactory nerve so that the victim may have no warning of exposure" (MOE 2005). Whereas low-level hydrogen sulfide may cause irritations in mucous membranes and the respiratory system, high-level exposures result in more neurological and pulmonary symptoms, including possible loss of consciousness. Very high concentrations lead to cardiorespiratory arrest because of brainstem toxicity (ibid.). Several researchers point out the corresponding correlation between ambient air pollution and elevated hospital admission rates for respiratory and cardiovascular disease in London, Ontario, 100 kilometres east of Chemical Valley (Fung et al. 2005). In 2005 citizens and stakeholders met to discuss their concern about the impact of pollution on health and wellness within Lambton County. As Chapter 6 discusses in depth, by 2008 they had formed a board of directors and commenced the Lambton Community Health Study.

Tourism literature and accolades from the Chamber of Commerce tout Sarnia, population 73,000, as a beautiful and desirable place to live and work. Located within the county of Sarnia-Lambton, it is part of a gorgeous region affectionately referred to as Bluewater Country (Tourism Sarnia-Lambton 2011). With a total population of 128,204, headquartered in Wyoming, Ontario, the Corporation of the County of Lambton encompasses eleven municipalities and the four regions of Sarnia and Point Edward, St. Clair River District, Lambton Shores, and Central Lambton (Statistics Canada 2006). This is truly a rich place in material and natural beauty. The reported 2005 median income for couple households with children was $90,929, approximately $3,000 higher than the average Ontario income level (ibid.). Adjacent to Lake Huron, the county boasts miles of scenic waterfront, sandy beaches, and breathtaking sunsets. It is a place to "discover your inner explorer"; "experience a festival of fragrance"; and "escape to a place that puts it all in perspective" (Tourism Sarnia-Lambton 2011). In under an hour, Sarnia citizens can escape to Pinery Provincial Park, host to the last remaining oak savanna in North America, or continue fifteen kilometres to reach the stunning site of Ipperwash Provincial Park.[8]

In addition to boasting a relaxed waterfront lifestyle, Sarnia is a hotbed of industrial activity. Oil was first discovered and produced in the area during the 1850s, which spawned the emergence of an oil boom and industrialization. Imperial Oil Limited soon followed. The affectionately coined "Chemical Valley" moniker emerged after the Second World War, during which time the

Crown corporation Royal Polymer came into being, effectively starting an empire of rubber manufacturing. It even graced the country's ten-dollar bill (Bellamy 2007). Sarnia's central position within the Great Lakes waterways and its accessibility to the United States make it an ideal location for industrial development. With deep-port access on the St. Lawrence Seaway, it is an international water corridor. Moreover, Lake Huron and the St. Clair River cater to the industrial sector, connecting it to the waterways for processing, cooling, fire protection, marine docks, and effluent discharge. In addition, Sarnia is serviced by the Canadian National Railway and the rails of CSX Transportation, as well as by the Chris Hadfield Airport. Chemical Valley's industrial complex in South Sarnia contains an extensive network of hydrocarbon raw materials, such as natural gas, crude oil, ethylene, and natural gas liquids (SLEP 2011). It is a world leader in plant construction, process engineering and operations, metal fabrication, sustainable energy production, and environmental technology and management. Sarnia is also at the forefront of petrochemical production and its relevant spinoff industries. For instance, when the Gulf of Mexico oil spill disaster hit, British Petroleum turned to a Sarnia firm to "mop up" the devastating mess (Dobson 2010). However, Sarnia's own cleanup efforts remain a matter of dispute.

After nearly a century of heavy industrial manufacturing and refining, and following the 1985 "blob" incident at Dow Chemicals – the release of perchlorethylene, a dry-cleaning solvent, into the St. Clair River – this stretch of sixty-four kilometres along the river was identified as an "area of concern" in the Canada–US Great Lakes Water Quality Agreement (Environment Canada 2012). This designation rode the coattails of Dow's legacy of releasing mercury into the river for many years. Prior to the introduction of environmental legislation, regulation, and standards in the 1970s, some Aamjiwnaang residents played with and collected mercury during childhood. In 2002 Dow began dredging to remove methyl mercury from the riverbed. In 2005 Pollution Watch added three Chemical Valley industries to its list of the top ten respiratory polluters (Ecojustice 2007a). As these environmental concerns began making waves, Environment Canada, the Ontario Ministry of Environment, and the US Environmental Protection Agency met to discuss a remedial action plan. Shortly thereafter, wetlands, wastewater treatment sites, and various restoration projects appeared on the landscape.

Local residents residing in this area face a large pollution problem. Dow Chemical is but one facility among sixty-two located within twenty-five kilometres of Sarnia and Aamjiwnaang (Scott 2008). Community-based participatory research between members of the Aamjiwnaang First Nation and the

Occupational Health Clinic for Ontario Workers – Sarnia (OHCOW) has revealed a range of health concerns within the community, including headaches, diabetes, thyroid issues, asthma, skin rashes, high cancer rates, neurological, reproductive, and developmental concerns, and a declining male birth rate, in addition to a loss of cultural practices on the land (Ecojustice 2007a; Hoover et al. 2012; Mackenzie, Lockridge, and Keith 2005). With the help of OHCOW, these concerns were tracked on large "body maps" with colour-coded stickers and shown to the community (see Chapter 4). In addition to bodily concerns, industrial sources of air pollutants pinch the reserve on all sides and are located directly across from the band office, the church, the cemetery, a resource centre, and until recently, the daycare centre (Ecojustice 2010). Lead levels beyond acceptable MOE guidelines were found in Talfourd Creek, which weaves through industry and the burial grounds and into the St. Clair River.

Red-lettered signs with a skull and crossbones that tell people to "KEEP OUT" demarcate Talfourd Creek's course in Aamjiwnaang. Figuring out the composition of the creek's contamination requires sustained monitoring sanctioned by the reserve in partnership with government officials and researchers. Although the testing continues, questions are still being raised, and concrete answers are few and far between. Despite the signs with the skull and crossbones, as life goes on, many citizens swim, fish, and play in the waterway.

These living conditions are unsatisfactory to several community members and activists. To raise awareness, residents like Ron and Ada often provide public "toxic tours" (Garrick 2015). In 2009 Ron and Ada requested a legislative review under the Environmental Bill of Rights. Upon receiving no response, these individuals had to resort to the court. Soon thereafter, I participated in one such "toxic tour" and ended up in Sarnia.

My Place

> Aaniishnaa
> Sarah, dizhnikaaz
> Vancouver, ndoonjibaa
> Niizhtana niizhwaaswi niin doonsibboongis
> Anishinabek nigee ndaw.[9]

During my time residing in Sarnia, I joined a weekly Ojibwe class. We spent the first few weeks discussing the meaning of introductions. As my teacher continuously emphasized, who you are connects to where you are from. While attending and participating in many events and ceremonies, I learned that community members often used Ojibwe words to introduce themselves to each other. I introduce myself as such here and explain how I came to live in Sarnia to research environmental reproductive justice in Canada's Chemical Valley.

While I was growing up in British Columbia, Indigenous concerns were always part of the political landscape, aesthetic, and life of the province. The ongoing treaty process exemplifies this reality today. My analysis is motivated by an effort to think through our inherited political histories and spaces. To investigate politics, we must look both elsewhere and nearby. I grew up in the village of Belcarra on a body of water called Indian Arm just outside of Vancouver in Tsleil-Waututh territory. As a youth, I spent many summers volunteering as a "beachkeeper" to inform park visitors about "environmentally friendly beach behaviour," working as a day camp leader, and enjoying recreational activities in Belcarra Regional Park. Only as a graduate student at the University of Victoria did I come to realize the importance of this park for the Tsleil-Waututh people. Years later, while meeting with a member of the Tsleil-Waututh band council, I learned about the ceremonial uses of both the park and the island across the bay, a stretch of water that demarcated my home from the reserve. The island was once a burial ground, and the park was a residential area. Today the island is filled with waste, and the park is open for public use while the Tsleil-Waututh look on from across the bay.

While I was a research assistant at the University of Ottawa doing work on contested illnesses such as multiple chemical sensitivity and fibromyalgia, a CBC documentary film entitled *The Disappearing Male* caught my eye. It drew my attention to Aamjiwnaang and the ongoing struggles for environmental reproductive justice. The film pointed me toward an environmental movement there, premised upon corporeal health concerns and ongoing challenges to various regulatory authorities. I became curious about the ways that citizens within the movement organized, articulated concerns, and sought redress. Health policy and environmental policy are both domains of Canadian governance that fall within shared provincial-federal jurisdiction according to the constitutional division of powers. When the twin issues of environment and health impact citizens on a First Nations reserve, responsibility for this *policy assemblage* is even more opaque. If there is a normative motivation present in these pages, it is both to reduce the obfuscation of the qualities of this policy assemblage and to put forward a plea that we take seriously environmental reproductive justice in Canada in pursuit of a more equitable, decolonial policy in Canada.

In Chemical Valley citizens of the Aamjiwnaang First Nation reside on "Crown" land set aside for them – a reserve – with their exposed bodies at the fence line of an industrial complex that has the densest concentration of petrochemical manufacturing in the country. Examining contemporary power relations extends beyond sovereign spectacle and transcends into the tentacles of government, executed through practice, on the ground. In Canada's colonial present, when Indigenous citizens' bodies are continuously exposed to chemical contamination such as in Aamjiwnaang, the politics of life itself are at stake. Questioning the administration of life as a relation of power is one of the most compelling intellectual challenges of our time. Following Rabinow and Rose (1994, 25), this task must not be undertaken by claiming that there is some "deep hidden secret of modernity to be revealed"; rather, it requires meticulous attention to life's grey matter, namely the details and practices of life and death that we construct, inhabit, and contest. This task is simultaneously banal and profound.

Contrary to visible practices of corporeal violence in the public domain, citizen bodies live at the forefront of pollution exposures. The everyday, chronic penetration of these toxins remains out of immediate sight and out of mind for governments, neighbouring industries, and most Canadians. Thus it is a kind of "slow violence" (Nixon 2011). The placement of their bodies in this precarious place continues below the radar of public consciousness. As a result, residents here face a dilemma that reveals the multiple edges of citizenship. On the one hand, they are forced to respond instrumentally to environmental violence. On the other hand, they voice a strong, relational attachment to this place. Citizens' practices, activities, actions, and resistances expose this dilemma as a paradox of freedom and draw attention to the deeply interconnected relationships between their bodies and this place that they call both prison and home.

Facing this dilemma, citizens of Aamjiwnaang refuse to be complacent. Following over a century of cultural distillation and a decade of aggressive activism, latent concerns propelled members of this community forward in a movement for environmental reproductive justice. Aligned with Schlosberg (2013), this research contributes to an emerging body of scholarship enhancing and reframing the discursive dimensions of environmental justice in theory, method, and practice. It goes beyond recognition of environmental injustice and beyond a discussion of the inequitable distribution of risks and goods to include consideration of the more-than-human world as a condition for social justice. Critical scholars must pay attention to the ways that the body is central to ongoing struggles and that experiential knowledge is a core conduit for justice. Thus it is clear that reproductive justice cannot be separated from environmental justice. Hoover and colleagues (2012, 15) claim that environmental reproductive justice entails the right and ability to reproduce in culturally appropriate ways:

"for many Indigenous communities to reproduce culturally informed citizens requires a clean environment" (see also SisterSong 2013). Here, empirical research on the community's struggles and on the corresponding assemblage of policy responses and encounters forms the ground for theorization of justice from below. These encounters provide new ways of thinking about the political subjectivities of citizenship. Achieving environmental justice, when understood through a feminist and prismatic biopolitical focus on politics of the body, requires an intersectional and placed treatment of reproductive justice. Thus our legislative and policy processes must adopt an affective and situated approach to *sensing policy* that begins with citizens' *lived experiences.* These processes both generate and encounter *situated bodies of knowledge.* A sensing policy approach must entail a *multilayered analysis,* scaled from the global to the local through *geopolitical location.*

Intersectional Policy Analysis: Insights from Feminist Biopolitics and Geopolitics

Thinking about the body politically is not new. It has always been part of the art of politics. "Bodies" formulate bounded systems. Literally and figuratively, bodies construct boundaries between self, mind, and the outside world. For Aristotle (1962), participation in the civilized political community – the polis – required *bios,* or qualified life, which was distinct from *zoe,* or bare apolitical existence. Superior to the bare, unqualified life of *zoe,* the cultivated life form of *bios* led to citizenship. In this political depiction, the body was considered to be a separate entity from the natural uncivilized body. Hence notions of political community operated within an exclusive logic.

Contending with gendered systems of meaning draws attention to the body. As Massey (1994, 4) highlights, Western dualisms have "coded masculine" predominant ways of thinking, privileging a "disembodied, free-floating generalizing science." Western thought predominantly continues to maintain primacy of mind over matter. Best known for a mechanistic view of the body, seventeenth-century French philosopher René Descartes put forward the idea "cogito ergo sum" (I think, therefore I am), which still holds traction in our current time. This conception treated the body as inferior to the mental faculties of the cultivated mind. The body functioned as a system of parts, as matter constructed of bones, nerves, muscles, veins, blood, and skin; it moved only through an act of will. This dualistic depiction of the body created a mechanistic and determinist model that separated body as "matter" – associated with the physical, private, and natural world – from the superior rational mind.

Consequently, there has been an overemphasis in political thought and practice on the primacy of the rational individual, where the body is considered to be an organism that is distinct from the mind and separate from nature and place. This bodily ordering bears upon the meaning of citizenship today, which merits interrogation.

Classical political thought treated the body as emotive and thus outside the reasonable public realm of political life. As Young (1989, 254, 253) notes, women have been conventionally relegated to the private realm as guardians of "need, desire and affectivity," whereas the public arena remains filled with masculine "discourse framed in unemotional tones of dispassionate reason." Citizenship, following a long line of liberal political thought, functions as an "expression of the universality of human life" and as a "realm of rationality" that is distinct from need, interest, and desire, which are designated feminine (ibid., 253). This role of citizenship has considerable implications for the private "apolitical" domain of existence – where classical political thought tends to (dis)place femininity, the body, and desire. A relational approach to citizenship and democracy conceives of this public-private relationship otherwise.

Life in a democracy is far from smooth. Contending with this demarcation draws attention to the emotional, conflictual, and affective dimensions of "the political" as such. Drawing attention to the paradoxical nature of modern liberal democracy, as well as informing the orientation to radical and relational democracy in this manuscript, Mouffe's (2005b, 28) critique of "rationalist" political life sheds light: "the theorists who want to eliminate passion from politics and argue that democratic politics should be understood only in terms of reason, moderation and consensus are showing their lack of understanding of the dynamics of the political." Discussing embodied dimensions of politics aligns with both Young and Mouffe. Advocating for *sensing policy* chimes with Mouffe's (2005a, 11) call for a "life politics," which reaches into the areas of personal life to create a "democracy of the emotions." Doing so problematizes the superficial dividing lines between the public and private, the masculine and feminine, and the rational and corporeal realms of "the political" to carve out new space for thinking differently about citizenship, subjectivity, and belonging.

Interrogating biological subjugation is central to feminist political thought. Matter – bodies and the "natural" world – has conventionally been considered something to control, to tame, and to temper. Feminist analyses tackle the separation between mind and matter, seeking to bring the body "in" to political analyses in material and discursive ways (Brown 1988; Butler 1993). Early waves of feminist thought – concerned with suffrage and with social and legal equality – are largely credited with making the personal political. Although respectful of these motivations, the argument advanced here is not about "making room" for women in politics or directly about critiquing gender-based assumptions about political behaviour and action. Rather, this study offers a discursive account of the body as a site of political analysis uniquely situated in Canada's Chemical Valley. Following Brown (1988), this methodology is about interrogating the gendered nature of political life. Citizenship, as a defining feature of political life, is a gendered concept at its core. According to Gabrielson and Parady (2010, 375), "written into the very concept is a privileging of the epistemic that constructs political space through the reinforcing dualisms of mind/matter, nature/culture, reason/emotion, men/women, public/private and so on." A biopolitical feminist approach to citizenship thus contests any notion of a disembodied citizen.

The most obvious manifestation of the gendered nature of political life is the persistence of Cartesian dualism. Grosz (1994) eloquently inverts these dualisms by building upon "postmodern" theorists, including Friedrich Nietzsche, Michel Foucault, Gilles Deleuze, and Félix Guattari, to demonstrate how subjectivity can be thought otherwise.[10] Challenging the egocentricism of liberal theory's rejection of the atomistic body in political thought and practice advocates for a relational body to examine, interpret, and assess citizen agency in Canada's Chemical Valley. At the heart of this approach is an interpretive and intersectional attempt to dissect the body-mind and body-place dualisms that continue to dominate Western philosophy and science.

Bodies are personal and they are political. In fact, the body is powerful and regenerative. The body is a "force to be reckoned with" (Grosz 1994, 120). A body is no simple "thing." Bodies are "the centers of perspective, insight, reflection, desire and agency" (ibid., xi). Bodies give life; they are productive and they are placed. Bodies interact, they produce, and they act and react, generating what is "new, surprising and unpredictable" (ibid.). Bodies challenge rigid demarcations between private and public life, merit political inquiry, and tell us about the constitution of political life itself. Such understanding deconstructs or displaces the inadequacies of Western, liberal thought that demarcate between body and mind, nature and culture, and human and environment.

To decentre the primacy of a rational, atomistic individual charged with mastering an unruly body, and to situate the reproductive body in *place*, this approach to citizenship and policy contributes to a fledgling field of "intersectionality-based policy analysis" (Gabrielson and Parady 2010; Hankivsky 2012; Hankivsky and Dhamoon 2013; MacGregor 2006). As discussed elsewhere, there are three central types of gendered approaches to citizenship: formal, substantive, and discursive (Wiebe 2010). Although components of each are present in various stages of the analysis here, the discursive, corporeal, and felt dimensions are brought front and centre as a means to discuss emergent forms of citizenship.

To avoid a discursive overemphasis on "lifestyle blaming" for wound and injury in Aamjiwnaang, and consistent with an environmental reproductive justice framework of inquiry, individual subjects should not be considered place*less* individuals. Ontological questions of *place* draw insight from scholarship in feminist geopolitics (Dixon 2014; Dixon and Marston 2011; Dowler and Sharp 2001; Massaro and Williams 2013; Sharp 2011) and respond to Western, liberal notions of rationality and "individual responsibility" for the management of land and life. The feminist and intersectional body of scholarship provokes a turn away from institutional dimensions of power relations and an examination of embodied and situated knowledges that ground discourse and practice in place. Although indeed concerned with the intersection of geography and politics, feminist geopolitics is to be distinguished from conventional notions of "geopolitics," which as a field of study tends to examine international relations and the geographic, economic, and political forces confronting state boundaries. Feminist geopolitics examines power relations through the hidden workings of everyday life. Thus it focuses our attention on local practices and embodied struggles for knowledge. A feminist geopolitical lens scales from the global to the intimate. It interrogates the impact of macro-level policy assemblages on individual bodies as they encounter these situated, placed ensembles of political forces.

Places are affective; they entail strong emotional commitments and visceral feelings. Whereas space is broad and abstract, place is specific. Although it can range conceptually between the macro and micro levels – from "nation" to "home" – this analysis hones in on place and place-making practices that are rooted and local. Moreover, acknowledging and respecting the cultural knowledge of place is a core axiom of reproductive justice analysis. "Place" is a centre of meaning constructed by experience. Following Tuan (1975, 159), I emphasize that shared meanings and feelings produce "bodies of knowledge." Knowledge forms as individuals interact with place through experience. Relationships between individuals and places disrupt rational accounts of individual subjectivity that hierarchize individuals above place. Humans are directly involved with place through a phenomenal encounter. Places are sensed, felt, breathed, and lived. Bodies encounter places over time and through spaces that are mediated by daily life and experiences. As bodies guide us into place, we encounter cultural knowledge. Whereas "space" is a broad and general category, place is relational and particular.

Places give character to people who inhabit or dwell in them. Thus the characteristics of people and places are intertwined. Those who inhabit places come to share features with the local landscape, but they also mark land in particular ways. Bodily encounters, actions, and positions – such as posture, word, sensation, memory, image, and gesture – shape and inform place through common engagements and configurations. Places are never coherent or fixed (Massey 2005); they are relational and multilayered like a mille feuille cake. By engaging with places, one can gesture toward generating local knowledge, which can challenge, unsettle, and dispel overarching generalizable terms. Aamjiwnaang's location, intruded upon by Canada's Chemical Valley, entails no set number of representations or categorizable "Truths"; there are numerous articulations.

The fleshing-out of place is made possible by piecemeal snapshots, read through an analysis of citizen practices and conversations with Indigenous knowledge carriers who graciously shared their teachings with me. These carriers form a diverse group, including elders, community members, artists, and poets. According to John Borrows (2010, 242), for many Anishinabek, the earth "grows and develops or dies and decays because it is a living being subject to many of the same forces as all other living creatures." Many Anishinabek people characterize the earth as a living entity with thoughts, feelings, and agency. In this respect, the earth has an animate personality, which is a notion in stark contrast to much of Western political thought. Caution is important here. On the one hand, this claim may appear to construct a single "Truth" and to generalize about Anishinabek ontology. That is not the aim. Although reality is diverse and there is no one "Truth," there are also some sophisticated metaphysical teachings illuminated by an Anishinabek ontology that speak to the heart of tensions between contemporary Western life and an alternative way of being in today's world.

Furthermore, a desire to understand the subtle and not so subtle violences and injustices that citizens encounter provides the ideational and institutional motive for this theoretical undertaking. Following Shaw (2008), the unfolding discussion contributes to a conversation about how our inherited circumstances constitute and legitimate some forms of authority and marginalize others. Why study the plight of Indigenous peoples in a precarious place? One should not take on a social justice project for particularly noble or just motivations. Such situations are neither markedly deplorable nor righteous. These situations reveal core issues of "our" contemporary colonial politics, illuminating relations of power between the state, the Canadian public, and residents of Chemical Valley who are citizens of the Aamjiwnaang First Nation. Moreover, the situation for many Indigenous peoples is especially revealing about the character of modern politics because many reside in political states and spaces that are defined by colonial settlement: "Our own identities are constituted partly in relation to" Indigenous peoples, "our economies and political communities are enabled by resources colonized from them," and "their situations reveal most profoundly the violences inflicted by our own modes of life and understanding" (ibid., 5). The experiences of Indigenous peoples in Canada are a condition of possibility for our all-too-settled existence.

The claims made by many Indigenous peoples and movements seek to profoundly unsettle the sedimented foundations of Canadian sovereignty. In the process of developing an understanding of what motivates Indigenous mobilization – inequitable distribution of resources, in addition to structural, discursive, ontological, and epistemological conditions – the acknowledgment of this unfavourable context is not a licence to "solve" their struggles; rather, these tensions offer a stark reminder that we must understand uneven social conditions and power relations to conduct a critical ontology of ourselves and our contemporary political life.

Chapter Overview

This body of work – a corpus – unfolds sequentially through seven anatomically correspondent chapters. Chapter 1 highlights the ongoing, slow-moving, and latent yet viscerally penetrating pollution problem as a matter of environmental reproductive injustice in Aamjiwnaang. It advances the central argument that policy in pursuit of environmental justice in Canada must account for reproductive justice and, in doing so, offers a *sensing policy* approach that entails four intersectional analytical facets: *multilayered analysis, lived experience, geopolitical location*, and *situated bodies of knowledge*. By locating concerned citizens' bodies in *place*, Chapter 1 underscores the implications of these struggles for environmental justice policy, for the concept of citizenship, and for political life itself. An intersectional and prismatic biopolitical analysis informs the overall theoretical orientation of sensing policy.

Chapter 2 explains and fleshes out the nuances of a sensing policy framework for analysis. It situates citizen narratives in *place*. To make sense of ongoing struggles, it outlines the theoretical and methodological approach undertaken, as well as setting the stage for the interpretive unfolding inquiry, grounded within an *affective* intersectionality-based policy analysis. This chapter also contributes to ongoing scholarly debates regarding environmental justice and citizenship studies in Canada and beyond. Using an interpretive and intersectional method, this section explains the qualitative approach undertaken, namely in-depth interviews, archival research, political ethnography, and community-engaged scholarship. I discuss the relationship between engaged research, lived experience, and decolonizing methodology, which inform the empirical chapters that follow.

As Chapter 3 draws into focus, Canada's official treatment of Indigenous peoples reveals biological beliefs and values across macro (federal), meso (provincial), and micro (community) layers of policy making. This chapter discusses the numerous institutional and discursive ways that the Canadian state has regulated the bodies of "Indian" citizens in Canada and Aamjiwnaang. It reviews both official and unofficial policies of the state that affect Indigenous bodies. Illuminating the multifaceted dimensions of Indigenous environmental justice, Chapter 3 presents three components of this policy assemblage: *institutional configurations, discursive fields,* and *citizen practices.* Specifically, the chapter assesses the changing governance structure and citizenship policies for First Nations – or "Indians" – in Canada through an analysis of the Indian Act, as well as broader policy initiatives. This section concludes with an assessment of the paradox of freedom that is created by the dilemma of citizenship and with an account of the related policy implications. Citizenship is thus at once disempowering and empowering, as citizens assume responsibilities for the management of their land and life as disciplinary stewards, while advocating for a radical form of recognition and belonging embedded within the more-than-human world.[11]

Inspired by Foucault's genealogical method, the treatment of history builds upon a textual analysis to investigate the shape-shifting nature of this policy assemblage, which entails relevant laws and policies, jurisdiction, and governance for on-reserve environmental health. According to Adkin (2009, 298), "when citizens become involved in environmental struggles, they very quickly find themselves enmeshed in a much broader web of relationships and issues." These webs can be understood as assemblages, ensembles, or regimes of power that define the limits of our contemporary democratic existence. Following Mouffe (2005a, 18), counter to purely instrumentalist terms for liberal democratic theory, we can think of modern democracy as a "regime." This political form of society considers the wider context for democratic life, including the symbolic ordering of social relations in site-specific places.

Drawing directly from interpretive and ethnographic observations, Chapter 4 highlights citizens' lived experience as expressed by residents of the

Aamjiwnaang First Nation. It engages with everyday lived experiences articulated by citizens in their own words. It presents a discursive analysis of concerns about the experienced and sensed pollution problem in Aamjiwnaang and a discussion of the various ways that citizens and stakeholders in Aamjiwnaang and Chemical Valley practise citizenship. They articulate a simultaneous disdain for and attachment to the place they call both prison and home, where they live with their bodies on the frontlines of toxic chemical exposure, with limited state intervention. Chapter 4 introduces the experiential knowledges employed by citizens and stakeholders who mobilize their bodies as they seek recognition of environmental health concerns. Following Orsini and Smith (2010), I emphasize that contrary to conventional modes of public policy analysis, which explore the ways that problems are to be "solved" by accessing or shaping the healthcare system, *sensing policy* begins from the view that citizens are active agents who mobilize distinctive knowledges. Aligned with Foucault (1977, 59) and Tuan (1975, 159), we can understand these as "bodies of knowledge."

Adding to the personal interviews, published materials, and archival documents, Chapter 5 highlights a "regulatory gap" in on-reserve environmental health and the ongoing problem of jurisdiction (Mackenzie 2013; Moffat and Nahwegahbow 2004). It subsequently explores some of the continuities and discontinuities of official citizenship policies and practices in Canada as they affect Aamjiwnaang's specific geopolitical location. It traces historical links between citizenship, Indigenous governance, and the body. In doing so, Chapter 5 provides an overview of the historical formation of the Aamjiwnaang First Nation's social location through official public policies at the federal, provincial, and municipal levels. The material reviewed includes regulations, policy statements, and media articles to examine the multilayered effects, techniques, and strategies of biopower from Canada to Chemical Valley.

Chapter 6 anchors a discussion of *situated bodies of knowledge,* while highlighting relationships between citizens, expertise, and knowledge in various forms of activism. These bodies of knowledge can be categorized as *experiential, external,* and *engaged.* Focusing on how these struggles play out in an ongoing countywide health study, this chapter demonstrates how the community seeks recognition of its environmental and reproductive health concerns in this politically charged and deliberative process.

The final chapter is both a closing and an opening. Chapter 7 looks at continued citizen involvement in Idle No More, at Attawapiskat chief Theresa Spence's high-profile hunger strike, and at the final report of the Truth and Reconciliation Commission of Canada (2015). Moving forward, rather than offering closure, this chapter weaves together implications of each action as part of an ongoing movement for justice, democracy, and citizenship. It includes a distillation of the previous empirical chapters and offers directions for future environmental justice scholarship in Canada, beginning with the lessons and teachings offered by Aamjiwnaang. Bringing the findings into conversation with selected literature on Canadian politics and policy, citizenship studies, and environmental studies, Chapter 7 draws attention to how sensing policy is both practically and conceptually crucial to the formation of environmental reproductive justice. The chapter closes by pointing toward the promising potential of collaborative and creative arts-based approaches to environmental reproductive justice as an avenue for addressing many of the themes and concerns taken up in the book. Throughout the writing journey, by collaborating on this project with artists both inside and outside the community, I sought to share voice, knowledge, and power. Ongoing involvement with the Aamjiwnaang Green Teens through collaborative photography and with the Kiijig Collective through participatory community filmmaking exemplifies this objective, as does my collaboration with international photojournalist Laurence Butet-Roch, whose brilliant and arresting images illuminate and visualize the text.[12]

Conclusion

Setting the atmosphere and location of Chemical Valley surrounding the Aamjiwnaang First Nation provides a sense of place that informs the following chapters. With the intention of situating ongoing citizen struggles for environmental reproductive justice in place, this book advocates for a different way of thinking about citizenship and policy. A *sensing policy* lens, which entails four components – *multilayered analysis, lived experience, geopolitical location,* and *situated bodies of knowledge* – presents a new vantage point and framework for analyzing complex policy assemblages such as Indigenous environmental justice. Creative photographic works enhance this textual lens to illuminate themes of atmosphere, daily life, and cultural resurgence while drawing into focus lived realities in order to diversify representation and ultimately democratize knowledge.

2

Sensing Policy
An Affective Framework of Analysis

Examining and Reimagining Citizenship in Canada

Reimagining citizenship requires a new vision that begins with relationships. The Two Row Wampum model is one of the oldest treaty relationships between the Onkwehonweh (original people) of Turtle Island (present-day North America) and European immigrants. It goes back to an early agreement between the Dutch traders and Haudenosaunee (Iroquois) people in Kanien'kehá:ka (Mohawk) territory (Keefer 2014). It is to be distinguished from a patriarchal and colonial relationship. As per the custom of recording events of significance, the Haudenosaunee created a wampum belt out of purple and white quahog shells to commemorate the treaty agreement. The wampum belt represented two vessels travelling down the same river together, or two nations existing together without interfering in each other's internal affairs, customs, or legal traditions (J. Borrows 2010; Keefer 2014; Tully 1995). It is a symbol of reciprocity, peace, friendship, and respect, a foundational philosophical principle of "non-domination, balance and harmony between forces" (Keefer 2014). The wampum thus offers a relevant and decolonizing perspective on treaty relations today.

Scholars of the liberal citizenship tradition in Canada worry that the "nation-to-nation" approach outlined by the Royal Commission on Aboriginal Peoples (RCAP 1996) will weaken the idea of common belonging. In contrast with the Two Row Wampum model, these scholars emphasize the role of the individual in society. Despite recognizing the importance of Aboriginal rights and title, liberal approaches to citizenship demonstrate concern with the "oneness" of the Canadian nation (Cairns 2000, 200). In this respect, liberal *ontology* – worldviews, categories of being, and relations – contend with Aboriginal values and beliefs. Flanagan (2000, 194) goes so far as to call the commission a "stop-sign for human progress," pursuant of an "Aboriginal orthodoxy." At the turn of the twenty-first century, intending to take a progressive step forward, Cairns (2000) resurrected a historic policy document, the 1963 Hawthorn-Tremblay Report, to advocate for a "citizens plus" lens on Canadian-Indigenous relations. This conception of citizenship attempts to mediate between collective and individual identities without forcing Canada to be a "container for international nations" (ibid., 199). According to him, a coherent and unified nation requires Indigenous peoples to maintain special rights while respecting individual responsibilities and obligations to fellow Canadian citizens through civic duties. Aligned with Flanagan, Cairns presents a vision for the accommodation of Indigenous citizenship in Canada that draws upon a civic form of Western possessive individualism. The federal government responded to the Hawthorn-Tremblay Report in 1969 with its "White Paper" (Government of Canada 1969), which failed to recognize Aboriginal title and rights. Many saw the paper as a mechanism to further assimilate Aboriginal peoples into the colonial Canadian state. It was a wide departure from a "citizens plus" vision. Despite the inclusive promises of citizens plus, even this conception of citizenship fails to address the inherently Western, Eurocentric assumptions upon which the notion rests.

Furthermore, institutional approaches to the study of citizenship articulate hope about the capacity of Canada's configurations to recognize and accommodate diverse multinational claims within existing structures. Papillon (2009) exemplifies this optimism about the opportunities for Indigenous peoples within the Canadian federation by suggesting that federalism itself does not cause the exclusion of Aboriginal people; rather, the historical expression of federalism is to blame. From this perspective, federalism is not merely a set of institutions but also a normative ideal.

This societal approach to federalism – comprised of both institutions and ideas – goes a step further to move our attention away from the formal parameters of institutional configurations and toward the practical realm of public policy. As Papillon (2009, 406) highlights, although we are not in a "postcolonial" arrangement, important developments that merit political investigation are occurring across the political landscape in the "realm of everyday governance within Aboriginal nations and communities" and are also apparent in "interactions between Aboriginal, provincial and federal governments in the design and implementation of public policy." This malleable discussion of federalism takes us in two directions: toward "executive federalism" and toward "daily governance." However, although emergent spaces and tactics may operate within an opportunity structure for Aboriginal peoples on macro and meso scales, this account conflates executive legitimacy with the diversity of community perspectives and experiences on the ground at the micro level. Although Papillon highlights the executive approach to addressing the concerns of Aboriginal peoples, the analysis reads as unfinished with respect to the informal realm of "daily governance." In this regard, the discussion of federalism "from below" ends within the institutional dimensions of executive Aboriginal leadership – it eclipses community-level experiences. Although his analysis of federalism may be "from below," it is certainly not one rooted in the daily experiential practices of governance at the local, community level.[1]

Informed by Tully (1995), Papillon (2008b, 137) suggests that we should conceptualize federalism as a "normative framework to facilitate the constant negotiation and struggle over the definition of communities." Approaching federalism in this manner – as a means to recognize distinct identities for various groups internal to the federation – provides an opening to reconfigure Canada's formal arrangements. However, analytically, liberal and institutional approaches alike remain fixed to structural scales of political inquiry without substantive regard for, or *recognition* of, the lived experiences outside of these formal sites.[2]

As we can see, many debates about Canadian citizenship and policy assume the liberal primacy of inclusiveness and coherence without problematizing the more informal forms of internal exclusions. Canadian scholars frequently hail Canada as one of the most open-minded, hospitable, inclusive, tolerant, and even "postmodern" societies in the world (Ignatieff 2009; Kymlicka 1989, 1995, 2004; Simeon 2004; Taylor 1994). A more critical account contends that in a postmodern society, oppressions and violence are increasingly subtle and invisible, taking shape through a "fluid confluence of politics, economics, psychology and culture" (Alfred 2005, 30). There are cracks and gaps within our institutions that impact minority communities and challenge our existing democracies. A focus on community experience accentuates an understanding of these failings. There is also a gap between democratic theory and the impacts of our constitutional configurations on communities fighting for justice. Examining grassroots practices of citizenship through an intersectional lens grabs abstract democratic theory by the throat and grounds it within the minutiae of everyday life.

Taking a different turn, postcolonial scholars attempt to trouble Canada's colonial grip on Indigenous citizenship. Colonialism within this framework is not seen as a dead artifact of the past; rather, its sustained force impacts people's everyday experiences. In general terms, postcolonialism is an approach that is hopeful about the potential of Canadian policy making to address claims for recognition and reconciliation. It aims to move toward progressive social and institutional working relationships with marginalized members of society in pursuit of living in a time of peaceful coexistence in a decolonial world. According to Tully (1995), in contrast to a modern constitutional politics that seeks to impose uniformity in the name of unity and power, the way forward for Canadian-Indigenous relations is through "strange multiplicity" and constitutional dialogue. Tully (ibid., 24–25) argues that we can take the metaphor of a vessel, namely Bill Reid's sculpture *The Spirit of Haida Gwaii,* as a way to think about bringing a multiplicity of needs into a constitutional conversation. He introduces the concept of a "multilogue" – an ability to change perspectives, to see and understand aspectually through multiple vantage points, which takes place through participation in intercultural dialogue. In contrast to Cairns's notion of two societies travelling in separate vessels while sharing the same river but not interfering with each other's choice of direction, Tully (ibid., 24) puts multiple nations within the same vessel:

> As you walk around the canoe you soon realize that it is impossible to take it in from one comprehensive viewpoint. It defies this form of representation. Rather, you are drawn to see it from the perspective of one passenger after another, and their complicated interrelations guide you to see the whole now under one aspect, now under another. Since recognition is never definitive, the particular Constitutional arrangement of the members of the canoe is presumably not meant to be fixed once and for all. Constitutional recognition and association change over time, as the canoe progresses and the members change in various ways. A Constitution is more like an endless series of contracts and agreements, reached by periodical intercultural dialogues, rather than an original contract in the distant past, an ideal speech-situation today, or a mythic unity of the community in liberal and nationalist Constitutionalism.

By listening to the many stories others tell, and by in turn providing stories, participants in a "multilogue" come to see common interwoven histories from a multiplicity of paths and perspectives. This decolonial approach aligns with Anishinabek thought and the wampum belt vision, premised on reciprocity and respect (J. Borrows 2010; Doerfler, Sinclair, and Stark 2013). As membership and participation in the canoe are not meant to be static, it serves as a useful allegory for thinking about ongoing treaty relations and citizenship as a relational practice.

It is imperative to make clear that there exists no singular postcolonial voice in Canadian political thought. Notably, Alfred (2009) argues that Canadian sovereignty does not work for Indigenous peoples; in fact, he contends that the formal institutional terrain insufficiently accommodates difference. Like Tully, Alfred argues that the future of Canadian-Aboriginal relations does not lie within a fixed vision of a unified nation-state; yet he goes further than Tully to argue that the future of Canadian-Indigenous relations requires a return to spiritual and ancestral teachings outside of Canada's institutional confines. Canadian sovereignty, according to Alfred, produces a patronizing, false altruism, which forces Indigenous peoples to live as co-opted artifacts. Thus the state, he argues, cannot and will not accommodate Indigeneity, no matter how pliable. This ontological stance fundamentally challenges liberal and institutional conceptions of citizenship.

Furthermore, a critical, intersectional approach to citizenship highlights the patriarchal formulation of "Indian" citizenship. In doing so, it draws social location into focus to account for race, class, and gender in both policy and practice (Hankivsky 2012; Hankivsky and Christoffersen 2008; Hankivsky and Dhamoon 2013). Constitutional struggles for recognition have particular resonance for Indigenous women. Canadian citizenship has always been a gendered concept (Fiske 2008).[3] Feminist approaches to postcolonial thought bring questions of gender into the study of Canadian citizenship and politics. An intersectional, feminist, postcolonial approach invites scholars to think critically about the interacting ways that Canadian citizenship broadly – and Indigenous citizenship specifically – continue to be shaped by race, class, and gender (Fiske 2008; Hankivsky 2012; Hankivsky and Christoffersen 2008). The Indian Act and subsequent struggles for recognition continue to affect Indigenous women in particular ways.

Contributing to the theory and practice of decolonization, an intersectional approach to policy making emphasizes the lived and gendered effects of power relations, social location, diverse knowledges, and multilayered analysis. It also maintains a commitment to social justice (Hankivsky 2012). Intersectional policy analysis treats policy as an "art of government," which prompts critical reflection beyond institutional parameters within the capillaries of community, where power relations are sensed through everyday life. Expanding upon intersectionality-based policy analysis, the aim of *sensing policy* is to take Canadian and citizenship studies further by examining how citizens are *affected* by policy. Similar to Anderson's (2014, 3) approach, an intersectional analysis of policy accentuates the ways that "affective life takes place and is organized." To address the following questions, this book invites the reader into a conversation about citizen encounters with institutions, discourses, and knowledges that shape and constrain struggles for justice: What are the affective dimensions of citizenship in Canada's Chemical Valley? How do policies both impact and shape citizens? What does policy feel like? How can we make sense of policy, and how can affective policy make sense to policy makers?

Governmentality: Approaching Policy as an Art of Government

An affective approach to policy employs an interpretive methodology. Thus it takes as axiomatic that discursive and structural forms of power, authority, control, and oppression are interconnected and overlapping. Moreover, this approach contends that theorizing must be connected to lived experience on the ground. An interpretive inquiry seeks to open up possibilities for politics by creating avenues for multiple voices to come to the fore. The investigation begins with the understanding that we live in a world of multiple intersubjective social realities. This assumes that humans move through the world experientially and that "embodied," experiential knowledge is full of multifaceted meanings. The normative impetus for accessing this knowledge gestures toward a possibility that it may generate alternative, *situated bodies of knowledge*. Based upon particular practices or forms of expression, these bodies of knowledge may ultimately speak truth to power or prompt the development of more widely representative and inclusive policy making.

Rather than addressing questions about the state's effective or efficient function in governing a healthy *demos*, a focus on the state's appendages or capillaries reveals how certain thoughts, practices, and subjectivities become established. This "governmentality" approach to political analysis, when coupled with ethnographic methods, draws into focus the effects of power and the "lived experience of subjection" (McKee 2009, 474; see also Brady 2011, 266; Foucault 1994a). Governmentality can be understood as an ethos of investigation and as a way of asking questions not only or necessarily about *why* things happen but also about *how*. Drawing on the work of French philosopher Gilles Deleuze, Darier (1996, 601) underscores governmentality's utility to political scientists not as a "truth" concept but as a toolbox to assist us with the continuous process of resisting truth claims and the effects of power. It is a way of approaching policy that accounts for modern and neoliberal subjectivity at the nexus of struggles over power and knowledge from the macro, or state, scale through to the micro, or individual, level. This approach "emphasizes variation and context" and seeks to reveal the "messiness and complexity in the struggles around subjectivity" (McKee 2009, 479). Governmentality studies offer a lens through which scholars can examine the effects of power as mediated by actors or agents – citizens – in particular places.

In contrast to policy approaches that centre on the state or the individual as a core axiom for analysis, a governmentality approach begins with regimes, or relations, of power, which are shaped through discursive fields. How one speaks about an issue is inherently tied to questions about what frames the contours of "the political." A governmentality lens examines the effects of institutions or structures on political behaviour. Coined by French philosopher and social theorist Michel Foucault during his lectures at the Collège de France in 1977–78, the term "governmentality" refers to dealings with the state but reaches beyond the realm of institutions to include its apparatuses, administration, and citizenship, revealing power relations through the extension of the state's tentacles into the spaces and practices of everyday life. This view rejects the notion that "government" is coterminous with formal or official institutions of power, known as "the state." Rather, "government" encompasses a multitude of processes and practices within and outside the state that shape individuals and communities toward desired ends (Murray 2004). This extension of state power operates through the "art of government" and raises questions about how to govern oneself, how to be governed, how to govern others, and how to become the best possible governor (Foucault 1994a). The art of government twins two poles: hierarchical modes of governance and the internal power relations among citizens themselves. Thus citizens act as agents who are active carriers and producers of knowledge. Humans – citizens – are not "objects" but rather agents who actively and collaboratively construct and deconstruct meaning.

Governmentality studies illuminate the paradox of freedom: although liberal theories of governance cling to the notion of individual choices, actions, and responsibilities contingent upon free will, this rational, self-disciplined ethic is simultaneously a linchpin for market-based commodification in a democratic capitalist society. A governmentality framework considers the characteristics of liberalism as a mentality of government, one that entices citizens to become self-regulating, culpable, and active individuals through gentle means, without the state's striking "sting" (Foucault 1994a, 227). The ruler governs through the productive practices of agents at a distance rather than through overtly repressive, bloody, and spectacular means.

Studying political science and public policy in terms of governmentality illuminates the plurality of forms of government and activities that (in)form state-citizen relations. Although governmentality studies may focus on the capillary domains of power and knowledge, where the "king's head" has been cut off, the state is not excused from this analytical framework. The state is only one sphere among others whose examination reveals the ways that power relations emerge and take form (Murray 2007, 163). Foucault (1994a) refers to analyses of governmental power and authority as a kind of topology, which includes the multifarious layers of power and its reach beyond institutions to individual citizens. Governmentality helps us to examine the intermixing of *institutional configurations, discursive regimes,* and *citizen practices.* As Rutherford (2011, xxiv) observes, discourse emerges from multiple sites and can be thought of as inherently unfinished since it is "continuously renegotiated, re-articulated and resisted." Furthermore, it is too simple to draw any rigid dividing line between an external sovereign authority and internal citizen practices. Thus there is a continuity of government both upward from citizens to the state and simultaneously downward from the state to citizens. Well-governed states require well-disciplined citizens to perpetuate productive political and economic relations. Approaches inspired by governmentality examine the play between the "inside" and "outside" of the political boundaries that separate states and citizens, public and private spheres, and government and freedom. Governmentality scholars examine the functioning and expression of political authority and ask not just *who* governs but also *how.*

Viewed through a governmentality lens, governance of the state's population – its *peoples* – operates in sync with individual self-management as a form of "biopower." Biopower is productive. Power produces things: pleasure, forms of knowledge, and discourse. It operates as a productive network that runs through society (Murray 2007). Biopower takes shape in a positive sense, premised upon the assumption that individuals are autonomous and rational beings who have the capacity to govern their own lives and well-being. The rational, liberal logic of the state is transposed upon citizens themselves. The crux of biopower refers to the simultaneous management of populations and individuals. Control over a well-disciplined citizenry or population requires two manoeuvres: mastery of territory and the construction of individually responsible and productive citizens. Biopolitical analyses examine the ways that subjectivities are produced and ordered both at the local level of communities or individuals and, more broadly, at the national level of populations. This critical governmentality-inspired lens thus moves toward an ethnographic approach to policy that is concerned with the everyday and experiential manifestations of power relations on the ground and with their discursive fields.

The Arts of Engagement: Encountering Experiential Knowledge

Researchers are not external to the worlds in which they investigate. Scholars committed to community-engaged scholarship examine their views about the world by seeking to render visible both the macro- and micro-level aspects of our societies that are inexorably linked to broader socio-political forces, which may be invisible to mainstream society. To examine, evaluate, and comment upon these forces, critical scholars conduct what Rabinow and Rose (1994, viii) refer to as "fieldwork in philosophy," which takes thinkers outside of the armchair, laboratory, or classroom and into the materially and discursively constructed social world. It is a kind of applied philosophy, a logic of inquiry that moves beyond the conventional positivist "scientific method," wherein one articulates hypotheses, defines concepts, operationalizes variables, establishes relationships, and "tests" these for validity, reliability, and generalizability (Schwartz-Shea and Yanow 2012, 1). Interpretive research focuses on situated meanings and actors' meaning-making practices in particular *places*.

Turning to Aamjiwnaang, for instance, the name itself pertains not only to a geographical area where the rapids meet the shore but also to a spiritual connection that Anishinabek people have to this locale. As Plain (2007, 1) discusses, "Aamjiwnaang" is a word with no English equivalent; it is descriptive of a unique characteristic of territory, meaning "place where mahnedoog [spirits] live in the water." The territory once covered a much larger area on both the American and the Canadian sides of the border; today, the name "Aamjiwnaang" has become localized to one small reserve. It is a unique place, unlike anywhere else. Acknowledging this is crucial to situating my own social location as a researcher who came from elsewhere. As an engaged scholar, I worked alongside the community to understand and document ongoing injustices in the spirit of participatory-action research with the intention of contributing to the decolonization of research and knowledge.

I am mindful that this research took place on Indigenous land. Thus my research approach is motivated by an attempt to work toward decolonizing methodology (L.T. Smith 1999). From my perspective, this means that the principles of reflexivity, respect, reciprocity, and relationship building are central to the project design, delivery, and dissemination (Native Women's Association of Canada 2009). This approach to research stems from a collaborative, participatory, community-engaged model. Participatory research seeks to connect research to practice by sharing knowledge and authority about the research project with community members through their involvement in all stages of the process. Thus community members were included in critical stages of the project's development, planning, design, analysis, and results dissemination. Such a participatory approach to research requires working *with,* not speaking *for,* the community. Moreover, the members of a community-based advisory committee acted as "cultural navigators" to facilitate a culturally appropriate research design.[4]

It is widely known that Indigenous peoples suffer from research fatigue. They are considered some of the most studied peoples in the world (L.T. Smith 1999). Conducting a meaningful, culturally appropriate, and compassionate investigation that also benefits the community is thus crucial. Even the word "research" contains colonial and negative connotations for many First Nations communities. Aware of this colonial legacy, I took efforts to share knowledge with members of the community throughout the entire process in pursuit of action research to *democratize knowledge* (Hall et al. 2013). I endeavoured to adopt culturally appropriate behaviours, including offering tobacco along with an honorarium for individuals who participated in an interview. Whereas the interviews shed light on certain kinds of knowledge, informal interactions and conversations over coffee, at community events, in public locations, or in people's homes provided in-depth knowledge about people's lived realities.

Engaged research emphasizes community participation in the process and invites the community into the formation of the body of work itself. This approach stems from a belief that the tasks of shaping and controlling research must be shared between the academic and nonacademic communities. Each partner is involved in an ongoing and emergent process of knowledge exchange. This model seeks collaborative partnerships in all phases of the research to foster shared learning. Moreover, it aims to find balance between research and action. Such an approach emphasizes the importance of bringing local, relevant, and ecological perspectives to the fore and acknowledges and integrates a variety of perspectives into the policy-making process. It also endeavours to produce transparent, cyclical, and iterative research, where findings and knowledge are shared with and disseminated to participants along the way and at the end of the study period.

Moreover, it is also crucial to be mindful of community realities, notably that community participation is time- and resource-intensive. Some community-based research models stem from the assumption that moving toward full community participation and engagement is optimal, necessary, and advantageous. This form of research builds upon the strengths and existing resources of communities, including supplemental funds, training, employment opportunities, and shared power relations (Israel et al. 2001, 184). With a community-based approach to research, there exists a normative belief that research will be of direct benefit to the community.

In practice, this ideal faces some challenges. Often the very communities in question are underresourced and overworked, and they may have little time for and interest in the details of academic research. Furthermore, there is an assumption within the notion of "community-based research" itself that "community" represents a coherent identifiable unit (Israel et al. 2001). The reality is that communities are often representative of a variety of perspectives and interests. It is important to be conscious of these concerns, challenges, and divergences before embarking upon a community-engaged initiative.

Participatory research is appealing, as it encourages an open and nuanced methodology. As identified by scholars of Community-Based Research Canada, this approach emphasizes the following core principles: *community relevance, research design, equitable participation,* and *action and change* (Ochocka and Janzen 2014; Wiebe and Taylor 2014). This flexible community-focused approach seeks to be transparent about what one is looking at and for as well as about how and why one is looking. It commits to a continuous exchange of knowledge and ideas, with the aim of social change and action. The most suitable way to think about this kind of participatory research is as a committed and engaged supporter, without trying to guide or steer activism within the community. The iterative process of knowledge exchange itself is a productive enterprise, which seeks to highlight and address public policy gaps while calling into question dominant discourses and practices that marginalize communities.

In addition to making theoretical and methodological contributions to scholarship, pressures emerge to make policy-relevant and policy-meaningful recommendations and interventions in the spirit of social action. I sought to share knowledge with the community by providing a policy brief to the Aamjiwnaang Health and Environment Committee on the ongoing Lambton Community Health Study and by volunteering with the Aamjiwnaang Green Teens, an environmental youth group, through various activities, such as grant writing, event organizing, and supporting this group's work with the Kiijig Collective to create a collaborative documentary film project. My research findings were presented to the community in December 2012. These findings are thus aimed at addressing policy gaps in Indigenous environmental justice in Canada to speak *with,* not *for,* this community in our shared effort to co-create a collaborative approach to *sensing policy*. Although I have formally left the field, the field informally follows me. During numerous return visits, I continue to discuss environmental politics and strategies with community members of all ages, and I support ongoing community-building initiatives, including the preservation of traditional plant use. This relational, intersectional, and interpretive method seeks to contribute to the democratization of knowledge production by moving beyond the "expertise" of technical researchers in order to include the situated voices and stories of those directly affected by ongoing injustices. These relationships extend well beyond the end date of the specific research project.

Resistance to dominant discourses, practices, and operations of power is a crucial feature of critical, interpretive policy analysis. The role of an engaged scholar is not to spearhead a social movement. Perhaps an engaged researcher is best suited to call into question structural and discursive forces that constrain movement and agency. In such an approach, it is not the role of the academic to say, "It is imperative to revolt, do you not realize that your world is intolerable?" (Rabinow and Rose 1994, xxvii). The scholar's role is not to tell those experiencing injustice what to do and not to do or what to strive for and what to reject. Rather, the engaged scholar seeks to criticize the present without "anaesthetizing" those who must act within it, as well as to make conventional actions problematic while opening up space for movement. Furthermore, these aims must be achieved without slipping into a prophetic posture that makes it not only impossible to act but also more, not less, difficult to know what to do (ibid., xxviii). Social science researchers need to recall that actors have voice and agency; they are not helpless or passive. As Latour (1999, 19–20) suggests,

> Actors know what they do and we have to learn from them not only what they do, but how and why they do it. It is us, the social scientists, who lack knowledge of what they do, and not they who are missing the explanation of why they are unwittingly manipulated by forces exterior to themselves and known to the social scientist's powerful gaze and methods.

To investigate the practices of power relations within communities, scholars may find themselves situated "in the field" of those relations.

Ethnographic studies are crucial to the exploration of inclusion and exclusion in any political community. This aligns with an interpretive methodology, which requires the researcher to navigate the relationship between official discourses, situated narratives, and local knowledges that have grown out of daily practice and interactions. Such a method expands and explodes the boundaries of "the political" to examine peoples' lived realities (Kubik 2009; Schatz 2009). It is furthermore a disorienting enterprise for the researcher, which unsettles prior assumptions or truths that a scholar brings to bear upon the field of investigation. It assumes a considerable loss of control and involves "interactive observation" rather than "objective observation" through a one-way looking glass (Schwartz-Shea and Yanow 2012, 54). An ethnographic approach to the study of (in)justice provides a vehicle through which researchers can examine the location of power in unfamiliar places, like Canada's Chemical Valley.

Ethnography brings you exceptionally close to your "data." In many ways, the field can guide the research design, plan, and methodology. Interactions with "data" and "research participants" occur through ongoing and continuously evolving learning. It requires significant flexibility, openness, and comfort with accepting a loss of complete control over the entire structured research process. Flexibility in the field is a conscious, intentional strategy: "It applies not only to the need to respond in the moment to things said or done, but also to how the research process may be changing initial research designs and questions" (Schwartz-Shea and Yanow 2012, 55). Thus research design in this setting is not necessarily linear. The research question often comes into focus in unexpected ways through hermeneutic encounters that can send the researcher off in multiple directions. It is a circular approach and therefore iterative and recursive, with "each of its parts informing and folding back on the others, enacting the same sense-making spiral that characterizes the conduct of interpretive inquiry" (ibid.). It seeks to open up rather than to hone in on its subject, emphasizing iteration over controlled design.

Delineating between "participant" and "observer" in the field falls within a constantly shifting continuum. Like many locals, while residing in Chemical Valley, I also smelled peculiar odours and noticed when the stacks flared larger and burned brighter at night, and I too wondered about the impact on those living close by. As many locals did, I kept a record of the various leaks, accidents, and spills from Chemical Valley on a large calendar. Sometimes these were reported in the media – radio, print, or television – but most times they were not. I connected to an online alert system that would – in theory – let me know about such releases via email and cellphone text messaging. Conducting research in this manner involves engaging in practices of daily life that resemble those of local residents. Thus the only escape, or break, tends to be physical removal from the site itself.

Immersion in the field is an embodied, emotional, and affective research strategy. The researcher places his or her body in what can be a foreign or unsettling context, allowing it to experience a range of impulses, feelings, and emotions, which may (re)shape the research design. These are registered and unregistered – conscious and unconscious – drives that motivate the project's formation. Generally speaking, "affect" refers to the registered, yet unconscious, experience of feelings or emotions (Wiebe 2013). It is part of the body's reaction to external stimuli and may deal with gut feelings and visceral impulses and their relationship to cognition. By living in a new environment, one's relationships and habitus, or mode of operating in a particular setting, become shaped by the field. Thus this kind of research is as much personal and emotional as it is political. Furthermore, in such a new and emergent setting, power relations are never absent from the research context. In addition to physically immersing one's body in the field, the separation between external expert researcher and internal community member becomes somewhat blurred, although it is never completely erased.

From an interpretive approach, the exploration of research questions is intimately tied to a particular setting. Situating oneself within that setting and thinking reflexively about one's positionality is crucial. I am cognizant of my position of privilege as a young female researcher with access to technology (e.g., car and computer), the ability to pay honoraria, mobility to and from the site, and an identity as someone who is not native to that place yet is interested in studying the experiences of others living in a precarious setting. Upon entering the field, I was motivated by conceptualizing my own experience as a "researcher" in the spirit of what Yanow (2003) refers to as "passionate humility" and willingness to revisit my own, sometimes hidden, assumptions. This kind of passionate humility aligns with a commitment to conducting an ontology of the self as part of "personal decolonization" (Irlbacher-Fox 2009; Rabinow and Rose 1994). A critical questioning of one's "self" is not a search for universal values or truths; rather, it calls into question, problematizes, and dismantles assumptions.

The overall approach to *sensing policy*, as interpretive research coupled with a commitment to a participatory and decolonizing methodology, aligns with critical scholarship and concretely seeks to contribute to social justice (Burnham et al. 2008; Madison 2005; L.T. Smith 1999). The intention here is to share voice, knowledge, and place with those who shared their experiences with me rather than to create "traveller's" tales that I take back to my privileged academic community (L.T. Smith 1999). By writing and recording extensive field notes to document my own thoughts, interpretations, and reflections, I continued to evaluate the views and values that I brought to the study with the intent of challenging my assumptions in order to make space for new meanings, ontologies, and epistemologies.

Specifically, my immersion in Aamjiwnaang involved repeated formal conversations and encounters with community members over a two-year period, although my relationships with community members are ongoing as the struggles continue. In January 2011 I relocated to Sarnia, Ontario, approximately 720 kilometres away from Ottawa. This followed a year of work as a research assistant at York University for Dr. Dayna Scott, who had an established relationship with the community based upon her environmental justice efforts with citizens of the Aamjiwnaang First Nation. During this research, I developed relationships with and ties to the community. Following numerous trips between Ottawa and Sarnia, it became apparent that if I wanted to commit to understanding struggles for environmental reproductive justice, greater proximity would be both simpler and necessary. Guided by my intuition and my commitment to this study, I relocated to an apartment in downtown Sarnia for an indeterminate period. My intention was to split my time equally between Sarnia and Ottawa. Trips to Ottawa became less frequent as Sarnia became my adopted home.

The motivations for this uprooting were threefold. First, it reduced travel time between Ottawa and Sarnia, which made attending public meetings much more feasible. As part of my participant observation methodology, I attended monthly board meetings of the Lambton Community Health Study (LCHS) starting in January 2011. Prior to that, in 2010, I attended each of the five open houses for the LCHS community consultations, during which I listened to community concerns, took notes, and observed how the facilitators captured these concerns and presented them to the board. I paid attention to the articulation of power, knowledge, expertise, and authority. The public meetings in Aamjiwnaang included industry open houses, community consultations, environmental information seminars, and Aamjiwnaang Green Teens meetings. Residence in Sarnia made conducting sixty-one in-depth interviews over this period possible. Interview questions were approved by the University of Ottawa Research Ethics Board, by a community supervisory committee, by the Aamjiwnaang Health and Environment Committee, and by the chief and council. Participants were recruited by means of a flyer in the community newsletter, the *Chippewa Tribe-une;* and I conducted all the interviews myself, either at the E'Mino Bmaad-Zijig Gamig Aamjiwnaang Health Centre, at a coffee shop, or in the comfort of someone's home.

I conducted semistructured interviews with sixty-one participants over a year-long period. Thirty-five of the interviewees were citizens of Aamjiwnaang, and twenty-six were policy makers or public officials at all levels of government.[5] Public officials included LCHS board members, municipal representatives, provincial and federal policy makers, and community policy makers. I spoke with past and present members of the Aamjiwnaang First Nation Health and Environment Committee and with the chief and band council members, although not all agreed to an interview. Pseudonyms are used for all participants, unless they provided consent for their name to be recorded. Every attempt was made to ensure confidentiality in accordance with both academic and community ethical protocols. I took notes during each interview while also recording them (with consent) on a handheld audio recorder. I then transcribed the interviews. These transcriptions, along with policy documents, reports, speeches, and legislation, were coded based on subject themes. I looked for patterns, dissonance, and disjunctures between textual documents and oral narratives. The results are discussed at length in Chapters 4 and 6, where I present an interpretive analysis of the findings.

My second motivation for relocating to Sarnia was the need to immerse myself in the "field" so that I could not only observe community events but also participate in them. Given my overall interest in supporting struggles for environmental reproductive justice, nearly everything in my surroundings became part of the research process. I continued to volunteer with the Aamjiwnaang Green Teens, to attend community meetings on and off the reserve, and to plug into the local Sarnia art and social scene. Community engagement was marked by on- and off-reserve relationship building. Involvements led to the creation of an arts group, the Kiijig Collective, which is a collaborative enterprise with the mandate to share knowledge about First Nations values and beliefs among its members through creative forms of expression. In 2012, while writing up my research findings, I continued to reside in Sarnia and subsequently took on the role of "executive producer" of a documentary film entitled *Indian Givers,* coproduced by the Kiijig Collective and released for presentation at a local high school and on the reserve.[6]

Moreover, field relationships entail recurring interactions between "researcher" and "researched" and may extend beyond the formal research timeframe. The engaged nature of these interactions calls a researcher to attend to the humanity of those who give of their time and resources in helping the researcher gain "access" to, or greater understanding of, the research topic. Thus research participants are much more than simply "informants" or "data." This recognition consequently entails treating "research participants" in their full humanness rather than merely as a "means to an end" (Schwartz-Shea and Yanow 2012, 59). In doing so, I frequently joined Aamjiwnaang citizens at speaking engagements, participated in panel discussions, attended local consultation meetings with stakeholders, and and was available in Toronto and Ottawa to receive and offer advice on arising research concerns.

My third motivation for relocating to Sarnia was that it made possible a community-engaged research strategy, which involves sustained relationships. As stated, ethical, engaged research entails reflexivity, respect, reciprocity, and relationship building. Upon the suggestion of Dr. Dayna Scott, initial contact with members of the Aamjiwnaang First Nation took place offsite in Toronto. I explained my doctoral study interests and research assistantship with Dr. Scott to my first interlocutor, a local activist and Aamjiwnaang First Nation citizen. Shortly thereafter, I visited the community and participated in a "toxic tour" given by a member of the Aamjiwnaang Health and Environment Committee. I attended public information events in the community and began to develop a rapport with the Aamjiwnaang Health and Environment Committee. When the reserve committee's structure changed, I continued to work with Dr. Scott on building a positive relationship with the incoming committee members in order to support the Aamjiwnaang Green Teens while also co-organizing a Community Forum on Pollution and Action, held in Sarnia in February 2011. I maintained relationships with my initial interlocutors as informal community advisers and also requested the assistance of an elder and several other community members to guide and support the overall structure and framing of my project. Community advisers were offered an honorarium for their continued time, advice, and support. Moreover, I presented all recruitment and research materials to the Health and Environment Committee and subsequently requested and received approval from the chief and council to conduct my research. On an ongoing basis, I maintained contact with my advisers as well as the Health and Environment Committee.

Finally, an interpretive approach to policy is not a matter of saying that things are or are not right. Rather, this approach seeks to uncover what kinds of assumptions remain too familiar and unchallenged. It deconstructs or unpacks modes of thought, circuits of management, and practices that we accept as given; the "truth will not set you free" (Murray 2007, 162). Interpretive research opens things up to problematize – not to close down, complicate, simplify, or police – the boundaries of any body of work. It aims to multiply lines of investigation and possibilities for thought. Thus *sensing policy* as an affective framework of analysis reveals multiple dimensions of any oeuvre, narrative, discursive field, or body of knowledge and its correlate appendages. Opening up that which constitutes "the political" moves scholars toward providing visibility of certain aspects of their invisible, normalized, everyday experiences, which are thus made profoundly political themselves.

Situated Bodies of Knowledge

Drawing upon the 1986 explosion of the Chernobyl nuclear reactor in the Ukraine, Petryna (2002) examines how wounded individuals organize and make claims to the state based upon their biological condition. She discusses the ways that individuals who are living with uncertainty band together and forge (in)formal networks. Petryna refers to this as an emergent social practice, where the damaged biology of a population becomes the grounds for social membership and the basis for staking citizenship claims. Her analysis exposes how the forms and terms of engagement, struggles for resources, and rationalities go beyond traditional notions of citizens as bearers of formal legal rights. Instead, she offers "biological citizenship" as a way of bringing the body forward as central to the nature of contested forms of inclusion and exclusion in a political community. Thinking about citizenship as a practice in this regard reveals informal – lived, affective, visceral – aspects of power relations.

Aligned with Petryna, Rose (2007) expands upon the notion of "biological citizenship" to explore the connection between nation building, colonization, and ideas about desirable citizens based on their biology. Life itself becomes a political object. Much public health discourse reveals how humans are expected to take an active role in shaping their bodily functions, to promote life and vitality, and to activate an interest in their own health. The bodies of citizens are of prime value to the enforcement and regulation of state authority, governance, and control. Consequently, citizens are expected to take responsibility for exercising "biological prudence" on behalf of themselves, their families, and the state (ibid., 24). As responsible individuals, citizens become concerned with managing their livelihoods and are expected to inform themselves about what appropriate actions to take in order to adjust their "lifestyle" in accordance with living a positively healthy and viable life. Individuals are called to fulfill this life responsibility in relation to oneself and others in pursuit of being a good biological citizen. This "responsibilization" appears in all kinds of public health policy and programming in Canada, which emphasizes "health promotion" (Orsini 2007). Such positive reinforcement has a flipside: it produces categories of unruly, unworthy citizens, seen to be unable to manage their own well-being.

Rather than thinking solely about the makeup of citizens imposed from "above" by hierarchical state authority, an analysis of biological citizenship also focuses on the languages and aspirations employed by individuals who understand themselves and relate themselves to others. These understandings, meanings, and framings, oriented around citizen agency and biology, constitute expressions of identity formation and biosociality. Informed by Rabinow, Rose (2007, 134) discusses "biosociality" as a way to characterize forms of collectivization organized around the "commonality of a shared somatic or genetic status," which draws attention to emergent technologies that are assembled through the categories of corporeal vulnerability, suffering, risk, and susceptibility. Individuals congregate around a sense of shared corporeal status and engage in a kind of activism to refute dominant modes of governance and biomedical expertise.

Consequently, individuals become experts of life itself. As engaged corporeal experts, responsible for self-care and prudence, citizens become active agents who pioneer a new ethic of the self, a "set of techniques for managing everyday life in relation to a condition, and in relation to expert knowledge" (Rose 2007, 146). Biological citizens are thus obligated to engage in activism and become responsible to live through a series of calculations and choices in order to manage and preserve their livelihood. In examining the relationship between politics and life itself, Rose does not aim to call for a "new" philosophy of life but to explore how citizens embody an ethic of responsibilization for biology and the management of vitality. Challenging Rose, this analysis moves away from thinking about corporeal management or stewardship and toward a more place-based ecological understanding of the body.

"Government" refers to much more than "sovereign authority" or the "state." Governmentality turns our attention toward this "more than" quality of government and includes the multifaceted ways in which society itself becomes governmentalized. Thus techniques of government, adopted by citizens and communities, permit the state's survival. Governmentality conceptualizes "liberalism" as a mentality of rule that cultivates state survival through its creation of, and dependence upon, free subjects. Governmentality approaches examine the outcomes of the multiple thoughts and practices that shape assumptions about what government is and how it operates. These outcomes can be understood as discourses, or bodies of knowledge, that limit the agency of the actors who are embedded within them. Thus language, speech, and communication carry and transmit relations of power.

Moreover, this critical, biopolitical lens draws into focus how the manifestation and articulation of power relations occur at an arm's length from the state and how they can be situated within and upon the body. As critical policy scholars note, politics and policy increasingly occur across different spatial horizons (Orsini and Smith 2007). Examining the practices of citizens engaging in struggles for environmental reproductive justice in Aamjiwnaang entails a consideration of how embodied power relations are sensed in a particular place. Field research offers a compelling method for developing a nuanced understanding of experiences, emotions, and activities on the ground and for advancing a detailed understanding of how citizens ascribe meaning to their daily lives. This approach also offers a means through which the researcher can examine and evaluate discrepancies between expert (or elite) knowledge and local (or situated) knowledges (Haraway 1991; Yanow 2003). Power is diffuse and takes multiple forms to constitute fields of knowledge. Actors operating within these discursive fields are constrained by practices that frame the parameters of speech and thought. Chapters 4 and 6 elaborate upon these struggles for knowledge in greater detail.

Furthermore, biosocial identities emerge when the vitality of a community is in question. For example, we can take a look at the experiences of victims in Chernobyl, Bhopal, and Love Canal, among others, which reveal how life acquires a value whose violation must be recognized, redressed, and compensated for. In these examples, and as will be explored with respect to the Aamjiwnaang First Nation's experiences, the damaged biology – and moreover *ecology* – of a population forms the basis of its vital rights and belonging, expressed by injured citizens.

Intersectional Geopolitics, Prismatic Biopolitics

Space is fundamental to the exercise of power. Historically, the colonial doctrine of discovery adopted a notion of *terra nullius,* a term derived from Roman law for land considered to belong to "no one." This "unowned" or "unoccupied" land was considered "no man's land," propelling a policy for the expansion of colonial empires whereby "sovereign" states claimed "empty" territories as their own. For Indigenous peoples today within what became Canada, the conditions of possibility for the sovereign Canadian state continue to facilitate a spatial politics of demarcation and segregation that manifests colonial power in the present reserve system. These colonial power relations have local, lived effects. Thus, rather than offering a monolithic study of Indigenous environmental justice, an intersectional focus offers an opportunity to nuance a biopolitical reading of governmentality through an orientation to *social location* (Braun 2007; Hankivsky 2012; Rutherford 2007, 303). An attunement to spatial geopolitics – geography and location – intersects with human experience through time and space (Massey 2005). It reveals the prismatic and multifaceted ways that individual citizen bodies are embedded within "a chaotic and unpredictable molecular world" that is connected to broader "networks and pathways, movement and exchanges" (Braun 2007, 15; Lynes 2013). Rather than producing a strictly global focus, as the term "geopolitics" conventionally infers, the application of a feminist geopolitical lens to the biopolitical analysis of social location can help us to visualize how power relations take shape in particular places between human and more-than-human lifeforms. Specifically, through the daily activities of its citizenry, the Aamjiwnaang Reserve, a unique geographical site, produces meanings that reveal "place."[7]

Interpretations of meanings about environments, or spaces, create site-specific practices of everyday life. Informed by scholarship in feminist geopolitics, I emphasize that broader power assemblages can be connected with the particular site of Aamjiwnaang's geographic and political formation (Dixon 2014; Dixon and Marston 2011; Dowler and Sharp 2001; Massaro and Williams 2013; Sharp 2011). As discussed by Bertram (2011, 170), a site reveals the "complex effects" of power. The formation of this site as a geopolitical place comes into being over time and through space. It is also uniquely experienced within communities.

A place orientation brings time and space together so that we can examine how people construct meanings, attachments, and identities in particular locales. Thus examining histories as well as the ongoing practices in place makes stories spring to life and showcases how citizens make sense of and hitch meaning to their environments. Following Thornton's (2008, 6) observation that "to understand places, one must understand the people who inhabit them," we can think of place as a network of relations produced out of the interactions between bodies and territories. A placed account of citizenship is simultaneously corporeal and territorial. It is something rooted, particular, and enacted through bodily practice. Examining citizen actions in specific places brings corporeal individuals into space-time, as a chronotope, where "time takes on flesh" (ibid., 17). Places situate time and space by setting human bodies in a local habitat. These settings constitute meaningful experiences, knowledges, and feelings, derived through perception, emotion, and imagination. The body, as an ultimate "arbiter" of human interaction with the environment, takes on ecological consciousness based on sensuous experience. The body continually takes one into place. It is an agent and vehicle as well as an articulator and witness of being-in-place (ibid.). Living, moving, practising bodies structure and configure senses of place.

Distinguishing between "space" and "place" is crucial to understanding contemporary struggles for environmental reproductive justice on an Indigenous reserve. Reserves are places with thick and textured histories. They are also spaces that keep people in place. As discussed at length in Chapter 3, Canadian sovereignty is predicated on the historical and present (dis)placement of Indigenous peoples within Canada in pockets of their traditional territorial land bases. In addition to displacing Indigenous peoples from their territories and emplacing them on reserves, early settlers appropriated their land by effecting exclusive jurisdiction over their territories, which were opened up to resettlement and to Western traditions of land use, namely farming, resource exploitation, and capitalist development. The long-term effects of this (dis)placement included overcrowded housing, welfare dependency, limited education, health issues, and high rates of unemployment. According to Razack (2002), in precarious zoned-in spaces like reserves, marginalized bodies appear almost transparent, forgotten, left behind as a part of earthy debris. Making this image strikingly clear, one simply has to tour the perimeter of the Aamjiwnaang First Nation Reserve in order to see landfills, disposal sites, and waste treatment facilities, in addition to the numerous chemical facilities surrounding the small portion of initial treaty land that this First Nation retains. Conversations with residents reveal the history of repeated dumping of toxic waste on land that had already been deemed "wasted" due to Indigenous occupation.[8] Thus, space is inextricably linked to power.

Opening up space for settler interests to the detriment of Indigenous peoples in Canada has long been an essential manoeuvre for external authority and control. According to Alfred (2009, 45), the regime of European settlement produced a vacuum, or "empty space," thus making Indigenous peoples available for exploitation and making their domination within Canada possible. As a result of the colonial perpetuation of the notion of *terra nullius,* Indigenous people were not seen as civilized masters of the land. *Terra nullius* produced an "empty zone," or space, to be fortified through state boundaries. Consequently, Indigenous peoples were reduced by the settler society to natural savages who were to be controlled and contained. This (mis)conception of land as an empty space has long permitted its colonization (Taussig 1987). A precontact notion of *terra nullius* justified European settlement and moving Indigenous peoples onto reserves (Razack 2002). Today, it justifies filling these spaces with toxic waste.

An intersectional lens takes us beyond the structural configurations of space and into the experiential dimensions of place. Spaces tell stories. They communicate values, meanings, beliefs, and feelings and are locations for "organizational acts" (Yanow 1998, 215). Spaces are structures created by society. As such, they are social productions, not merely an "environmental context or container for society" (Soja 2010, 91). Spaces are much like characters that constitute part of the plot; both contain and carry messages. As communities change over time, so do their interpretations and meanings. Built spaces are not passive. They are at once "storytellers and part of the story being told" (Yanow 1998, 215). In addition to the literal dimensions of space, boundaries can be metaphysically and socially constructed through linguistic and discursive policy arrangements. For example, a name such as "Chemical Valley" is imbued with meaning. Interpretive geopolitical investigations look at values, beliefs, aesthetics, affect, and the feelings that these factors evoke in order to ask about the stories that spaces tell.[9] Notably, as Aamjiwnaang's experience interacting with Chemical Valley reveals, land means more than simple geography. As is the case for many Indigenous communities across the country, land and territory are "the root of their spirit, belonging and way of life" (Suleman 2011, 11). Counter to a static notion of space, land is place-specific, relational, and central to *being*.

Assessing Policy Assemblages through Multilayered Analysis

Governmentality studies examine "ensembles of power," an amalgam of *institutional parameters, discursive fields,* and *citizen practices.* As Hankivsky (2012, 35) emphasizes, attending to the multilevel effects of power and where these relations are situated requires an interrogation of multiple scales, locales, and sites, from the global to the local. Given Canada's constitutional configuration as a federation, a multilevel approach to policy making is increasingly the norm, especially in an emergent policy area such as Indigenous environmental justice.

As Chapter 3's discussion of Canada's *policy assemblage* for Indigenous environmental justice explores at length, governmentality includes the assemblage of institutions, procedures, analyses, and reflections, as well as tactics, that allow the exercise of a specific and complex form of power to take shape (Foucault 1994a, 244). An assemblage is much like a bricolage or constellation. Moreover, a biopolitical policy assemblage hones in on Canada's *body politic* to evaluate power relations across social and physical bodies. As Deleuze and Guattari (1987, 88, 505) explain, an assemblage entails *content, expression,* and *relations*. Content encompasses order encoded in laws, policies, and institutions; expression in the form of language, discourse, and framing; and relations whose forces and flows shape and constrain the intermingling of bodies where and when citizens encounter both content and expression. As elaborated in subsequent chapters, these relations are simultaneously material, corporeal, and territorial. This prismatic lens sheds light on the effects and affects of biopower. As a multilayered lens, it reveals how power is generated both from the state downward to society and from the ground up through productive means. Thus a biopolitical analysis of power relations, tuned into the manifestations of power's micro forms, also visualizes different kinds of relationships between power, authority, and knowledge across multiple scales. In Chapter 3 these are referred to as *institutional configurations, discursive fields,* and *citizen practices.*

This mode of analysis creates some wedging, or openness, into dominant operations, formations, and expressions of hierarchical power relations. Knowledge about multiple nodes or sources of power relations beyond the strict parameters of state-centric practices may open up opportunities for alternative voices and concrete social action. In this sense, knowledge is a powerful force for change. According to Rabinow and Rose (1994, ix), "In anatomizing the detailed ways of thinking and acting that made up our present, and constituted ourselves in the present, Foucault asked us to consider the possibility that we might invent different ways of thinking about and acting on ourselves in relationship to our pleasures, our labors, our troubles and those who trouble us, our hopes and aspirations for freedom." Following suit, I draw inspiration from Foucault's "governmentality" approach to social science research, combining ethnographic and interpretive methods to investigate how meanings are ascribed to citizens' encounters within discursive fields – bodies of knowledge – in Canada's Chemical Valley in their struggles for justice.

As Chapter 4 presents, citizens in Aamjiwnaang bear the responsibility for monitoring their own well-being in a climate of state withdrawal. Community members are called upon to practise self-care for their livelihood and habitat; consequently, governance of land and governance of life become fused. Citizens of this community are disciplined into becoming first responders to ongoing spills, accidents, and releases as active and responsible "environmental citizens." This circumstance presents a dilemma and reveals the multiple edges of citizenship. Citizens respond to their polluted landscape as managerial stewards, while also practising an Anishinabek way of life.

Thus environmental citizenship is to be distinguished from ecological citizenship. Ecological citizenship opens up creative possibilities of thought. It presents a kind of ecological thinking and aligns with a place-based relational Anishinabek approach to land and life that includes a strong awareness of the earth's animate "agency and personality" (J. Borrows 2010, 243; McGregor and Plain 2013). As John Borrows (2010, 248) discusses, Anishinabek law includes land rights through "political citizenship," which incorporates attentiveness to the character and sacred power of land. This understanding accentuates place and unsettles the "self-certainties of western capitalism" and its corresponding epistemology (Code 2006, 4). Ecological citizenship interrupts predominant liberal conceptions of citizenship in Canada and elsewhere. According to Code (ibid., 5), the "protagonist" in this story is both an ecological subject and a distant relative of the antagonist in this account, namely the "autonomous individual," who is paramount in Western, liberal political theory. Ecological citizenship requires thinking about epistemological grounding in place as a framework not only for reconfiguring knowledge but also for encountering and enacting place. In theory, method, and practice, ecological citizenship is a lens that helps us to think about how we, humans, can live well together with the more-than-human environment.

Locating citizen actions in the specific site of Aamjiwnaang allows for the development of a relational and placed account of the emergent practices of citizenship, engagement, and resistance, which constitutes a new way of prismatic and multilayered thinking about citizenship as "ecological citizenship." A considerable amount of the literature on green theory and on environmental-ecological citizenship emphasizes active citizenship.[10] Frequently, normative or moral arguments are put forward that justice should include notions of stewardship, responsibilities, virtue, and justice. Following Adkin's (2009, 4) criticism that much of this literature focuses on the dimensions of citizenship that are "normative" (i.e., duties and obligations) and "procedural" (i.e., institutional and deliberative), this analysis builds from the perspectives of community members in a particular place to create an argument about citizenship and justice through an account of everyday life. *Sensing policy* as a framework for analysis provides a lens through which scholars can ask questions about belonging, forms of knowledge, and the environments where they live.

The ontological stakes of citizenship are at the centre of tensions between Western individualism and Anishinabek thought. As explained in the chapters that follow, Western, liberal notions of citizenship that separate land from life and that blame individual citizens for their health and well-being diverge from Anishinabek values and beliefs. Conceptually, discussing an "Anishinabek" approach to citizenship, considered to be a *way of life,* highlights the multiple edges of ecological citizenship. Doing so is important for Indigenous and non-Indigenous scholars alike, who must jointly assume responsibility for making Indigenous knowledge part of the present and future (Alfred 2009). Within a spirit of reciprocity and intersubjective engagement, the unfolding discussion aligns with Alfred's (ibid.) call for academics to assist in this process of knowledge translation by creating some room for Indigenous knowledges and ways of being in the world within policy, contemporary structures, institutions, discourses, and practices. This spirit of mutual respect, sharing, and translation illuminates both this written text and the participatory-action approach to knowledge production.

Before I proceed, some caveats: there is no singular, identifiable "Anishinabek worldview." This term is used to illuminate some of the tensions between "individual" and "place-specific" notions of health and the environment based on relevant literature, field immersion, and interview results gathered throughout my research (McGregor and Plain 2013). Moreover, the mere act of "writing" about traditions comes directly into tension with an oral culture of knowledge translation and teachings. Many times, I was reminded that one cannot simply "read" about Anishinabek people; one also has to live, experience, and share knowledge that cannot be neatly transcribed as text. The culture under study must become part of a person's being (Doerfler, Sinclair, and Stark 2013; Johnston 2005; L. Simpson 2011). Written works reflect only a small proportion of the unwritten traditions and practices that form Anishinabek culture and life.

An Anishinabek way of being connects the incorporeal and the corporeal, including the physical world, such as plants, wildlife, and land. Notably, traditional teachings articulate that humankind was created from new substances unlike those out of which the physical world was made, thus connecting the corporeal and incorporeal. Traditions state that the human, a composite being, was created according to the fulfillment of the vision of Kitche Manitou (Johnston 2005, 119). Dreams, visions, and connections between the past, present, and future are central to understanding Anishinabek ontology, which contrasts greatly with Western, liberal ideology.

Western thought tends to place beliefs and concepts into easily accessible and manageable categorical schemes. It is easy enough for government officials, policy makers, and community members to consider "traditional knowledge" as something external to the individual self. Yet, as demonstrated by literature and by my conversations with community members, "traditional knowledge" is a concept that pins down thought, turning it into an object. For many who participated in the research process, such "pinning-down" of knowledge to create easily categorizable and immutable facts reduces the richness of Anishinabek culture. A more contextual, fluid, emergent, experiential, and practised understanding of Anishinabek life and language is considered to be more appropriate. This resonates with Alfred's (2009, 181) dictum, "Don't preserve tradition, live it!" Knowledge is not intended to remain an immobile artifact. Alfred argues that traditional knowledge is a way of living life. It is in this respect that thinking about ecological citizenship as a mode, practice, or ethic resonates with an Anishinabek ontology.

Anishinabek thought places citizens within their environment. Nature is not something *for* us; it is *part* of us. None of us can own our mother – the earth – in the present nor in the future (J. Borrows 2010; Johnston 2005, 25). This illuminates some tensions between Eurocentric notions of property, equal entitlement, and private ownership. An Anishinabek approach to land and the environment regards individual beings as part of the ecosystem. In this close relationship between people and the earth, we might think of the land not as a plotted "territory" but as an interpretive "place." From this perspective, the natural world is not merely a compilation of inanimate objects. For example, a tree is never merely a tree; it could be someone's grandfather (Bryan 2000, 27). The more-than-human world cannot be pinned down as a series of merely inanimate objects.

Counter to a technological view of society that constructs a sharp dividing line between humans and more-than-humans, according to Anishinabek thought these relationships are mediated through a matrix of relationships. Humans connect to an animate more-than-human world in flesh and spirit. This connection includes the corporeal and the incorporeal, as well as an articulation of being that illuminates a deep respect for plants, animals, people, and the spirit world. It connotes respect for Mother Earth and Father Sun. Although Anishinabek teachings discuss the principle that "all are related" and emphasize interconnectivity, there are four main orders within creation: the physical, plant, animal, and human worlds (McGregor 2009; Johnston 2005). Each intertwines to make up the richness of life's whole existence.

With fewer than the four orders or realms, life and being are incomplete and unintelligible. No one portion is self-sufficient or complete. Each derives its meaning from and fulfils its function and purpose within the context of the whole creation (Johnston 2005, 21). The place, sphere, and existence of each order is predetermined by great physical laws of harmony. Through the relationships of the four orders, the world generates sense and meaning. This Anishinabek approach to life offers a radically different notion of embodied and placed citizenship than does Western liberalism. As mentioned in Chapter 1, it is commonplace for individuals to introduce themselves to groups by stating their name and where they are from, as the latter (in)forms their being. "Nature," or the environment, cannot be owned. One is not superior to nature; rather, it is to be respected.[11]

Cultivating a respectful and relational way of being in connection with one's environment is central to many Anishinabek teachings. Citing one teacher, a research participant referred to "walking the Red Road" and to the notion that "we humans must come to a moral comprehension of the earth and air"; further, she stated, "we must live according to the principle of a land ethic." The alternative "is that we shall not live at all." When we spoke further about the meaning of this kind of Anishinabek "land ethic," she informed me that from her perspective, it referred to "respecting and giving value to all living things and the environment we live in; land, air, water ... Being grateful and giving thanks for everything, from the smallest organisms to the highest mountains" (written correspondence with Charlotte, May 17, 2011). Subsequent conversations with an elder about the meaning of "land ethics" as "environment ethics" illuminated the following:

> This teaching was given to all human beings from the time of Creation. I once was told, that the Medicine Wheel consists of 4 major colours of human beings. The Yellow people were to look after and make sure the Air was properly cared for. The Black human beings had the responsibility of the Waters. The Red human beings were to take care of the clean and respected Earth. The White human beings were to watch out for the Fire with great Respect. Fire is way out of control today. Fire is Spirit and Energy in all of Creation. This includes "Technology." See today, how it is out of control. It is the cause of all the pollutions we see today, along with the loss of our Original Teachings. We, all were, from time to time, supposed to come together and meet with each other to see that Air, Water, Earth, and Fire were looked after with Great Respect and Love. This has not been done in Hundreds and hundreds of years. Instead meetings are taken place to see how much more we can advance technology. It is almost too late for environmentalists to do any good to get on our original paths, of our Teachings. The Mayans knew this. So did we, the Red people. "Land Ethics????" Well, we can only try to get back to Land Ethics. (Written correspondence with Mike, May 19, 2011)[12]

Moreover, elders and community members continued to firmly state in our conversations that this "land ethic" is not based upon "traditional knowledge"; rather, it is to be considered a *way of life*. One gains knowledge through adopting this way of life. Much of Anishinabek knowledge production can be understood as an epistemology of lived experience. Acknowledging and respecting lived experience is an essential part of knowledge generation.

Conclusion

A *sensing policy* lens requires distinguishing the relational, intersectional, and interpretive approach to public policy from linear technocratic approaches to policy analysis. Informed by governmentality studies, this analytical approach emphasizes "affect" rather than "effect" as an *affective framework of analysis.*

Thus it places a high degree of importance on citizens' experiences and daily life, noting that power relations exist in a continuum between state authority and citizen practice. To understand these power relations, an approach to citizenship and policy is put forth that takes the scholar into discursive fields of power relations beyond textual and institutional parameters. This approach requires a combination of theoretical and methodological tools.

This critical and interpretive methodology brings theoretical concepts like governmentality and biopower together with political ethnography to assess how citizens are impacted by policy decisions or nondecisions at all levels of government, from the federal state to the intimate lived reality on the ground. Going beyond a mere understanding of citizens' lived realities decentres the primacy of Western, liberal theory, prevalent in literature, policy, and discourse, to make space for diverse ways of knowing, beginning with Anishinabek approaches to land, life, and citizenship. Making better policy requires thinking about different forms of citizenship, such as an ecological citizenship that is relational and place-based.

Chapter 3 next fleshes out the long, dark, and coloured history of Canada's biopolitical shadow. One of Canada's most notable public policies on "Indians" was the 1969 "White Paper," which sought to bring Indians "into" Canada's body politic as assimilated citizens just like everyone else. A governmentality lens makes clear that the many layers of Indigenous environmental justice comprise a messy, nonlinear, ad hoc policy assemblage arrayed from the top down and scaled from the state to the citizen. This lens makes possible an assessment of citizen encounters with the legal and policy parameters for on-reserve environmental health. These encounters are embroiled within structural and discursive fields of power, which shape and constrain access to justice.

3

State Nerves
The Many Layers of Indigenous Environmental Justice

> Descent attaches itself to the body. It inscribes itself in the nervous system, in temperament, in the digestive apparatus; it appears in faulty respiration, in improper diets, in the debilitated and prostrate bodies of those whose ancestors committed errors.
>
> **– Michel Foucault, "Nietzsche, Genealogy, History"**

A Made-in-Canada Biopolitical Assemblage

Bodies ascribe historically constituted meaning across time and space. Like a nervous system, which sends sensory information from the brain to the body's organs via neurons, politics extend from the head of state into the capillaries of society. An approach to settler-colonial relations that employs governmentality studies illuminates the inner workings of biopower and some of the ways that Indigenous bodies have always been at stake in practices of Canadian state making. As Martineau (2014) argues, settler-colonial rule operates through governmentality, a diffuse set of governing relations that structurally ensure continued access to Indigenous peoples' land and resources through neocolonial subjectivities that incite Indigenous people into becoming instruments of their own dispossession. Notably, with settler contact came diseases such as smallpox and tuberculosis, unsettling and threatening the vitality of Indigenous peoples. Alfred and Corntassel (2005, 598) observe that members of a settler society perpetuate the colonial legacy of their "imperial forefathers," who attempted not only to eradicate the "physical signs of Indigenous peoples as human bodies" but also to "eradicate their existence as peoples through the erasure of the histories and geographies that provide the foundation for Indigenous cultural identities and sense of self." A multilayered examination of the geopolitical connection between population management, bodies, territory, and culture reveals how biological beliefs are tied to Indigenous politics in Canada, how the Canadian state regulates the bodies of Indians,[1] and how this has changed over time both in and across space.

A governmentality lens draws into focus the operationalization of power through political assemblages. An assemblage, as a kind of "arena of rule," entails much more than the formal institutions of government (Dean 2010, 34). Assemblages take shape geopolitically in site-specific locales and include an amalgam of political forces and practices. As an "analytics of government," a governmentality approach examines the conditions under which particular regimes of practices, knowledges, laws, and policies emerge, exist, and change (ibid., 30). The amalgamation of these relations can be understood as an assemblage. This perspective acknowledges that governmental processes are neither seamless nor smooth and that state power takes shape through *institutions, discourses,* and *citizen practices*. It seeks to expose "truth" claims that are taken for granted and to lay bare how particular institutions, discourses, and practices emerge through specifically and "historically situated systems of rule" (Rutherford 2011, xxvi). More precisely, a governmentality lens does not treat concepts like the state, citizenship, or democracy as "ideal types"; rather, it highlights how institutional practices produce objects of knowledge. The particular emphasis in this chapter is on *how* the current policy assemblage of Indigenous environmental justice has come into being through a complex amalgam of institutional configurations, discursive fields, and citizen practices. Twinning the messy, ad hoc features of environmental and health policy, this chapter examines the functioning of Indigenous environmental justice as a *policy assemblage.*

Public health statistics all too often present an unflattering snapshot of Indigenous peoples' health and personal lifestyle choices, revealing high rates of smoking, drinking, obesity, and HIV, low life expectancy, and the fastest-growing population in Canada (Health Canada 2003). It is commonly known that Indigenous peoples in Canada suffer higher rates of injury, suicide, and diabetes than do most Canadian citizens (Health Canada 2011a). What this picture fails to capture is the long history of Canada's colonization, settlement, displacement of Indigenous peoples through institutional arrangements such as residential schools, and detrimental control over the social determinants of health, resulting in substandard housing, the persistence of boil-water advisories, widespread environmental contamination, and prejudice within the education system.[2] Contextualizing these unflattering statistics and unpacking some of the past injustices embedded within Canada's treatment of Indigenous peoples helps us to understand contemporary manifestations of both disciplinary and productive biopower. Related practices of population management undertaken by the state to regulate Indians in the country include monitoring their movement, restricting their bodily capacity, and tying them to often marginalized pockets of land that are mere fractions of their traditional territorial bases. Unsettling some of the settled assumptions that many Canadians take to be "Truths" paves the way for understanding the continuities of these discomforting practices that persist in the present.

Institutional Configurations

Since the assertion of British sovereignty in Canada, Indians have been subject to the principles of fiduciary law. The Crown's fiduciary relationship for Aboriginal peoples is unique (Boyer 2004). It operates on Aboriginal "beneficiaries" through the paternalistic, caring, and "protective" language outlined in the Royal Proclamation of 1763. The British Crown's successor, Canada, assumed these fiduciary responsibilities. Aboriginal peoples were placed in a guardian-ward relationship. Thus the Crown acted out of an authority that was "moral," not "legal," and the state was not administratively responsible for its actions: a "sacred political obligation" is discretionary and does not equate to a "legal obligation" (ibid.). This discretionary authority has practical implications with respect to the provision of healthcare.

Prior to Canadian Confederation in 1867, healthcare for Indians came through missionaries, Indian Agents, traders, and the Hudson's Bay Company. In the mid-1800s the Hudson's Bay Company, on "humanitarian grounds," began to inoculate Indigenous peoples against diseases such as smallpox. Rather than brutal force and military violence, a subtle yet similarly pervasive expression of Indian population management took shape through the humanitarian approach, carried out by an assortment of "semitrained" police agents, missionaries, and officers (RCAP 1996). As a technology of population management, with a mixture of "paternalism and contempt," surgeons of the North-West Mounted Police, acting as agents of the government, provided routine medical visits to Indians and played a role in quarantines to manage the outbreak of diseases such as tuberculosis, influenza, smallpox, and whooping cough (Boyer

2004; Waldram, Herring, and Young 2004, 150). Following the realization that the death rate of the Indigenous population in Canada was double that of the general population, Canada officially appointed Dr. Peter H. Bryce as its first superintendent general of Indian health in 1904 (Boyer 2004; Waldram, Herring, and Young 2004, 156). At the time, epidemics like tuberculosis were rapidly spreading, perpetuating the stigma that Indigenous peoples within Canada could not advance from a nomadic society to a modern one.

Historically, the Indian Act outlined various authorities for healthcare, although the jurisdictional responsibilities remained vague. Provincial medical officers in all municipalities and health districts were charged with the administration of provincial health regulations and were empowered to ensure their enforcement. The Act listed "places of detention" that pertained to health regulation: hospitals, sanatoriums, clinics, lockups, jails, reformatories, or any other place designated by the superintendent (Government of Canada 1978). The superintendent ensured the enforcement of Indian health, and persons with infectious diseases were required to place themselves under the care of the state and to undergo treatment prescribed by a medical officer or practitioner. During the daytime, the superintendent or medical officer could enter any dwelling or other premises situated on the reserve under his charge to inquire about the state of health of any person therein or to examine the hygienic condition of the dwelling or other premises (ibid.). The Crown's oblique fiduciary responsibility for the protection of Indigenous health continues to play a part in this *policy assemblage.*

Today, the healthcare of Indigenous peoples in Canada falls within a convoluted amalgam of jurisdictional configurations. Primary responsibility for "Indian" health remains at the federal level, whereas healthcare for most Canadian citizens appears largely under the rubric of provincial or territorial jurisdiction.[3] The federal government directly funds health professionals, including dentists, dental therapists, and optometrists who provide services to remote and isolated communities on a visiting basis, or it funds First Nations and Inuit people who travel to larger centres for specialized and emergency treatments. Funded services include dental care, prescriptions, medical supplies, and allied health services outside of hospitals (i.e., mental health, community-based preventative care, and homecare), and they are not provided by provincial governments to First Nations communities on reserves (Health Canada 2011a, 2011b). At the same time, First Nations and Inuit peoples obtain much of their care from the provincial and territorial health systems, including hospitals and physicians, as data are kept within provincial and territorial databases (ibid.). These costs fall under federal jurisdiction, administered by Health

Canada. Historically, health services have always functioned through a network, patchwork, or *assemblage* of service delivery mechanisms.

In 1867 Canada's constitutional structure established powers between the federal and provincial governments in Canada. At the time, the British Parliament omitted any mention of legislative power over health and healthcare. As a result, the subject of health does not expressly fall under the ambit of either the federal or provincial governments; provinces have jurisdiction over the administration of healthcare, whereas the federal government sets priorities and principles outlined in the Canada Health Act as a matter of policy through its spending power (Boyer 2004; Waldram, Herring, and Young 2004). This constitutional ambiguity is cause for heightened concern in the context of the treatment of Indigenous peoples within Canada. Jurisdictional squabbling between the federal and provincial governments frequently results in a convoluted system of health delivery for Indigenous peoples, including underfunded "hit or miss" provincial programs serving this population (Boyer 2004). Canada's fiduciary obligation toward Indigenous peoples, arising from Aboriginal rights and treaty rights, is poorly understood. These treaty rights stem from the Treaty 6 "medicine chest clause," although in practice, it does not apply evenly to all Indigenous peoples (Waldram, Herring, and Young 2004, 141).[4] Primary responsibility for this policy domain remains unclear (ibid.). The constitutional commitment to provide Aboriginal healthcare stems from judicial interpretations of the medicine chest clause.

Canadian healthcare falls under Section 92 of the Constitution as a provincial responsibility. Although provinces have jurisdiction over healthcare in the country, they do not have a "responsibility" for the provision of healthcare services to Indigenous peoples (Craig 1992, 3). Application of the "doctrine of paramountcy" gives federal legislation pre-eminence over provincial legislation (ibid., vi; Mackenzie 2013). For Indigenous peoples, health is a discretionary policy domain with multiple layers of responsibility. It is a "matter of policy" rather than a legal obligation; thus the government can alter services as it deems appropriate (Waldram, Herring, and Young 2004, 149). Consequently, the federal government often develops programs to support First Nations communities without establishing a legislative or regulatory framework for them. Therefore, for First Nations members living on reserves, there is a "regulatory gap" that has limited the creation of legislation to support programs in important areas such as education, health, and drinking water (Auditor General of Canada 2009; Mackenzie 2013; Moffat and Nahwegahbow 2004).

The overall lack of clarity on Canada's jurisdiction and responsibility for Indigenous health results in poorly defined services and confusion about the requirements for adequate federal funding. According to a 2011 auditor general's report, among the several structural impediments to adequate healthcare are ambiguity about service levels, an insufficient legislative base, an inappropriate funding mechanism, and a lack of organization to support local service delivery (Auditor General of Canada 2011). It is often unclear who is accountable to First Nations citizens to achieve improved outcomes or better services. The federal government generally claims responsibility for funding services but not for administering service delivery. Thus sometimes First Nations communities work more closely with provincial authorities (i.e., school boards, health boards, and social services), and sometimes they meet these responsibilities with their available resources and become actively engaged in policy development.

In Indigenous communities, healthcare services are delivered piecemeal, and many citizens struggle to address their healthcare needs. As Picard (2011) discusses, "it is shameful that our wannabe leaders do not have to explain why, in 2011, we tolerate entire communities living without safe drinking water and reliant on 'honey pots' – human sewage collected in buckets or plastic bags." The consistency of drinking-water advisories on reserves challenges the myth of Canada's pristine natural landscape, as it contradicts the common conception that Canada is one of the most desirable places to live. The tethering of health to environmental concerns further occludes the obligation to provide comprehensive healthcare to Indigenous peoples in Canada.

The predominance of provincial responsibility for environmental policy in Canada further complicates this *policy assemblage*. Ontario's environmental protection is governed through the Environmental Protection Act. This Act grants the Ministry of Environment powers to deal with the discharge of potentially harmful contaminants (MOE 1990). It contains a general discharge prohibition on "contaminants," and it requires "permits" for emissions in accordance with a certificate of approval issued by the minister of the environment (Scott 2008). These certificates are legally binding licences that set out the conditions under which a facility can operate. As Scott (ibid.) discusses, the approach is predicated on the development and implementation of standards, many of which were established more than twenty years ago. The standards determine the allowable emissions for each facility by using air-dispersion models developed to ensure that between the location of the stack and the property fence line ("the point of impingement," in the regulation's terms), the pollution becomes diluted to the point that it is below any applicable health threshold. Scott (ibid., 33) states, "The regulation seems to be based on the unlikely assumption that pollution never leaves industrial property." Furthermore, "cumulative effects" are not taken into consideration when the Ministry of Environment issues certificates of approval – an oversight that is of particular concern to the residents of Chemical Valley. This approach means that in conducting its modelling, each facility can assume that its background levels of contaminants will be zero, even though in Chemical Valley, for example, over sixty high-emitting facilities are clustered together, which makes the assumption blatantly false. Moreover, the prevalent human health harms in Aamjiwnaang – and adjacent to Chemical Valley, for that matter – remain "unintentional," despite the fact that pollution is a "fixed feature" of "modern economies" (ibid., 37). As a result, citizens thus take up the charge to keep their legislators accountable, and communities appropriate responsibility to manage environmental health.

Discursive Fields

As introduced in Chapters 1 and 2, biopolitics is a theoretical orientation that examines how the vitality of bodies is regulated, managed, disciplined, and produced. In addition to colonial state rule, which takes shape through the techniques and technologies of population management, biopower emerges through incentives and enticements. Species-wide population management and individual citizen responsibility alike are techniques that serve to achieve the political aims of life optimization. Health and the biology of a population or body politic are increasingly matters of individual responsibility (Braun 2007; Orsini 2007; Rose 2007). Activities such as actively investigating health conditions reveal assumed citizen responsibilities in a climate of state withdrawal. Studying the disciplinary manifestations of biopolitical power through the discursive field (i.e., the language, policies, and framing of the Indian body) that emanate from Canadian institutional configurations and examining changes in the techniques of productive biopower that have been brought about by the devolution of environmental health policy to communities and citizens can help us to understand their implications for citizens of the Aamjiwnaang First Nation specifically and for Canadian citizens more broadly. Citizen actions eventually become interpellated into this discursive field as a paradox of governance through freedom.

A turn to the past in order to consider where we have come from is necessary if we are to move in an alternative direction. The Royal Commission on Aboriginal Peoples (RCAP 1996) reminded us of the half-truth of our reputation as a "fair and enlightened society" given the "cache of secrets" embroiled within our historic and contemporary treatment of Indians. In 1876 the Indian Act consolidated all laws pertaining to Indians in Canada. Governing the Indian

Table 1
Pivotal policies toward Indigenous peoples in Canada

Legislation/Policy	Date	Approach
Royal Proclamation	1763	Nation-to-nation recognition with the British Crown
An Act to Encourage the Gradual Civilization of the Indian Tribes in This Province, and to Amend the Laws Respecting Indians	1857	Assimilation
British North America Act	1867	Federal protection of Indians and land reserved for Indians
Indian Act	1867	Government administration of Indian life
An Act for Conferring Certain Privileges on the More Advanced Bands of the Indians of Canada, with the View of Training Them for the Exercise of Municipal Powers	1884	Known as the "Indian Advancement Act," focus on eastern Canada, promotion of municipal-style government
Indian Act (revised)	1951, 1960	No federal vote for Indians until 1960
Hawthorn-Tremblay Report	1966–67	Citizens plus
Statement of the Government of Canada on Indian Policy	1969	Known as the "White Paper," assimilation
Charter of Rights and Freedoms	1982	Constitutional recognition of existing Aboriginal and treaty rights (Section 35)
Bill C-31	1985	Reinstatement of Indian women who lost their status under the *Indian Act*
Report of the Royal Commission on Aboriginal Peoples	1991–96	Nation-to-nation recognition
First Nations Lands Management Act	1999	Addresses matrimonial real property interests and rights on reserves

Note: See also Leslie (2002). For a detailed list of all Acts enacted by Parliament, see Aboriginal Affairs and Northern Development Canada (2014).

"body" has always been part of its regulatory constitution (see Table 1). Section 2(1) of the revised act states:

> "Band" means a body of Indians
> (a) for whose use and benefit in common, lands, the legal title to which is vested in Her Majesty, have been set apart before, on or after September 4, 1951,
> (b) for whose use and benefit in common, moneys are held by Her Majesty, or declared by the Governor in Council to be a Band for the purposes of this Act.

Historically, the Act defined Indians as "all persons of Indian blood, reputed to belong to the particular Body, or Tribe of Indians interested in such lands and their descendants" (Government of Canada 1978). The Act has always been orchestrated by the federal minister as superintendent of Indian affairs. In addition to this explicit declaration of bodily surveillance and management, the policies first put in place under the Act pertained to tracking the Indian population through a census register, referred to in the Act as an "Indian Register." Being Indian required registration with the band and with the federal government; the membership of this population was highly managed, tracked, and observed. The minister retained authority to form and dissolve bands, approve land use, appropriate "public land" at will, survey and subdivide reserves, regulate burial grounds, establish schools, enact health initiatives, determine the location of roadside construction, manage sales and transactions, offer certificates of possession for on-reserve housing allocation, and set the parameters for the bylaws and governance of band councils (Government of Canada 1985). Subsequent sections of this chapter assess the emergent ways that citizens take up the responsibility for self-management in a climate of state withdrawal. These activities can be understood through a biopolitical lens as responsibilized practices of self-care.

Biopolitics, Population Management, and Disciplinary Power

The 1876 Indian Act reflected past and present efforts to expand frontier society through land ownership, regulation, and integration of Indian peoples into mainstream Canadian citizenship. Canada envisioned that enfranchisement would entice Indians to accept good civic responsibility, aligned with nineteenth-century beliefs in progress and modernity. "Good Indians" were incited to give up their land for the right to vote, own property, and sit on juries. To be a serious-minded individual meant to be a responsible property owner, which conflicted with many Indigenous values and beliefs toward land and ownership. The white-settler society, through regulatory tools and instruments, encouraged Indians to adopt local government structures resembling those of the "developed" communities in pursuit of progress and advancement (RCAP 1996). This was most clearly reflected in the Indian Advancement Act of 1884, which outlined the authority of the Indian Agent to preside over band councils. Indian Agents were de facto sovereign doppelgängers – "petty sovereigns" – acting out the will of the federal authority in Indigenous communities across the country (Butler 2004, 56). If Indians wanted to leave the reserve, they required written permission from the Indian Agent. Every move of an Indian was thus regulated.

In 1894 biopolitical population management reached its zenith with the maturation of the residential school system. Despite being rife with disease and lacking proper medical facilities, these schools served to "re-form" Indian bodies (Waldram, Herring, and Young 2004, 156). At one point, federal health officials considered turning residential schools into sanatoria (ibid.). As Kelm (1998) explains, capturing minds required capturing bodies. Residential schools were conceived to Christianize Indian youth. They were run jointly by the state and by churches across the country. In the events leading up to the formal residential school policy, churches across Canada opened their doors to offer orphaned children sanctuary, thus providing them with a home away from an Aboriginal home life associated with dirt, disease, and death (ibid.). Native students were to adopt a good Christian lifestyle. Compulsory school attendance of Indian children did not require the consent of children, parents, or communities. The governor general of Canada implemented these provisions through an 1892 executive order-in-council that mandated the joint operation of industrial and residential schools, fusing church and state responsibility for biological control of Indian citizens. This undertaking was intended to "kill the Indian in the child" and would impose cultural conformity on Indigenous peoples for over a century (CBC 2008b). These schools were predicated on the basic notion that First Nations were "by nature, unclean and diseased" (Kelm 1998, 57). Children were forced to attend schools at a distance from their families and home, barred from the provincial school system (Government of Canada 1991). This policy followed the preceding trend of civilizing the Indian through the ways of the dominant settler society, sequestering Indigenous culture, and encouraging good Christian ethics. The church-run, government-led aggressive assimilative initiative expected that this adopted "lifestyle" would be passed on to future generations, as children were easier to mould than adults (CBC 2008a). As state doppelgängers, Indian Agents ensured their attendance.

Thus the residential schools were operated as a technology of rule to "modernize" the Indian. These schools had a two-pronged approach to assimilation and civilization: isolation and integration. Approximately 80 schools were open during the peak of their operations in 1931, and 130 schools were opened overall across the country, except in Newfoundland, Prince Edward Island, and New Brunswick (CBC 2008a). The last closed its doors in Saskatchewan in 1996, and about 150,000 Indian children went through the residential school system (ibid.). As a tool of civilization, these schools often punished students who spoke their Native language and practised their Native ways of life. Some students lived in substandard housing conditions and experienced physical and psychological abuse. Graduates did not "convocate" to the "waiting world of agricultural labour, but to the sanatorium, the hospital, and the grave" (Kelm 1998, 80). According to the Royal Commission on Aboriginal Peoples (RCAP 1996), "Residential schools were more than a component in the apparatus of social construction and control. They were part of the process of nation building and the concomitant marginalization of Aboriginal communities." Moreover, "marching out from the schools, the children, effectively re-socialized, imbued with the values of European culture, would be the vanguard of a magnificent metamorphosis: the 'savage' was to be made 'civilized,' made fit to take up the privileges and responsibilities of citizenship" (ibid.). Many children returned to their communities broken, unable to adapt, and ashamed of their Indigenous heritage.

During the interwar period, a more aggressive form of assimilation ensued, led by Duncan Campbell Scott, the deputy superintendent of Indian affairs from 1913 to 1932. In 1920, in response to the "Indian problem," he sought to amend the Indian Act, explaining that "the happiest future for the Indian race is absorption into the general population, and this is the object and policy of our government" (quoted in Titley 1986, 31). In his view, the Indian problem was cumbersome:

> I want to get rid of the Indian problem. I do not think as a matter of fact, that the country ought to continuously protect a class of people who are able to stand alone ... Our objective is to continue until there is not a single Indian in Canada that has not been absorbed into the body politic and there is no Indian question, and no Indian Department, that is the whole object of this Bill. (Quoted in ibid., 50)

The peak of the residential school system can be attributed to his vision of the body politic. In 1933 Superintendent General Thomas Murphy contended that the time had arrived for the government to take the "final step" in making "the

Indian a full citizen" so that the Indian could obtain "that degree of advancement which entitles him to the full responsibilities and privileges of citizenship" (Government of Canada 1978, 130). The superintendent general retained his role as an agent of the Crown, a "petty sovereign" stand-in, whereas the Indians continued to be treated as wards of the Crown.

Although in 2008 the prime minister formally apologized for the injustices of the residential schools, the process of reconciliation is an ongoing struggle, as "Indians" are required to rearticulate their corporeal harm to state authorities in order to prove their injury and seek redress in the form of a "common experience payment." The independent assessment process today "allows former students to tell their story in a private hearing – sometimes with the alleged abuser present" (Curry 2011). Adjudicators listen to the stories and approve compensation using a bureaucratic matrix that increases the payment based on the severity of abuse, including an estimation of long-term emotional impact. Cultural and human sacrifices are accounted for through a litigious system of monetary compensation for physical, sexual, and mental abuse.[5]

Sovereign state authority in Canada has always been tied to the regulation, surveillance, and management of Indigenous bodies. As Kelm (1998, 57) states, "The drama of colonization was acted out in Canada not only on the grand scale of treaty negotiations and reserve allocations but on the supple contours, the created representations and the lived experiences of Aboriginal bodies." The manifestations and expressions of this authority are changing.

Although the regulation, surveillance, and management of healthcare for Indigenous peoples within Canada has always been centralized, responsibilities for this policy domain increasingly operate through partnerships devolved from the state to communities themselves. Reiterating that the constitutional obligation to provide health services to Indians was ambiguous, the minister of national health and welfare tabled the Policy of the Federal Government Concerning Indian Health Services in 1974. With this policy, the government wanted to ensure "the availability of services by providing [them] directly where normal provincial services (were) not available, and giving financial assistance to indigent Indians to pay for necessary services when the assistance (was) not otherwise provided" (Health Canada 2011b). This policy sought to ensure that healthcare was available to Aboriginal people and that they had financial assistance to cover the cost of medical treatment. This policy recognized the need for "community development," as well as "a strong relationship between Indian people, the federal government, and the Canadian health system" (ibid.). This preceded a new policy in 1979 that would acknowledge the state's "special relationship" with Canada's First Nations and Inuit communities.

This special relationship flows from constitutional and statutory provisions, treaties, and customary practice (Health Canada 1979). Seeking to enhance the derelict health status of many Indigenous people, Health Canada implemented this policy to seek community engagement. The federal government acknowledged that "only Indian communities themselves can change these root causes and that to do so will require the wholehearted support of the larger Canadian community" (ibid.). In addition to stating that one's eligibility for uninsured benefits would now rely upon "professional medical and dental judgment," the policy outlined three pillars: community development, socio-economic development, and cultural and spiritual development. The second pillar acknowledged the federal government's role as an advocate of Indian communities, whose interests it conveyed to the larger Canadian society and to its institutions. This pillar also emphasized the federal government's role in promoting the capacity of Indian communities so that they could achieve their aspirations. The policy contended that "this relationship must be strengthened by opening up communication with the Indian people and by encouraging their greater involvement in the planning, budgeting and delivery of health programs" (ibid.). The third pillar called for an interdependent system of health management that would include enhanced public health activities on reserves, health promotion, and the detection and mitigation of hazards to health in the environment (ibid.). Thus this policy strongly encouraged "active" engagement with, participation in, and management of healthcare in Indigenous communities.

Biopolitics, Partnerships, and Productive Power

The language of health promotion took centre stage in Canadian public health policy during the 1970s. This was in large part due to policy perspectives and statements such as that of the 1974 Lalonde Report, which emphasized the role of individuals in improving health (Lalonde 1974). With respect to Indigenous communities, the 1979 policy strongly encouraged individual responsibility for health:

> Indian communities have a significant role to play in health promotion, and in the adaptation of health services delivery to the specific needs of their community. Of course, this does not exhaust the many complexities of the system. The Federal Government is committed to maintaining an active role in the Canadian health system as it affects Indians. It is committed to promoting the capacity of Indian communities to play an active, more positive role in the health system and in decisions affecting their health. (Health Canada 1979)

This policy, based on the principles of health promotion, community engagement, and partnerships, sought to combat the "tragedy of Indian ill-health in Canada" (ibid.). Similar to the 1974 policy, this policy also recognized the need for community development and for a strong relationship between Indian people, the federal government, and the Canadian healthcare system.

A new climate of rights, recognition, and responsibilities emerged in the 1980s. In 1980 a report by the Advisory Committee on Indian and Inuit Health Consultation – the 1978 Berger Report – recommended "methods of consultation that would ensure substantive participation by First Nations and Inuit people in the design, management and control of healthcare services in their communities" (Health Canada 2011a, 2011b). Berger imagined that the federal government would put an end to policies that fostered the longstanding dependency of Indigenous peoples on institutions. His report gave credence to the idea that Indigenous peoples could manage their own affairs; in this respect, "the report was radical" (RCAP 1996). Whether the report can be interpreted as a step toward empowerment remains a matter of continued debate.

Moreover, in 1982 the Canadian Charter of Rights and Freedoms promoted the protection of individual rights and freedoms, and pledged to guarantee Aboriginal treaty rights and freedoms under Section 35. In 1985 Bill C-31 amended the Indian Act with the aim of removing gender discrimination in line with Charter rights. Shortly thereafter, Health Canada's Medical Services Branch started to put plans in place to transfer control of health services to First Nations and Inuit communities.

Other initiatives soon followed suit. A 1983 report by the Special Committee on Indian Self-Government – the Penner Report – suggested that an essential element of a new relationship between the federal government and First Nations and Inuit peoples required recognition of "Indian self-government." The report identified health as a key area of this relationship. Between 1983 and 1986, Health Canada's First Nations and Inuit Health Branch encouraged community-based health initiatives with the intent of localizing control for health within First Nations communities. On a case-by-case basis, many communities across the country achieved greater ownership of healthcare. By 1986 the federal government's Community Health Demonstration Program had funded thirty-one projects, although many criticized the persistent paternalism set out in the parameters for funding arrangements (RCAP 1996). This process was imperfect. One tribal leader asserted, "This policy direction had been criticized as an attempt to abrogate treaty rights and have Indian people administer their own misery. Nevertheless, we entered the transfer process – but with our eyes wide open. We saw transfer as a way to achieve some of our objectives, and we felt we could look after ourselves in dealing with government" (ibid.). Just as the state decentred authority by transferring it to communities, so too did it decentre the overall policy area of Indigenous health. In 1986 Parliament passed the Sechelt Indian Band Self-Government Act. The following April, the British Columbia Legislative Assembly unanimously passed a bill to give the Sechelt community municipal status (Health Canada 2011a, 2011b). The Sechelt Indian Band signed the first self-government agreement in which a First Nation community assumed control of its health services. Two years later, Cabinet approved the transfer of responsibility for health to First Nations south of the 60th parallel. Canada's Treasury Board supported the transfer of Indian health services from the Medical Services Branch of Health and Welfare Canada (now Health Canada) to First Nations and Inuit peoples wishing to assume this responsibility. Formal authority was transferred to the Strategic Policy, Planning and Analysis Directorate (Health Canada 2011b). The Subcommittee on the Transfer of Health Programs to Indian Control was formed with representation from experienced First Nations health professionals. The subcommittee incorporated the experiences of the aforementioned community health projects and recommended a developmental and consultative approach to health transfer (ibid.). The policy framework for health transfer then drew from these recommendations. Several tribal councils soon thereafter signed on to the Health Services Transfer Agreement.

The 1988 Indian Health Transfer Policy reaffirmed the three pillars outlined in the 1979 Indian Health Policy. Its main focus was to "increase community participation in all aspects of the health program, and to encourage and support the transfer of control of health programs to Bands, Tribal Councils or other First Nation authorities prepared to accept such authority and responsibility" (ibid.). With respect to northern Indigenous peoples, the orderly transfer of health services to the territorial governments, in full consultation with First Nations and Inuit authorities, emerged as a core concern. The 1988 Indian Health Transfer Policy provided a framework for the assumption of control of health services by First Nations people and set forth a "developmental approach to transfer centred on the concept of self-determination in health" (ibid.). Throughout the process, decisions to enter into transfer discussions with Health Canada rested with each community. Once involved, communities had the option of taking control of health program responsibilities at a pace determined by their individual circumstances and capabilities.

Following the release of the 1996 *Report of the Royal Commission on Aboriginal Peoples,* the federal government released a new plan: *Gathering Strength – Canada's Aboriginal Action Plan.* This plan outlined Health Canada's commitment to diabetes and tuberculosis initiatives, to developing the Aboriginal Healing Foundation, and to a healing strategy that would address the legacy of Indian residential schools in partnership with the Department of Indian Affairs (ibid.). It emphasized renewing partnerships, strengthening Aboriginal governance, developing new fiscal relationships, and supporting strong communities, peoples, and economies. Previously, the "Treasury Board approved the Integrated Community-Based Health Services approach as a second transfer option for communities to move into a limited level of control over health services" (Health Canada 2011a). In 1995 the federal government announced the Inherent Right to Self-Government Policy. 1995 "saw the distribution and implementation" of the *Pathways to First Nations Control Report* (Health Canada 2011b). This report outlined the essential differences between transfer and the integrated approach. The integrated approach was understood as an intermediate measure that would provide more flexibility than contribution agreements but less flexibility than the Health Services Transfer Agreement (Health Canada 2005, 2011b).

Overall, the 1990s saw a period of public health policies that expected bands to expand, consolidate, and create new programs to improve health services, with more streamlined funding mechanisms in place based upon agreements between Indian and Northern Affairs Canada, Health Canada, and Indigenous communities. In 2000 the Medical Services Branch was renamed the First Nations and Inuit Health Branch (FNIHB) and remains housed at Health Canada.

Today, the multipronged jurisdiction over the effective management of Indigenous health involves government agencies, communities, and individuals. To effectively carry out its mandate, the FNIHB partners with First Nations and Inuit communities to gather information on population health status, health determinants, and risk factors. To this end, the regional offices collect and report information from various sources (Health Canada 2011b). Territories are not required to report vital statistics, as they have responsibility for primary healthcare, although mandatory reporting requirements are in place for FNIHB-funded programs, including communicable disease control and environmental health initiatives. Communicable disease control includes reporting on immunization levels using biomarkers such as age, sex, and antigen. For diseases with epidemic potential, provincial, territorial, and regional offices require notification within twenty-four hours. Legislation to support communicable disease control remains under the domain of provincial and territorial governments.

In addition, "environmental health" falls under Health Canada's "health promotion" initiatives for Indigenous communities. These efforts range from confronting the effects of mould and poor drinking water to improving nutrition and food safety, and they include fostering natural and human-built conditions that will improve an individual's ability to achieve and maintain good health. The FNIHB's website is filled with information about environmental health resources and with enthusiastic descriptions of "what you can do" (Health Canada 2010). Health Canada's public service announcements state, "We all breathe the same air"; "Don't smoke regularly in your home"; "Dust and vacuum regularly"; and "Follow water advisories" (ibid.). Thus individual citizens are encouraged to play an active role in environmental health management for themselves, their communities, and their homes.

The Paradox of Citizenship

Indigenous citizens living in Aamjiwnaang dwell between the tireless task of managing environmental risk and practising their way of life. Thus citizen actions mark the threshold of their existence. Caught between worlds, they are forced to reconcile with their ominous industrial neighbours, while pursuing life free from contamination. Citing German theorist Martin Heidegger, Weir (2006, 1) articulates that thresholds "mark the transition from inside to outside" and bear the "in-between" of light and dark, or truth and illusion. Thresholds make relations possible between people in places. They mark entry and exit, while undergirding a sense of transience or liminality. Encircled by Canada's Chemical Valley, citizens live here "in a bubble" – a geographic zone demarcated by their industrial neighbours and by a complex *policy assemblage* that governs on-reserve environmental health, while shaping and constraining avenues for Indigenous environmental justice (Luginaah, Smith, and Lockridge 2010). For those struggling to make sense of this bubble – their home – everyday activism requires a heightened sense of commitment, mobilization, and engagement in order to hold their industrial and government neighbours to account.

Applying a multilayered approach to the operation of biopower sheds light on the lived realities of citizens of Aamjiwnaang in this *affective*, toxic zone (Anderson 2014). As citizens encounter this landscape, they face a dilemma: resist or appropriate responsibility for finding the answers to the questions they have about their environmental health. Lessons from green governmentality literature demonstrate how such responsibility for environmental management shifts from the state to the population as "citizens are called up to take the mantle of saving the environment," which allows for the individual management, regulation, and surveillance of behaviour and for individual claims to "the kind of subjectivity that those who are environmentally conscious wish to have";

consequently, the governing of such subjectivity "does little to address the neoliberal order which contributes to environmental problems" (Rutherford 2007, 299). Through regimented, disciplinary activities, "good environmental citizens" appropriate responsibility for mitigating environmental risk with limited systemic change. Aligned with Hobson's (2013, 56) commitment to exposing green governmentality's "blind spots in prevailing environmental citizenship frameworks," Chapter 4 turns to the site-specific practices of citizenship in Aamjiwnaang. Citizens of Aamjiwnaang are not merely "green citizens."

In Aamjiwnaang, everyday practices in the ongoing struggles for environmental reproductive justice – monitoring spills, documenting releases, sheltering-in-place, conducting bucket brigades, body-mapping, and biomonitoring, to name a few – are practices of disciplinary, action-oriented activism. Simultaneously, they are struggles over both power and knowledge, revealing the dilemma of empowerment for these citizens seeking change to their surroundings and their health. This is the paradox of ecological citizenship.

At first blush, it appears evident that the practices of self-management in Aamjiwnaang demonstrate a hands-off approach by state authorities for ongoing contamination. Amid this limited state role, citizens pick up responsibilities for environmental and reproductive health in their struggle for recognition, redress, and justice. A biopolitical analysis highlights some implications of these practices for citizenship, justice, and ultimately democracy, as I discuss in Chapter 7. Concerned with the implications of disciplinary biopolitical subjectivity for citizenship, applying a governmentality lens to these practices of responsible environmental management and self-care sheds light on the ways that citizens become disciplined into compliance with technologies of rule as a kind of "environmental governmentality" or "green governmentality" (Darier 1996; Rutherford 2007; Tully 2008b). When coupled with biopower, governmentality as a mode, art, or mentality of rule illuminates how citizens in Aamjiwnaang struggling for environmental and reproductive justice mobilize their bodies and bodies of knowledge. This mobilization is a practice and a kind of activity that prompts a rethinking of citizenship itself.

A *multilayered analysis* reveals the operation of biopower as it takes shape through official policies and power ensembles, as well as on the ground as experienced by citizens. At once a population-maximizing strategy and an individual-management technology, biopower requires communities and individuals to manage human and more-than-human life across macro, meso, and micro scales – from (inter)national to local levels. In Aamjiwnaang, as citizens mobilize their bodies through practices such as biomonitoring, bucket brigades, and body-mapping to better understand the relationship between their human and more-than-human life and to protect their health and environment, we glimpse how life and land become objects for governance and administration. In this respect, citizens perform a kind of "active citizenship" to maintain stewardship over their bodies and land. On the one hand, while being responsive to their noxious environment, citizens are "constituted as subjects acting on nature" (Tully 2008b, 81). On the other hand, citizens here have longstanding traditions of relating to their environments in an ecological web of life. Their traditions and entire way of life are affected by their proximity to Chemical Valley. Without transformative policy change, this active form of responsible and disciplinary citizenship leaves systemic injustices intact. Thus, aligned with Tully (ibid., 83), new thinking about citizenship and policy as not only embodied and corporeal but also networked and rooted in the ecology of place is imperative for an "alternative that is ecologically sound and responsive to the legitimate concerns of those affected by the changes." Rather than thinking about biopolitical citizenship in purely instrumentalist terms, as a kind of appropriation of "green governmentality," an account of lived experiences that considers their ontological rootedness in place challenges an individualistic approach (Darier 1996; Rutherford 2007). This tension bears upon a crucial distinction between "green governmentality" and "ecological citizenship."

The notion of citizenship itself belongs to a longstanding exclusionary tradition. Chapter 1 discussed citizenship as a concept highly imbued with dualistic meaning. Demarcating between mind and body, male and female, reason and emotion, and public and private, citizenship has always marked the threshold between the inside and outside of political life. Such binaristic delineations feature prominently in contemporary green theory and environmental citizenship literature. Following Gabrielson and Parady (2010, 376–79), much of current green theory emphasizes Western, Eurocentric notions of "stewardship," "duties," and "obligations" and gives "epistemological privilege" to citizen responsibilities *for* nature as a kind of body-blind "ecological enlightenment" (Barry 1999, 2002; Dobson 2003). These conceptual configurations disembody citizens *from* their environment. Calling for corporeal citizenship, Gabrielson and Parady (2010, 376) seek to theorize a more inclusive version of citizenship that "allows for greater recognition of the diverse attachments individuals have to the natural world and better attends to claims of recognition and social justice." As both a feminist and environmentalist formulation, such a theorization calls for greater attention to bodily and material dimensions of citizenship and, moreover, of *policy*. Not only is this conception of corporeal citizenship embodied and attentive to the particularities of human difference, but it also recognizes humans' "inescapable embeddedness in differing social (discursive and material) contexts that shape subjectivity and consider our collective agency" (ibid.). Bridging corporeal feminism and green theory, an intersectional interpretation of citizenship troubles the aforementioned binaries and creates some epistemological cracks for rethinking the ontology of citizenship as inherently ecological (i.e., based on reciprocal relationships between human and more-than-human worlds) rather than instrumentally ecological (i.e., transactional, with humans being distinct from the more-than-human world in need of management), thus gesturing toward more radical avenues for environmental reproductive justice in theory, policy, and practice.

Moreover, citizenship debates that examine the politics at stake on the threshold between public and private life and between human and the more-than-human worlds interest feminist scholarship for several reasons. As MacGregor (2006, 5) aptly notes, and as elaborated upon in Chapter 1, citizenship is a deeply gendered concept. Furthermore, in the context of a declining welfare state and a period of neoliberal economic and political restructuring, the activities assumed by the "private" realm have particular meaning for the labour practices of women. It is also notable that women tend to be at the forefront of many movements for environmental reproductive justice. With respect to Aamjiwnaang, Ada Lockridge's experience as a busy, unpaid activist for her community in this regard is exemplary. Moreover, debates about identity and the performative dimensions of gender are inextricably linked to citizenship (ibid., 6).[6] There is no singular coherent vein of feminist, eco-feminist, or ecological approach to citizenship; however, it is undeniable that the meaning of citizenship in theory and practice has a lengthy and gendered genealogy.

Ecological citizenship's multiple edges become most apparent when considering not only citizen practices in Aamjiwnaang but also ontological perceptions of place, as Chapter 4 highlights. The ongoing activities and practices in Aamjiwnaang reveal "active citizenship," with citizens becoming self-disciplined subjects as first responders in cases of environmental catastrophe, as well as health experts at arm's length from the state. In these capacities, they are vehicles for the operationalization of governmental power. With limited state intervention, citizens assume the responsibility for bodily and environmental management. At the same time, citizens in this community articulate a radically novel form of belonging that is both corporeal and territorial: it is rooted in place-specificity. Thus the dilemma of ecological citizenship is that it can be simultaneously a tool of coercion and agency.

Lifestyle practices, choices, and responsibilities illuminate the crux of ecological citizenship's visceral edges. In large part, "green agency" is conceptualized as an "individualistic commitment to take rational control over the body and the private sphere through 'green lifestyle'" initiatives such as recycling, waste management, and community cleanup (Gabrielson and Parady 2010, 383). From a Foucauldian frame, we might think of citizenship as just another way to discipline citizens or to absolve the state of its responsibilities to care for those most vulnerable at the margins of society. Conversely, a radically different ontological view of ecological citizenship considers agency to be embodied and emplaced, as well as relational, situated, and intersectional.

Citizenship is Janus-faced: it simultaneously serves to define and demarcate populations, in addition to offering up a radical mode of belonging. Thus citizenship as both a community- and government-led strategy is "simultaneously coercive and empowering" (Cruikshank 1999; MacGregor and Szerszynski 2003, 7). Citizens are embedded within power relations. As Cruikshank (1999, 5) states, "the citizen is an effect and an instrument of political power rather than simply a participant in politics." Citizens are both constituted by power and agents with power. Rutherford (2007, 298) states that ecological citizenship can be read as fundamental to the "production of regimes of governmentality that create the conditions of possibility" for citizens governing themselves, their bodies, and their environments. Ecological management of health and habitat operates at the fulcrum of power-knowledge subjectivity.

To illuminate an affective, felt, lived, visceral approach to *sensing policy*, subsequent chapters examine the struggles for environmental reproductive justice through an interpretive lens, inspired by Foucault's concepts of governmentality and biopower. Beginning with people – citizens – and their lived experiences, these chapters focus on the ways that knowledge intersects with power relations, intertwined within a *policy assemblage* that informs and impedes avenues for justice. An examination of people's struggles for knowledge and power illuminates citizen concerns and practices as individual, responsible acts of self-discipline that are embedded within larger structural and discursive socio-political forces shaping and constraining their freedom and agency. Beginning with experiential elements highlights the significance of this place – or social location – to their values, beliefs, and senses of belonging. This connection to place problematizes the individualizing logic of governmentality and biopower. It further troubles conceptions of "ecological citizenship" as a global, transnational, fluid, and ever-shifting force (Barry 1999, 2002; Dobson 2003). Rather, drawing from struggles in Aamjiwnaang, ecological citizenship is placed, particular, and specific.

The logic of governmentality and biopower assumes a hyperactive subjectivity and atomistic individualism on the part of citizens. In this frame, "neurotic" citizens exist in a constant state of alert and must change their behaviour to be an environmentally responsible steward and thus a good environmental citizen (Hindess 2004, 305; see also Hindess 2002; Isin 1997, 2004). There is an assumption that individuals will manage their lifestyles and livelihoods in the private sphere. Consequently, citizens at the margins of society struggle for recognition by the state (Isin 2002). However, thinking about the neoliberal biopolitical subjectivity of citizens is an approach that has some limitations. There is a need to open up space for alternative ways of conceptualizing Indigenous citizenship acutely and citizenship more generally by considering a radically different form of ecological citizenship.

A multilayered approach to biopower simultaneously examines individual responsibility and broader structural and discursive socio-political forces, which manifest through civic action. Thus citizenship as a concept imbued with meaning makes a claim on political life. As Cruikshank (1999, 3) notes, "citizens are not born, they are made." As citizens mark the threshold between the inside and outside of democracy, a biopolitical lens interrogates how lines are drawn in making the distinction between public and private life to expose, critique, and disrupt the ways that "democratic modes of government entail power relationships that are both voluntary and coercive" (ibid.). Moreover, a biopolitical lens renders visible the ways that technologies of governance manifest through citizenship as well as through participatory, democratic societies and schemes. Operating according to a certain political rationality, citizens become at once effects and instruments of political power.

Both classic citizenship theory and contemporary neoliberal practices of privatization relegate corporeal activity to the private, bodily realm as an object of rule. Cruikshank (1999, 6) elaborates upon Mouffe's (2005a) and Laclau and Mouffe's (2014) discussion of "radical democracy," wherein emergent social movements interrogate and potentially dissolve the public-private distinction in political life. As is the case in Aamjiwnaang, translating these concerns into actions in the public arena poses both a hindrance to and an opportunity for citizen claims. With respect to the Lambton Community Health Study, struggles for reproductive justice led to the formation of a countywide health study; however, the situated concerns of this community remained unaddressed, thus exposing the limitations of deliberative public policy in this instance. Although the Lambton Community Health Study enlisted public participation, it led neither to actually carrying out a health study nor to responding to Aamjiwnaang's concerns. Transformative change therefore requires some kind of political translation from the private to public domain, beyond merely bringing citizens "into" political processes.

As will be discussed in Chapter 7, although citizen agency and resistance begin with bodily practices, a radically reformed public arena that makes space for participatory and placed expertise is equally significant. Responding to individual/private action through state/public action is imperative to *sensing policy* in pursuit of concrete social change. Demanding that citizens make lifestyle changes or assuming that they will do so is not enough to mitigate struggles for environmental reproductive justice. Calling citizens into participatory public forums as engaged and active volunteers is insufficient for radical political engagement. Placing the onus upon individual citizens to acquire knowledge about environmental and reproductive health harms does not meet the need to address broader social justice concerns that extend beyond individual autonomy and serves only to justify a limited public role. Thus attention to the relationship between individuals and broader public socio-political configurations is important. Shifting attention away from individual (ir)responsibility and toward systemic injustice flips the gaze back upon the formal political realm. To address the root causes of systemic reproductive and environmental injustice, change requires a practical shift toward public transformation and away from responsibilized activities – that is toward amended regulatory policies and away from actions such as calling 1-800 lines, managing emergencies with "personal emergency kits" (i.e., matches, flashlights, AM/FM radios, work gloves, hand warmers, water purification tablets, hand sanitizer, first aid kits, multitools, candles, and a plastic container), obeying the wisdom of climate change mascots like Disney's Olaf from the film *Frozen,* and self-reporting accidents, spills, and releases (Toledano 2015). This does not mean shifting "active citizenship" from the private to the public arena but rather a conversation that involves retooling the public arena itself to carve out space for situated knowledges at the interstices of the public-private split within political life.

Conclusion

The metaphor of the body politic both serves as an allegory and entails practical application in Canada. Politics move away from centralized institutions and policies, creeping into the nervous system of human bodies, where they are assumed by communities and citizens themselves. Biological regulation decreasingly takes place through overt, coercive power relations but is instead achieved through productive and inductive means of governance. As one Aamjiwnaang historian notes, prior to Confederation smallpox-infected blankets were given to Indians as "gifts" (Plain 2007, 35–36). This is an early example of biological warfare. At the time of white-settler contact, Indigenous health declined as a result of the onset of new diseases, loss of traditional lifestyle, imposition of new diets, depletion of food resources, dislocation, confinement to reserve land, and the residential school system (Boyer 2004; Kelm 1998; RCAP 1996; Waldram, Herring, and Young 2004). A biopolitical lens offers a glimpse into some of the ways that citizens confront an opaque *policy assemblage* for Indigenous environmental justice.

As the subsequent chapters reveal, although the provincial and federal governments share responsibility for environmental issues, the provincial government does not formally have a role in on-reserve health issues. This problem draws into focus the regulatory gap, where the federal-provincial division of powers produces a zone where environmental health issues become "lost in a limbo of inter-jurisdiction or layered jurisdiction" (Agyeman et al. 2009, 12; J. Borrows 2002; Mackenzie 2013; Moffat and Nahwegahbow 2004). The status of the reserve as a fiduciary federal responsibility adds another layer to this *policy assemblage*.[7] Consequently, all too often, the reserve becomes lost in jurisdictional battles over who has to foot the bill for those harmed in this liminal space.

Chapter 4 next takes us into the heart of a place, Aamjiwnaang, surrounded by Chemical Valley, home to over 800 Anishinabek residents. Based on in-depth interviews, this chapter documents the "slow violence" (Nixon 2011) associated with living in this "sacrifice zone" (Lerner 2010). Some of the thirty-five community members interviewed either had or continue to have an official role within the community as an activist, employee, or public official. The atmosphere their words conjure is both harrowing and homely. It begins with the ongoing impacts, turns to practices of resistance, and concludes by underscoring the significance of this place to citizens of the Aamjiwnaang First Nation as a matter of cultural survival. This chapter brings the implications of this policy assemblage for citizen mobilization into focus as a paradox of freedom: citizens of the Aamjiwnaang First Nation are bound up within hierarchical, disciplinary power relations in this polluted place, while affixing meaning to a place that they call home, which is central to their Anishinabek beliefs and being. No matter how polluted, it is both a site of distress and a profoundly radical place of belonging.

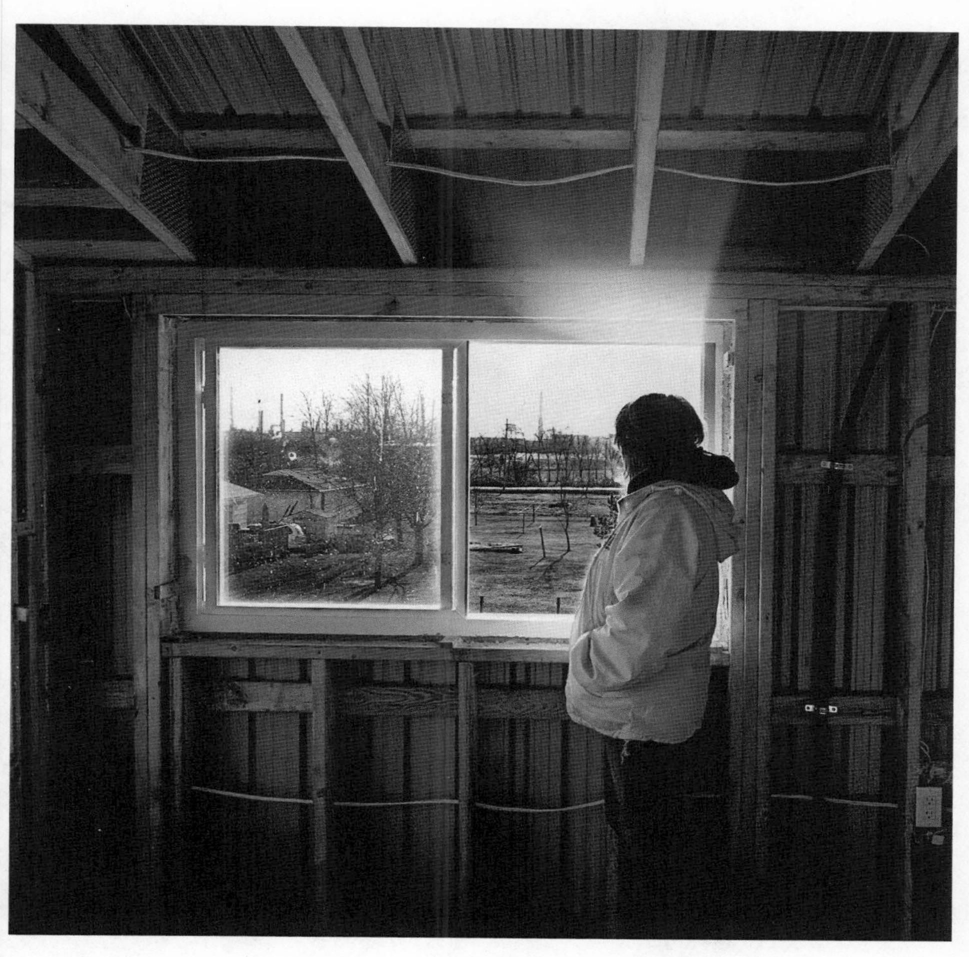

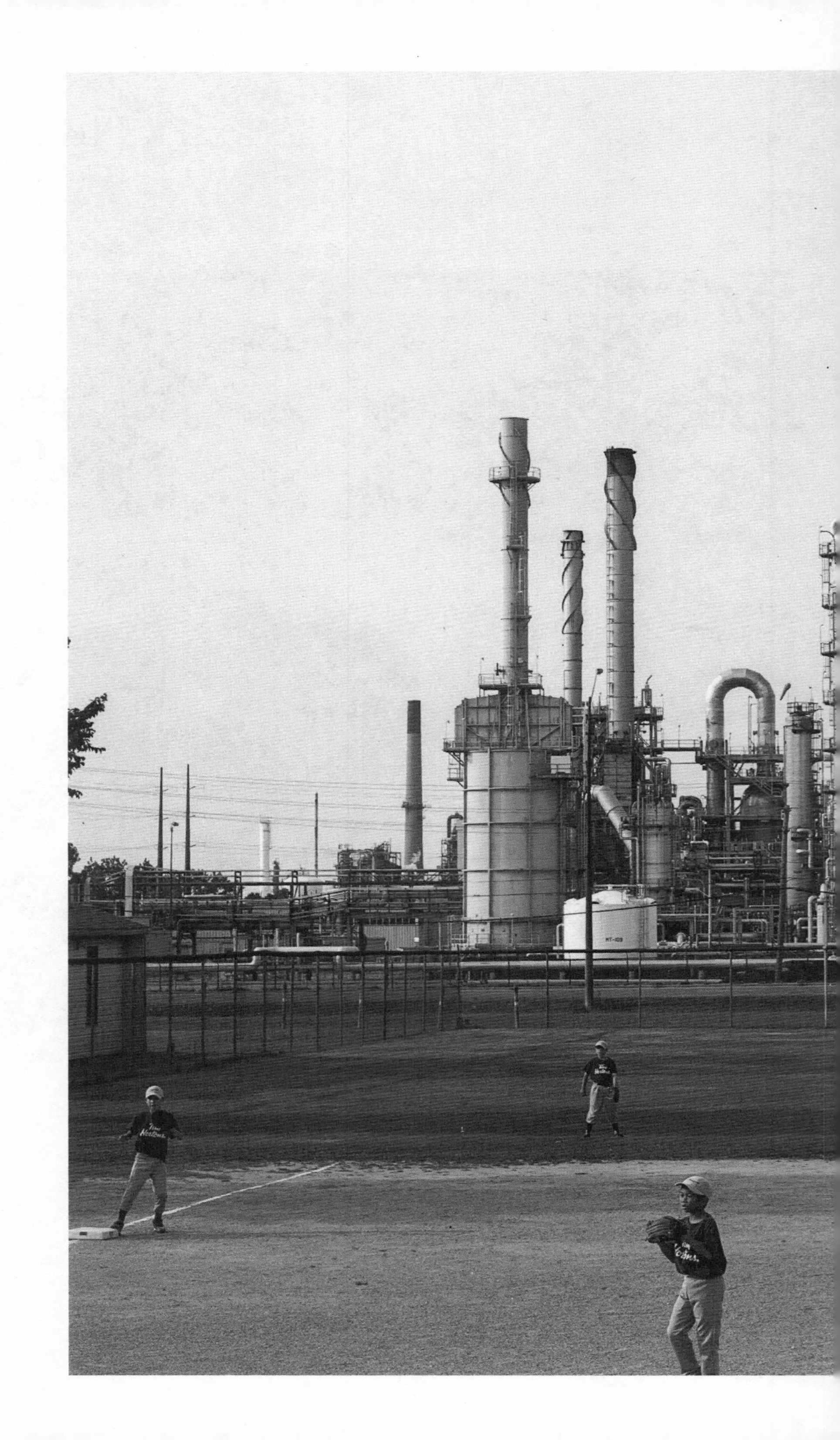

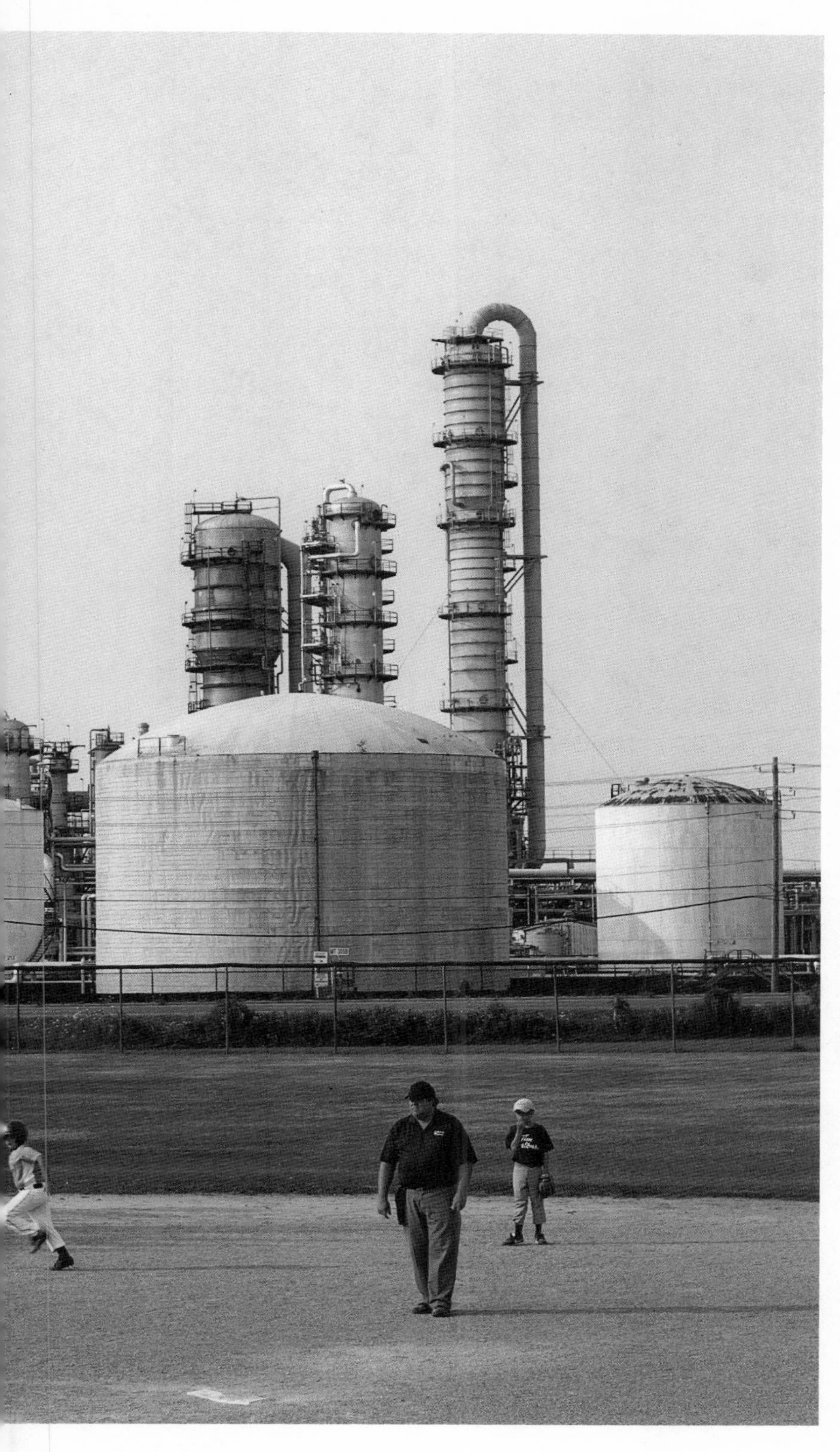

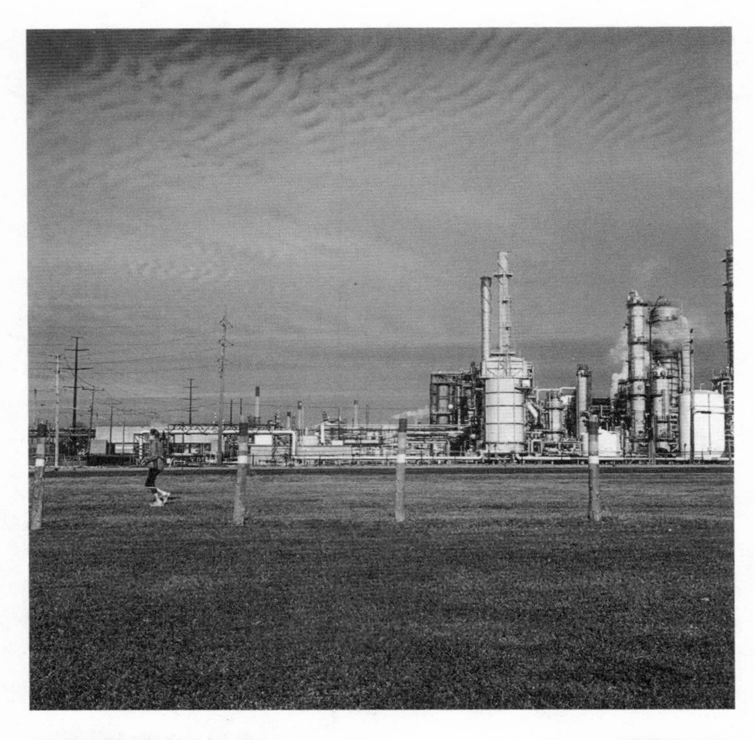

9

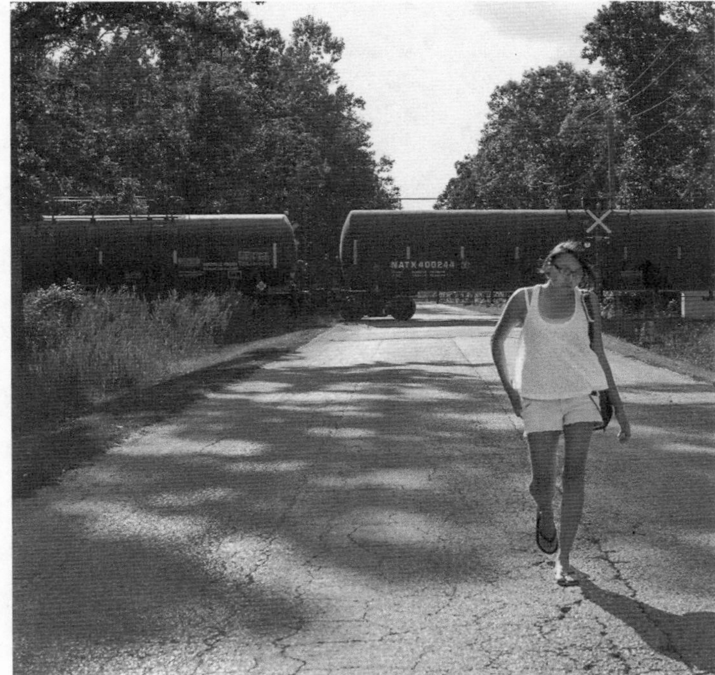

10

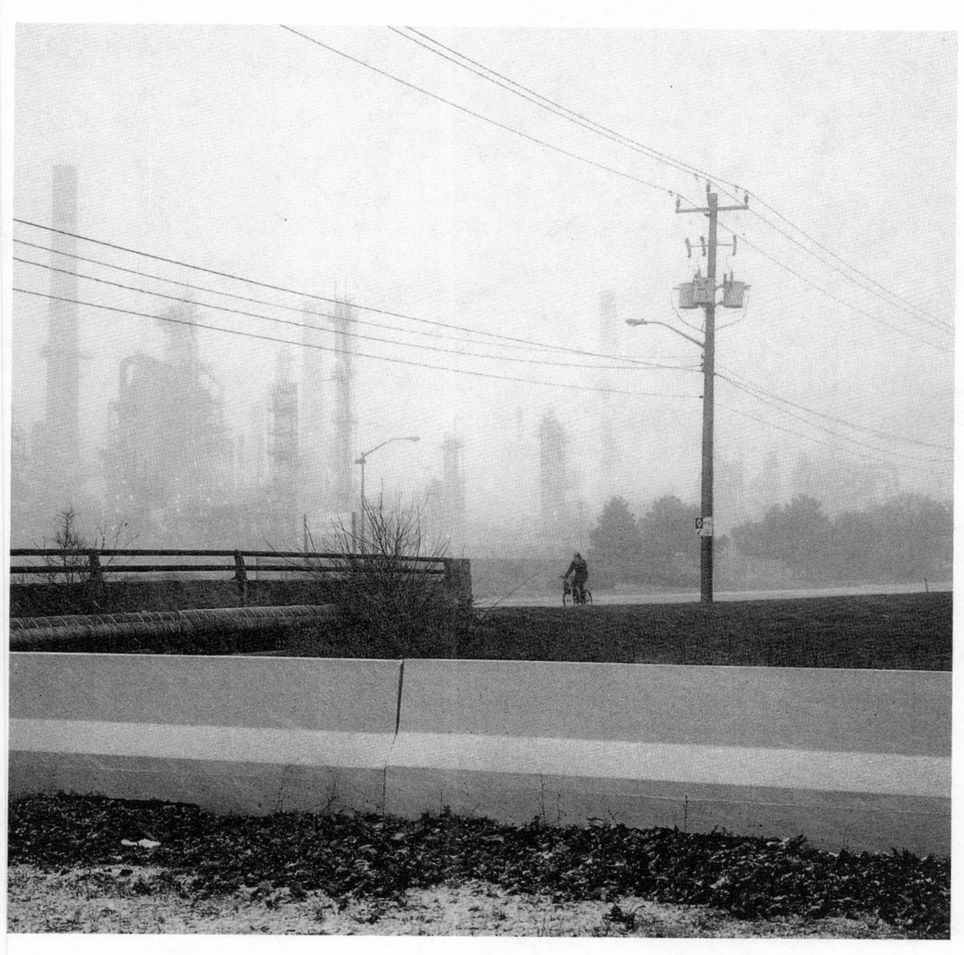

11

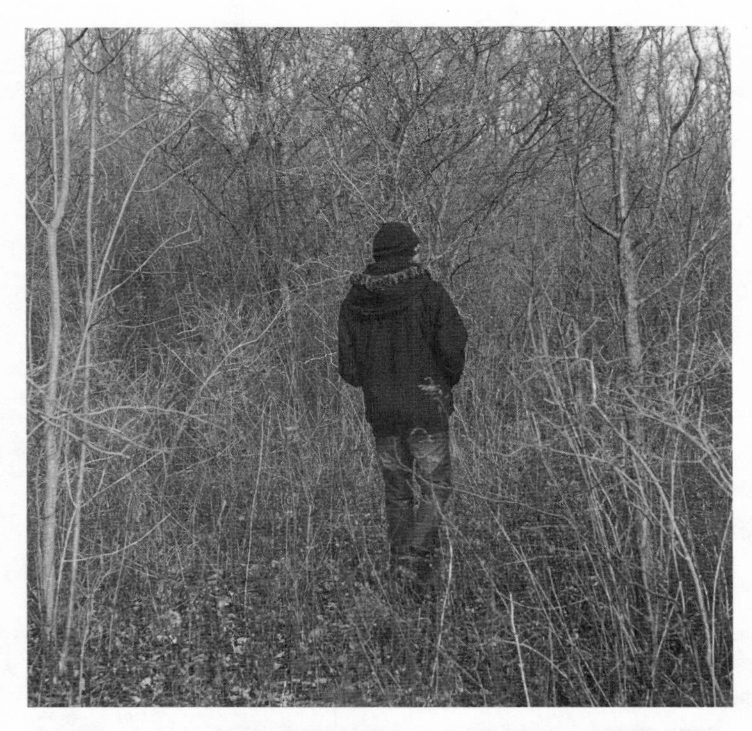

12

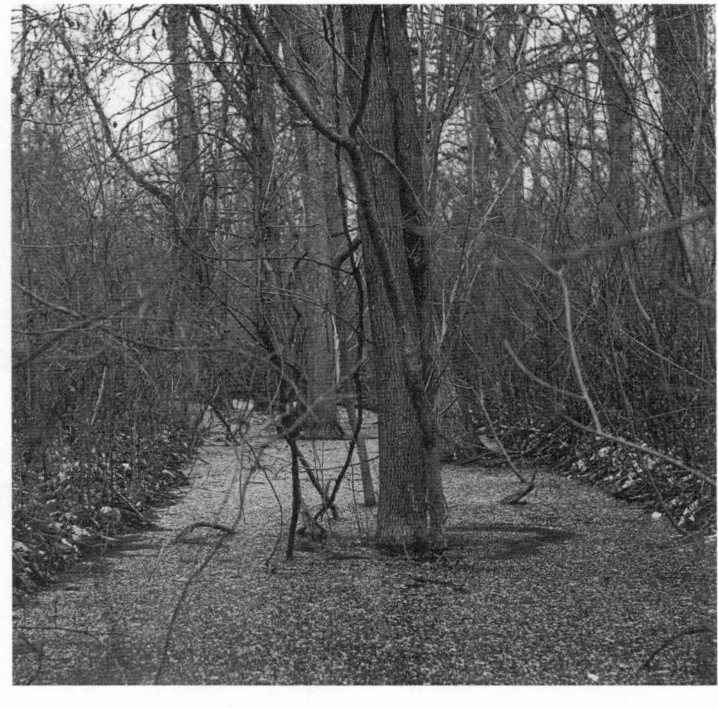

13

Life

In the shadow of "cloudmakers"

Along Tashmoo Avenue, the St. Clair Parkway, and Maness Crescent, in Aamjiwnaang most days go by quietly as they do elsewhere in Canada. Workers tend to their jobs, while kids go to school. Teenagers hang out in basements playing video games, while their younger siblings run around in the backyards. Meals are cooked and shared, and stories are told. Lights go out and dreams take over until the next day. Years pass. A grandfather turns fifty as his granddaughter graduates from high school. Young couples steal their first kisses, while breakups tear others apart. Football championships are lost, and baseball games are won.

All activities – the slumber parties, the bonfires, the family gatherings – take place in the looming shadows of chemical plants. Full of youthful imagination, children pretend that the smokestacks are cloudmakers. Worried parents sniff the air, hoping that no invisible substance is gliding by.

In 1985 a perchlorethylene "blob" poured into the St. Clair River, rendering the waterway an "area of concern." In 1992 a benzene leak threatened the safety of infants resting at the daycare, then located directly across from a polymer plant. They were promptly whisked away and taken farther afield. In 1993 a toluene release forced residents to leave their home at the break of dawn in order to seek refuge at Sarnia-based St. Clair High School. A decade later, in 2013, a mercaptan leak led community members to the hospital with nausea, headaches, sore throats, and swollen eyes.

These are but a few of the more serious releases that have happened in past decades. Every day, toxic industrial compounds seep into the air, water, and ground in and around Aamjiwnaang. No one is exactly sure of what might be the consequences of their gradual accumulation.

Entangled within this treacherous landscape, life goes on because it must: birthdays are celebrated, baseball tournaments held, and tales told (and retold). Throughout it all, beings continue to be honoured – from the songbird that wakes you up in the morning to the elder who keeps you on the right track.

CAPTIONS

7 Ada looks out of the window of her garage toward the Shell facility. In 2010, with help from Ecojustice, she brought the Ontario government to court. She contends that the province's ongoing approval of air pollution in Sarnia constitutes a violation of basic human rights under the Canadian Charter of Rights and Freedoms. December 2010.

8 Although the community centre and daycare have been moved farther inside the reservation and away from the plants, some leisure facilities, including the baseball diamond, are still adjacent to the factories. The Talons – Aamjiwnaang's team – play games against rivals from surrounding towns. August 2014.

9 Incessant pollution engulfs Aamjiwnaang residents as they continue to maintain a healthy and active lifestyle. Whether cycling, playing sports, or running, their environment serves as a continual reminder that they are surrounded by noxious chemicals. While citizens breathe the Chemical Valley air, they live with the unknown health effects of their everyday exposure to surrounding toxins in the atmosphere. Though a Lambton Community Health Study deliberated health concerns countywide, the specific ways in which Aamjiwnaang citizens are affected remain unexplored by public officials.

10 Gabby walks past a train carrying petroleum products during a "healing walk." Aamjiwnaang's residents and their supporters marched for three hours through the reserve to survey their land, honour Mother Earth, and bring awareness to the harm being done by the surrounding industry. August 2013.

11 Large industrial facilities create a barricade between the Aamjiwnaang Reserve and the city of Sarnia. The lack of readily available public transportation between the two further isolates the First Nation community and forces some to bike or hitchhike through the industrial complex. January 2012.

12 Mckay walks through the bush behind his home. As a kid, he spent much time in these parts, playfully pelting friends with pine cones, building treehouses, and engaging in paintball matches. Today, he spends his time wishing for brighter days, producing rap songs, and writing poems about his experience living in Chemical Valley. November 2014.

13 In Ojibwe the word "Aamjiwnaang" refers to the spirit of the water. Interpretations include spawning stream, meeting place by the rapid water, and braiding water. Pollution levels in the creeks today prevent many from enjoying them. November 2014.

Photos and text by Laurence Butet-Roch

4

Home Is Where the Heart Is
Lived Experience in Aamjiwnaang

Citizens of the Aamjiwnaang First Nation who reside in closest proximity to Canada's Chemical Valley experience a unique set of concerns vis-à-vis their Sarnia neighbours. Here, spills, leaks, chemical releases, and accidents are frequent occurrences. When such incidents take place, sometimes members of the industry are the first responders, and other times residents of Aamjiwnaang call the 1-800 line of the Ministry of Environment's (MOE) Spills Actions Centre, which collects concerned citizens' calls. At that time, a MOE environmental officer may opt to check out the event in order to determine an appropriate course of action. Sometimes the alert sirens may sound; however, more often than not, the sirens' shrilling is no more than an everyday occurrence. Most often, when a serious incident occurs, the Chemical Valley Emergency Coordinating Organization issues a code associated with the incident. Commonly, what results is an "information code 8," referring to an "internal non-emergency situation, that may be noticed by the public" (CVECO 2011). Frequently, these accounts accompany the statement that there is "no offsite impact" (*Sarnia Observer* 2011). Sometimes spills are not reported at all. Residents are expected to call the MOE 1-800 line if they smell something abnormal. Some citizens are alarmed by the normalcy of this situation for those living in Chemical Valley, whereas others have accepted that this scene is part of the everyday life of this place. A close look at the citizen's experiences of living in this sacrifice zone reveals the entwined impacts of this place on physical and cultural survival.

Living in a Sacrifice Zone

To the naked eye, smokestacks framing the reserve appear as majestic cigarettes, spewing up into the atmosphere. The bike lanes that trace the reserve's riverfront and then snake up along South Vidal Street leave much to be desired as the community's most accessible transit route. In the words of one resident, "When we go by Vidal Street, the air is really bad. It hits you in the chest. I'm always covering my face. I should just walk around with a mask" (Lily). Cognizant that "you can't go through your life wearing a respirator," individuals make the most of their environment (Olivia). Visions of citizens jogging along Highway 40, Vidal Street, or the riverfront illustrate the irony of attempting to manage a healthy and active lifestyle in Chemical Valley: "I like to go running, but it's hard to do. Oh, maybe I will hold my breath when I go by" (Heidi). Vidal offers the only viable bike route from the reserve to the town. Putting this scene into perspective, another citizen astutely stated, "I'd rather have pollution than get hit by a car" (Stew). Citizens carry on, living their lives much as citizens do elsewhere while trying to enjoy their surroundings.

The only reprieve – leaving – is a limited option for community members who consider this place home. From Sarnia, the glowing landscape on the horizon reminds citizens that their existence hinges on Chemical Valley's persistence. Moving to town provides little respite. Although some citizens have the means, ability, and desire to move off the reserve and into the city, they cannot escape the presence of smokestacks and plumes or the sound of sirens in their dreams (Tonia). As a result, citizens residing both on and off the reserve raise families and try to carry on while accepting the severity of their circumstances.

Living amid the hub of Canada's densest concentration of polymer and petrochemical industries is a matter of life and death. Citizens here dwell between light and darkness. As a community member recounted, a "nightlight" can be an ominous presence in Aamjiwnaang: "I remember being at my parents' house back near LaSalle Line, and the flare would light the whole room up – on Waboose Street. Even here sometimes it lights up everything" (Quinn). During the spring of 2011, one of Suncor's stacks lit up not only the sky but also the ground, as the gaseous ditch caught fire, startling citizens and regulators. MOE's "last ditch effort" to punish the perpetrators left Aamjiwnaang citizens perplexed, as little, if any, regulatory redress occurred.

At times, darkness marks the bodies of children in Aamjiwnaang. One individual recounted a serious event: "The supervisor from the daycare called me. There was black soot on the kids' clothes and on the ground, and I called MOE and they said they can't prove where it came from" (Nathan). At the time, the daycare was adjacent to Highway 40 and across from the former polymer plant, now replaced by Lanxess. With the support of industry, the daycare relocated to the heart of the reserve. Yet the band office, a resource centre, and a family services building remain in this location. Older community members recalled this sensorial scene: "There's a smell that comes off the styrene plant ... and it reminds me of being little, when I was there. It puts me right back. When I was in daycare" (Ken). As soot fell on the clothes of young children at the daycare centre and on homes, driveways, and cars, citizens assessed the damage: "There was a release ... it was on my car, on the trampoline, on my deck; it was all this black soot" (Quinn). The pittance of citizen compensation arrived in the form of $300 per exposed household. Monetary compensation is a stark reminder that citizens pay the price for both corporeal and community survival.

Children grew up with these facilities framing their horizon: "I remember my parents saying, 'Stay indoors and close the windows.' Not to swim in the river. I even heard, 'Don't eat the deer.' Everything was contaminated" (Quinn). The presence of these facilities even shaped children's games: "When I was a kid, we would play a game and scoop up mercury" (Billy). And it provided them with unique experiences: "It's like mercury. When I was a kid, our biggest thing was, you'd get mercury. Put mercury on a penny and you'd get a dime, use it to get candy" (Kirk). Eventually, this prompted some to ask, "So if it's on the shore ... what is on the bottom?" (Billy). Curious citizens have received few answers. Still today, parents speak of how toxic barriers frame youthful enjoyment of the landscape:

> You can't do too much with your kids. Sometimes it stinks. You don't know what's in the ground or waters here. At the powwow ... in the creek back there, there were a bunch of kids playing, and I thought, where are these kids' parents, why are they letting them play there, when there is a sign that says it contains toxic materials? When your kids go outside, you worry about them because you don't know what they are going to get into when they get out there. (Candace and Blair)

With the castle-like majesty of the smokestacks, some children find them enthralling, whereas for others they signal potential harm. As one mother shared, "My son always points it out too. He says it stinks. He knows they're not good for us; he's only three. He says, 'Put them in the garbage! It's stinky'" (Nancy and Bella). Enthrallment with the smokestacks reveals but one of the ways that the sights of Chemical Valley capture the imagination. Some in the community recounted that when gazing up at the sky, they would imagine seeing novel shapes in the fluffy atmosphere. At Christmastime, the twinkling stacks deceptively brighten the landscape:

> Something used to burn over there ... and you could see the smoke for miles and miles. The smoke was so big. I was a child. You know how a child will look at the clouds and say "that looks like a bear," or whatever ... The smoke looked like that. I would sit out there and never thought that smoke was going to hurt me. I don't know if they covered that up or what. They used to take everything back there ... at Christmastime, light it up. I thought that was really pretty ... They were bright, all different colours, like a bunch of Christmas trees. (Nancy and Bella)

The stacks that perforate the sky, these manufactured nightlights, affect the bodies of Chemical Valley's closest neighbours. Citizens feel and hear the rumble on a recurring basis (Quinn). These vibrations remind citizens that the rhythm of this environment is set by the beat of an industrial drum. Many community members worry about these effects on their children and future generations. One concerned mother said, "I still have a young daughter who is being exposed to a lot. There are leaks down here – benzene and whatever. So I think she's, you know, being exposed. The sooner I move her away, the better for her health" (Tiffany). Whereas some members noted concerns about their own health, many expressed frustration and sadness about the impact on the generations to follow.

And it was not only the adults who expressed worry. Families told stories of children speaking up during community consultation proceedings, simultaneously evoking rage and admiration that youth are propelled to voice their ongoing fears. "I've noticed our young people know a lot more because they are very concerned ... I get scared thinking, 'We're just surrounded.' It just takes one day ... for something to blow up and everything is gone" (Larry and Sonja). Worried about pollution's impact upon the creeks, trees, and deer, citizens refrain from catching game and wildlife on their land. Many spoke of experiencing a range of emotions, from "fear of mutating" to apathy (Stew), when sirens, evacuations, or shelters-in-place occur.

Citizens are frustrated with hearing from local officials that there is "no offsite impact." Impacts are felt, smelled, and feared: "They always say, when there is a spill or release, that there is no 'offsite impact' ... They think about their property but don't think about us living next to them" (Sam). According to one community member, "They say 'no offsite impact' ... That's a good one; it's not like the fumes or anything stop right at the gate line" (Tiffany). The persistent declarations of several facilities that their releases have "no offsite impact" infuriates some individuals: "That's the stupidest thing I ever heard. It's airborne. That stuff gets carried around for miles" (Edward). The plants cannot control the wind direction. Bright orange windsocks frame the reserve's perimeter, offering a symbolic and recurring reminder that at any given time, noxious fumes could be pouring over Aamjiwnaang.

In the case of spills, high-frequency emergency sirens alert citizens and prompt them to take action. There are three sirens situated within the Aamjiwnaang reserve's boundaries. Sounding at three-minute intervals – of five-second tones and a beat of silence – the sirens inform locals to head indoors, close all windows and doors, turn on the radio, and either shelter-in-place or evacuate. If a shelter-in-place is ordered, "The first thing you should be doing, unless advised otherwise ... it's like close the windows and shut the air off. Turn on the radio. It takes about a half hour more before you're notified. It could be all done with before the radio gets it. That's probably an emergency management point of view" (Tiffany). Some residents simply "turn the radio on ... and carry on" when the sirens sound (Candace and Blair). Citizens know the drill: turn on the television or radio and wait.

Aamjiwnaang citizens are constantly on alert. On Mondays at 12:30 p.m. sharp, the test sirens sound. As one resident explained, "I forget sometimes. That scares me. I'm always scared, worried, and still think some days, what if we all have to evacuate? Where are we going to go? Are we actually going to get out that fast?" (Larry and Sonja). For others, the frequent sound of the sirens, akin to the "boy who cried wolf," has had the opposite effect, causing them to grow complacent: "The thing about it is, it's normal. Really, when the sirens go off, I ignore them. I've grown accustomed to them. They honestly do not bother my children either. It's normal. It shouldn't be" (Elle).

Some community members claimed that when the sirens sound "it's not a big deal" and that there is no point "running around with your head chopped off" (Billy). These individuals laughed off community distress around this routinized sensorial existence. Characterizing the everyday normalcy of the sirens' presence in this place, community members described the perpetual chime that helps them keep time:

> Especially when you test them – every Monday at 12:30 – I set my watch to them. It doesn't bother me. I hear them go off and I know it's Monday. I don't know if any of their systems work all that well. There are different systems.

> One system would automatically dial residents' phone numbers. They do put it over Cogeco – I would get a test alert on Mondays. The idea is that if there is a real emergency, you turn on your TV ... If there was an emergency and I was supposed to evacuate, I don't know how I would ever tell. (Edward)

One plant worker described hearing the sirens "when you go for lunch break" (Frank). The shrilling sirens become a normalized part of everyday life in this environment.

Sirens, thunder, and lightning are common audible signals causing fear and anxiety among Aamjiwnaang citizens. Community members recalled being sent to neighbouring "safe havens" like the Holiday Inn, St. Clair High School, and the Lambton College cafeteria. Memories imprinted upon the psyches of the community's adolescents fuel their fears of potential strikes to the adjacent petroleum holding tanks each time a thunder or lightning storm occurs (Ken). As outlined in the Preface to this book, a 1993 incident resulted in a community evacuation when lightning hit an adjacent chemical holding tank. This event remains fresh in the minds of citizens living in Chemical Valley: "It was really traumatic for me. Ever since then, I've never trusted a lightning storm" (Elle). The explosive impact of this incident left a lasting impression on community members: "When a Suncor tank got hit by lightning, we got evacuated. It was scary. I was living near Esso, [and] I was worried about my mother and brothers" (Frank). Residents recounted, "I remember. I was fifteen when the one caught on fire. We had to leave. They tell you to stay inside. It's weird to live like that. We live ... being scared of your own ... Your home is like a refinery" (Edwin). As some discussed, if the plants were to "blow up," there would be a "chain reaction; all the plants would blow up, so that's what I think about too" (Candace and Blair). Concern with the possibility of a "chain reaction" event was a common theme: "Everything would be wiped out. I heard Sarnia is on the top-ten bombing list ... because it would cause a chain reaction if a bomb went off" (Candace and Blair). Understandably vexed about their livelihood and well-being, citizens asked, "We get blown up – who's responsible?" (Nathan).

The threat of evacuation remains constant. One elder recalled the past public service announcements – via megaphone – alerting citizens to leave their homes: "I have experienced a few ... There hasn't been sufficient protective gear" (Kimberly). Each time there is a thunderstorm or severe weather alert – as are frequent in Lambton County – many citizens cower in anticipation of the worst. Such circumstances have prompted some community members to ask, "What if we have a tornado and it hit those places: what would happen? Would we all

blow up?" (Nancy and Bella). For many, the end seems ne[illegible]
people are proud of their heritage and don't want to just giv[illegible]
my fear is that with everything going on in the world an[illegible]
closer to home, it's going to be the end with no warning, [illegible]
we can do to stop it" (Charlotte). Hope is a concept with li[illegible]
individuals struggling against such circumstances at the [illegible]
civilization. In its place, fear resounds.

Whether they are subject to the smell of rotten eggs or to the orange glow that glazes the sky, individuals living within the valley experience a stimulating and terrifying sensorial, aesthetic environment. Benzene exposure continues to be a visceral concern: "I've seen it. I've tasted it ... Workers were asked to dump coveralls in benzene. It would eat the oils right off"; moreover, repeated exposure has prompted speculation about whether it can affect one's reproductive health (Ken). Chemical Valley leaves a poor taste on this community's palate.

Over the years, fish consumption patterns have changed: "I grew up on it. You can taste the toxins. You can smell 'em when you're cooking them. You're used to it. We ate quite a bit during the fishing season. That was our dinner" (Ken). For many, it takes leaving the community to recognize the ongoing environmental health concerns. Some individuals noted differences in comparison to the neighbouring Kettle Point Reserve: "When I used to come to Sarnia before [from Kettle Point], it just stunk. After living here, you just get used to those smells" (Tiffany). Others described their appreciation of nature when vacationing. For example, one community member said, "I was looking at a palm tree [while in Florida]. I'm going to take a picture of that. It just looks so nice. I realized it's because there was a blue sky ... We never get to see blue sky. It's always grey with smog" (Tanya). In Chemical Valley living in a constant state of alarm, continuously on alert, has become a routinized, everyday experience.

Many community members feel helpless against the plants' presence in their everyday lives. Moving away provides little solace. After moving her family off the reserve, one mother said, "I don't think I can change things. So I don't think about it. It's not something you think about when it's there every day. So you just lay down and take it. It's all you can do" (Tonia). She said that being stuck, weighed down, and helpless can feel like "an arranged marriage gone wrong." Few are compelled to voice their discontent: "I probably could [speak out], but it doesn't do any good. If Shell is going to expand, or Suncor, or whoever, or build a new plant or a new plant comes in, there's not much we can do about it;

can't say, 'We don't want you here, you're killing us.' They say, 'But the money! Look at the jobs we provide'" (Edward). At the same time, several individuals remained unfazed by their surroundings: "Right now, when you catch this ... your body either stops it or it doesn't. There's nothing they can give you" (Kirk). What to some would be upsetting or distressing is to others just another daily occurrence, another experience, another instance of a toxin impacting their life.

Accountability to Aamjiwnaang citizens for industrial releases is not a transparent process. Sometimes the reserve's boundaries are policed: "We call it the 'yellow canary.' We say there is a strong odour coming from an area, can you go see what it is? What happens if you go there [to the site of a release] ... There is a strong odour, but you don't get out of there; they don't prepare you for stuff" (Quinn). Some chemicals cannot be sensed at all.[1] This "sniff test" is but one tactic employed by those charged with addressing issues of environmental concern. Those who are employed to police the plants worry too about their health. Exposed to benzene, one individual sought compensation, only to be brushed off: "What do you do? Someone says seek legal advice? It's a billion-dollar [industry] ... I don't have the money for a lawyer ... so I never did" (Quinn). Benzene is but one chemical released here.

Although some citizens used to believe that the government was protecting them, they are increasingly less certain: "I know we've lost a lot of our people from some kind of cancer ... Whatever is coming out, you breathe it in. But they don't realize, someday down the road ... They never come to the rescue" (Sam). There is an acknowledgment that the environment is harmful and a concern that nobody – neither the government, nor industry, nor media – monitors the plant activity closely enough:

> Sometimes they don't tell us or whatever when there's like a chemical spill or whatever. They don't say and they're supposed to ... It seems they keep it right out of the media or something. Like when you had that flare, it landed in that ditch on Vidal [Street], and that wasn't even in the media. But people took pictures of it. But after it was out, it was burnt. Great big burn marks on the grass. (Nancy and Bella)

Distrust of both the industrial facilities and neighbouring regulators is an ongoing issue. The flare's dominance does not go unnoticed. At night, "you can really hear the flaring. I don't think that's normal. To me, they are not informing the public about what they are burning" (Evelyn). Moreover, "with the smokestacks you can constantly see them flaring, and I don't think that's normal ...

With the flaring, they are releasing something but they are not telling you what they are releasing. They are so high at times" (Evelyn). There is confusion around who is to blame for this situation. Perplexed, individuals struggle for governmental recognition of their concerns:

> It's mind-boggling how the plants, they can get away with it. I don't know if it's the government or what. Somebody's got to step in and say it's affecting peoples' health. People in the plants have health concerns. But they need the money to pay for their mortgage or put their kids through schooling. So they risk their health for that benefit. That's not right. (Evelyn)

Community members feel trapped, and that they are at the mercy of limited state protection for their health and environment.

Despite the harrowing, swirling, and nauseating landscape of Chemical Valley, it is home and it is familiar. The deeply affective familiarity of this place is at once felt and smelled. According to one community member, "That's how I knew I was home ... You get that 'home feeling' from that nasty chemical smell" (Bob). And what do you do when you smell something out of the ordinary? There are some – limited – possibilities: "First thing is look the way the wind is blowing. If the wind is blowing the other way ... I don't think you have to move. If you smell something ... you should take shelter. Even if you can ... if there's an offsite leak, you can't prove it. The wind will blow it away ... They are like, 'What? We didn't do nothing'" (Bob). Some citizens stand their ground. If there was another evacuation announcement, not everyone would be hasty to leave the reserve "vulnerable and defenceless" and thus subject to foreign occupancy (Bob). You have the option to evacuate your home; you cannot evacuate your body.

Citizens' everyday experiences reveal a multiplicity of sensorial relationships to this place they call home. The atmosphere evokes light and dark, fear and hope, smell, taste, and touch. It is a region enabled by policy decisions and nondecisions. Bodies encounter, interact with, and bear direct witness to these decisions. Responding to this alarming sense of place, Aamjiwnaang citizens do not sit idle. In their ongoing practices of resistance, they access, deploy, and articulate experiential knowledge as they mobilize for justice. The next section discusses citizen agency and these actions as forms of resistance to ongoing toxic exposure. It then assesses the intersection between physical and cultural survival in Aamjiwnaang, which is directly affected by the reserve's geopolitical location within Chemical Valley.

Bodies Exposed: Taking Action

For many local community members, Chemical Valley is a sickening environment. One heartbreaking incident entailed a family's rude awakening when their son rose one morning with a bloody nose and his body covered in bruises. After he was diagnosed with leukemia, his swift passing rocked the community. Family members began to take action. They participated in numerous studies and mobilized knowledge to protest their toxic exposure – from body-mapping, to biomonitoring, to blockades – hoping to make their environment and home a safer, better place for future generations. Sickness abounds:

> As long as we are living in this area, we are always going to be sick. No matter how much they reduce the emissions from the smokestacks. You can see it. You can smell it. It affects the breathing, your sense of smell ... We're always going to be sick people ... I just don't think it's fair that we're sick. It shouldn't have to be that way. (Elle)

Citizens living in this community worry about a range of health issues, including physical and mental ailments. Some individuals reported difficulty focusing and noted that many children in their community grow up with learning disabilities (Elle; Ken). As one community member stated, "I've noticed the younger generation, teenagers and that, have commented that they all have ADD or ADHD: 'You name it, we've got it.' They're all on pills for some kind of condition they believe was due to the environment. I found that kind of amazing that so many were diagnosed with learning disorders" (Tiffany). Widespread psychological and physical health concerns affect the community.

Reproductive, respiratory, cardiovascular, and cancer-related illnesses are commonplace health concerns in Aamjiwnaang. Frequently, citizens connected these ailments to the environment: "I've seen many people die from complications from whatever comes out of these releases; there's been a lot of cancer; we're loaded down with asthma" (Sam). Residents expressed concern about the breadth of health concerns in this community, from thyroid issues and fibromyalgia to arthritis and a declining birth rate (Kimberly; Stew). Cancer is so present that it prompted some to say that "good health" in Aamjiwnaang can be reduced to being free from cancer (Edward). There was a common sentiment that Aamjiwnaang is facing an "epidemic of cancer" (Ken). Many feared that residents are not dying from "natural causes" internal to the body, such as heart failure, but are passing away from external factors, such as contaminants penetrating citizen bodies (Candace and Blair; Elle; Nathan; Tiffany). Mention of the omnipresence of cancer prevailed: "This year, if I took a number of people who've passed on, 99 percent is health related somehow to the environment in this community ... I've yet to see a natural death. That's a concern" (Nathan). As a result, citizens have begun to mobilize for change in order to raise awareness about the health circumstances plaguing the community.

Frustration with this noxious environment has propelled many citizens to assume responsibility for safeguarding their lives. Thus they are interpellated into being citizens on alert. They keep spill calendars, document the frequent releases, smells, and accidents, experience shelters-in-place, close their windows at night, evacuate, monitor wind direction and speed, and assess general air quality. These citizens have employed a variety of tactics and strategies for seeking recognition of their concerns. To increase awareness, with raised voices, community members have joined various environmental campaigns, which periodically receive flurries of local, national, and international media attention.

At the turn of the twenty-first century, while numerous local and national environmental initiatives garnered attention, Aamjiwnaang began to take a more active role in approaching and engaging with government and industry associations. Thus local citizens pick up responsibilities where government authorities fall short. By 2002, under the leadership of Ron Plain, the Aamjiwnaang Health and Environment Committee formed in response to Suncor's desire to establish Canada's largest ethanol plant just metres away from the community's band office.

In 2004 a flurry of outside interest regarding the high volume of accidental releases in Chemical Valley poured over the community. Aamjiwnaang's new emergency response planner, Nathalie Nahmabin, claimed that community members felt like a big "sitting duck" in Aamjiwnaang (Mathewson 2004b). Members of the Health and Environment Committee wrote to the Ministry of Environment, Natural Resources Canada, Environment Canada, and Health Canada to protest the federal government's provision of $22 million in funding for Suncor's site expansion as part of Canada's Ethanol Expansion Program. The community refused to be idle. "Enough is enough," they said, and a roadblock ensued in protest. The protest placed Aamjiwnaang on Canada's media and geopolitical landscape. Industries, government officials, and researchers began to notice ongoing concerns.

Angry sentiment persisted in February 2004 when Imperial Oil released 150,000 litres of solvent into the river, followed by a Suncor release of 44,000 litres of crude oil (Poirier 2004b, 2004c). In communication with the Sarnia Police Department, Suncor asked Aamjiwnaang residents to shelter-in-place.

A few months later, Suncor spilled 140 litres of gasoline, benzene, toluene, and other chemicals into the St. Clair River. Drinking water downstream in Wallaceburg, Walpole Island, and Stag Island was shut off for the fourth time in eight months, and radiator fluid was detected in the water both on Walpole Island and in the city of Wallaceburg (Mathewson 2004c). Finally, provincial officials took action.

Following this increase in the number of detected spills, Environment Minister Leona Dombrowsky and the ministry's thirty-member Industrial Pollution Action Team conducted a year-long sweep of regulatory compliance within Chemical Valley between 2004 and 2005 (MOE 2005). The high-profile team inspected thirty-five facilities,[2] finding all but one to be noncompliant with one or more of the regulatory requirements (ibid., ii). The sole compliant facility, a chemical plant, merely stored products and off-specification materials. Common deficiencies included a lack of spill-contingency and spill-prevention plans; no certificate of approval (COA) for wastewater collection and treatment or for air-emission control and treatment; altering equipment, systems, processes, or structures contrary to the COA for air or waste; and improper chemical handling, storing, and identification. Overall, 260 instances of noncompliance with environmental as well as legislative and regulatory requirements were identified. As the MOE team conducted its activities in Chemical Valley, environmental and human health issues caught the media's attention. In February 2004 CBC's *Disclosure* broadcast a series that investigated health impacts in the valley following a recent Imperial Oil spill (Mathewson 2004a).

The sequence of spills, accidents, leaks, and explosions caused community members to look at their local environment and their own bodies with alarm. Aamjiwnaang citizens mobilized to learn more about the impact of toxins within their community. In addition to emergent environmental concerns about toxins in Talfourd Creek, which swirls through the reserve, ongoing research documenting both the presence of "gender-bending," or endocrine-disrupting, chemicals in the nearby waterways and the impact of hormone-mimicking chemicals on wildlife, such as intersex fish, feminized amphibians, and other reproductive abnormalities, has caused citizens of Aamjiwnaang to look at their own population and birth patterns with raised eyebrows (Scott 2009; Weisskopf et al. 2003). Endocrine-disrupting chemicals – PCBs, cadmium, arsenic, and lead – were detected in Talfourd Creek. For years, this creek served as a drainage ditch for industries like Suncor, Praxair, and Dow.

Members of the Aamjiwnaang Health and Environment Committee teamed up with the Occupational Health Clinic for Ontario Workers – Sarnia (OHCOW) to conduct a door-to-door body-mapping survey of ongoing health concerns in Aamjiwnaang. As Scott (2008, 319) discusses, body-mapping is an epidemiological technology that pools the collective complaints of a community to identify patterns. This technique makes community concerns visible by affixing colour-coded sticky dots on human-size body maps to visually reflect symptoms (see Figure 3 below).

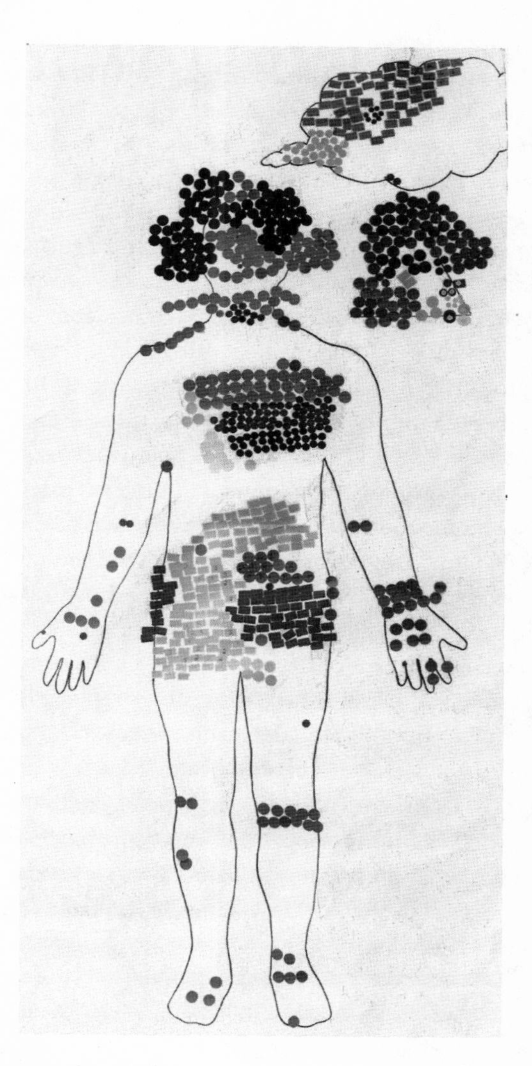

Figure 3 Body map

At the same time, a team of researchers, including OHCOW and Aamjiwnaang community members, engaged in community-mapping, a participatory research strategy to document community health concerns. Community-based researchers tracked birth ratio data over a twenty-year period, noting that between 1999 and 2003 eighty-six girls and forty-six boys were born, thus illuminating a birth ratio of nearly two females to one male (Mackenzie, Lockridge, and Keith 2005). The study revealed that since 1993, the male birth rate had declined significantly. News that women were giving birth to a disproportionate number of girls received national media coverage (Mittelstaedt 2004, 2005). These findings caused considerable fear about the potential loss of culture within the community and elsewhere. Consequently, a movement for environmental and thus also reproductive justice was born.

Shortly thereafter, recognition of Aamjiwnaang's situation within Chemical Valley began to reach policy makers at various levels of government. Emergent concerns regarding the twin issues of *health* and the *environment* on a First Nations reserve illuminate the nebulous, ad hoc dimensions of multi- and trans-jurisdictional policy making. Aamjiwnaang citizen Wilson Plain and his family participated in the ongoing national biomonitoring study Toxic Nation, which uses blood and urine samples to determine individuals' body burdens across the country (Dobson 2006b). In response to Aamjiwnaang's birth ratio study, a former president of the Sarnia-Lambton Environmental Association, the mayor of Sarnia, and Lambton County representatives called for a federally funded, comprehensive public health study focused on Lambton County (Dobson 2006a). Health Canada agreed, provided that local health authorities would play a leading role. Negotiations between local stakeholders regarding the establishment of a governance structure ensued.

Meanwhile, Ecojustice published a revealing report, *Exposing Canada's Chemical Valley,* which highlighted the results of the community-based body-mapping activities and detailed ongoing health concerns in Chemical Valley (Ecojustice 2007a). Community-based participatory activities continued, including "toxic tours," biomonitoring, body-mapping, participation in nearly a dozen documentaries, and community-based air-monitoring initiatives, such as bucket brigades, with the help of the California company Global Community Monitor. The bucket brigade

> allows residents of contaminated fenceline communities to actively participate in environmental monitoring and regulation. In essence, those residents are equipped to sample the ambient air in their communities at times and locations of their own choosing. The team consists of "sniffers" and "samplers" in

> a coordinated network using low-cost grab samplers that are explicitly designed to be inexpensive, easy to use, and made of materials that can be found at a local hardware store. (Scott 2008, 336)

Bucket brigades are a form of citizen-based epidemiology, or citizen science, a frequent strategy in Aamjiwnaang. Global Community Monitor showed Aamjiwnaang citizens how to collect air samples when a spill occurs using a plastic bucket approved by the US Environmental Protection Agency.

Residents thus take samples, log the time and wind direction, document physical sensations and any smells, and subsequently send the samples to a California lab to be tested for toxic chemical composition. According to one community member, "The bucket brigade picked up stuff ... but the Ontario government doesn't recognize that. We got this information from California. It was a lot of money to send down a sample to pay for it. They said, 'No, it's American. It's no good in Ontario, Canada'" (Sam). The ongoing costs of the bucket brigade fall upon the reserve. When community members detect any smell above a six – on a "stink scale from one to ten" – they are advised to take a sample (Sally). Citizens wonder about the chemical composition in the air around their cemetery. They are frustrated with the government's response to their environmental health concerns: "They keep saying it's our lifestyle factors ... choices that come into factor" (Sally). From smoking and drinking to using carpets, fabric softeners, cleaning products, and makeup, "lifestyle factors" or "choices" are targeted as health matters of personal responsibility. This response offends community members because it decontextualizes and distorts their lived realities.

In the years that followed, Aamjiwnaang citizens employed a variety of strategies to raise awareness about their corporeal and environmental concerns. In 2008 Health Canada funded a health symposium held in Sarnia. Although it drew an international crowd, Health Canada representatives refused to speak publicly about its fiduciary responsibility for Aamjiwnaang's environmental health. That year, Aamjiwnaang received its own air monitor, which remains located adjacent to the band's health centre.

The regulatory instruments available to them appear in a context of what the ministry calls an oversaturated airshed. According to Ontario's Environmental Bill of Rights, when industries wish to change their operations, the public is entitled to a thirty-day window for submitting comments and objections to be reviewed by the ministry (Government of Ontario 1993). Given the high concentration of facilities adjacent to Aamjiwnaang, staff responsible for providing input and feedback on the bill's website stated that "this does not work for

Aamjiwnaang" (Tina).[3] Consequently, the community has sought an alternative, nonstandard notice procedure and consultation arrangement.

Refusing to be idle, community members become accidental activists in response to their environment. At one community event, Ada Lockridge described her experience learning about her neighbourhood:

> I didn't know that we had a say on what goes on in the plants. I didn't know what was being released, or how much, or the known health effects from it. I didn't know to call the Ministry of Environment's Spills Action Hotline to report any unusual smells or happenings or to ask for a copy of the incident report. I didn't know that when there is an evacuation, that I should check the wind direction and know which plant it is so I can take the safest route away ... I didn't know that it wasn't safe to play here, in the river, or the pond, or the ditches. I didn't know that it wasn't safe to eat the fish, or the deer, or the rabbits here. I didn't know that I should keep my windows closed at night since the flares from the stacks mostly burn at night, so as not to bother so many people. I didn't know which government is responsible for what ... I didn't know that when Suncor was digging their first flare stack, they were digging up human remains. I don't know what they did with them ... These are some of the things that I didn't know, but I do know now. (Lockridge, Field Notes, First United Church, Waterloo, Ontario, April 6, 2011; Kiijig Collective 2012)

Officials frequently disregard residents' claims as speculative, unrepresentative, and unscientific. Although this community lies beyond the technical point of impingement by industrial emissions, residents occupy a middle ground, living with their bodies on the line between the insecurity of these "unknowns" and the security of what they "know" about their homes, bodies, and environments (Wiebe 2012). Citizens thus assume the responsibity for serving as stewards of land and life.

For some, it wasn't until joining community organizations that they began to notice their surroundings: "When I got on these subcommittees, I started realizing this" (Sam). Citizens situated in this place share knowledge and join together as they articulate harm. Political mobilization includes joining committees and organizations such as Victims of Chemical Valley, participating in door-to-door health studies, and sharing information on issues arising within the community through Facebook groups like Aamjiwnaang and Surrounding Area against Chemical Valley as well as Save Aamjiwnaang Forest and Ecosystems. Youth also mobilize creative voices to raise awareness about everyday life and to defend their home and land. Through groups such as the Aamjiwnaang

Green Teens and the Kiijig Collective, they organize to raise awareness, share knowledge, and seek social change.

While alive, citizens here do their best to survive. Many seek knowledge about their corporeal condition. As one community member noted, Aamjiwnaang officials, particularly the Health and Environment Committee, "are trying to get blood samples" of its citizens in order to gain a better understanding of the community's body burden (Kirk). Some community members continue to seek answers about their biological makeup: "I'd like to take a blood sample or something" (Sam; Sonny; Walter). Citizens participate in biomonitoring studies with the hope of better understanding the chemical composition of their biology for a variety of reasons. As one individual stated, "Knowing all these things are here, to me, just means I'm closer to the fight. I can keep working to try ... You may not ever get these plants and chemicals out of here, but you can at least make people aware and smarten up" (Walter). Those community members taking action and mobilizing for change are living on alert, trying to keep their industrial neighbours accountable. Citizens often cite the importance of keeping an eye on Chemical Valley to ensure that authorities follow appropriate standards and regulations (Sally; Walter). Engaging in biomonitoring studies is a recurring activity in Aamjiwnaang.

Whether or not the results of biomonitoring will be enough to achieve regulatory redress is a topic for future analysis. There exists a common fear that without the ability to generate credible, scientifically proven data that link one's biological makeup to harmful chemicals attributed to specific chemical refineries, environmental health concerns will not be an immediate policy priority and that report findings will continue to be silenced by officials and policy makers (Sonny). These individuals thus fear that it continues to be easy to discredit such data as merely "experiential" – unscientific and unproven.

Charged with calling MOE regulators and government officials to address environmental health concerns, citizens grow weary of living in a state of alert. The onus of environmental monitoring on the reserve is tiresome: "All the work that we do, we have to search and find everything before they take action. Why are they making me do this and making my body like this? I can feel the stress. When I do hear the sirens, I do feel my body tense up. I try to find which way the wind is blowing" (Sally). Hearing the shrill sirens is but one deeply felt lived experience.

Stress and bodily impacts are constant. The visceral effect of the sirens is an ongoing affective dimension of everyday life here: "When it turns towards you and hits you, the sound wave hits you, hits me; I could feel it vibrating my entire body from inside out" (Steve). According to another, as the plants burn off excess gases, "You can feel it; you can actually hear it because it's so loud" (Evelyn). Citizens mobilize, articulate their corporeal injury, and await response.

Mental health impacts cannot be understated. Finding solace among the chaos of contamination remains a challenge for community members trying to cope. Citizens note that on excursions into the bush, they are not exempt from Chemical Valley's sensorial residue, as the constant whizzing of the stacks accompanies hunters and gatherers on their expeditions deep into their territory. To find a healing place, community members will park along the reserve's service roads or drive into the community of Corunna, which is a town south of the reserve, and not within the reserve itself. One resident explained, "It's not just the visual and the smell. It's the sound, the noise pollution. There's no real place to be in solitude, no matter where you go. Even if you're in the middle of the bush, you can hear the trucks go by, flames, cars going down the 40 highway. No real peaceful place" (Charlotte). Citizens residing here try as they might to turn a blind eye – or ear, or nose – to Chemical Valley.

Many cope with this slow-moving, latent catastrophe by carrying on and living their lives: "You know it's there. You have to drive right through it. Not look to the left or right. And sometimes you smell that crap ... I just stay in my house. It's sad because it gets depressing when you have to lock yourself up" (Charlotte). Living like this functions as a kind of self-imposed shelter-in-place. As a community member noted, "There's no way you can deal with pollution. It's around us. You're going to go outside and walk around and breathe in pollution. What can you do? Put on a mask and walk around Aamjiwnaang?" (Mike). Feelings of helplessness coincide with apathy, despair, and loss. Despite this overwhelming situation, the community continues to survive as a distinct group of Indigenous peoples and to practise an Anishinabek way of life.

From sheltering-in-place to documenting spills and releases, biomonitoring, body-mapping, and bucket brigades, members of the Aamjiwnaang First Nation assume responsibility devolved from external authorities for protecting their health and local environment. The current regulatory environment, formalized through procedures such as the Environmental Bill of Rights, expects citizens to be on alert and to respond to ongoing noxious releases. For communities like Aamjiwnaang, these processes do not adequately account for cumulative effects and cumulative affects: citizens' bodies in this place are subject to exposure unlike that experienced by their Sarnia-based neighbours. Many ask why they do not leave. As stated, the Anishinabek people have a long history in this place, having established treaties with the Crown prior to Canadian Confederation. It is their home, and their territory is central to being Anishinabek.

A Matter of Cultural Survival

> I wouldn't move. No way. We are in the heart. The whole heart. You know Turtle Island? Aamjiwnaang is the heart of Turtle Island. North America is shaped like a turtle, we are where the heart is supposed to be ... It's the heart ... You can hit every major artery; every town that was booming back in the day you could hit from here in a day's travel.
>
> **– Bob**

Pollution profoundly, physically, and culturally affects the inextricable link between health, home, and habitat in Aamjiwnaang. In the words of community members, "Once that pollution's in our bodies, it's not going to leave, ever ... [So] your body must become immune to it ... [We're] used to it" (Larry and Sonja). Citizens of the Aamjiwnaang First Nation are thus frequently asked, "If your land is so toxic, and your health suffers, why don't you just pack up and leave?" Their responses to this question resounded with resignation: "For our future, healthwise it's definitely going to be a lot healthier for our community if we move" (DJ). In the words of another community member, "I'm already thinking that if they don't move the reserve, I'm going to move myself eventually. I don't want to move. I don't want to live in this cloud of pollution. I don't want to expose my kids to this when they don't need to be. I don't want this for them" (Diane). Fear of losing their connection to the people, community, and land deters residents living both on and off the reserve from leaving this area: "I would consider moving [but] I want to stay. I have a dedication to the Friendship Centre and to help out the people that way, but also being a pipe carrier, and this community doesn't have too much culture or faith keepers, so I have to go away to learn those things" (Frank). Some stay and many leave. Some return.

Moving away is a possibility always confronting citizens of Aamjiwnaang. Individuals living in this environment suspect that things will be better elsewhere. In Aamjiwnaang there is a concern that "people live here for a few years and get asthma ... They move away and aren't angry anymore ... They live here and start to get nosebleeds" (Elle). Relocation is a possibility that receives mixed reviews within the community. The question of why people do not move evokes a variety of responses. Notably, one resident said, "Well, this is my home. Why don't you make it safe?" (Kimberly).

Mobility, leaving, and relocation may be ideal in theory; however, freedom of movement is a concept imbued with privilege. Citizens are torn: "I love my community, but at least one time per week, I want to move off Aamjiwnaang. But I feel helpless. This is our home. We shouldn't have to go off where we grew up. It angers me – a lot" (Elle). Despite what citizens do or say, there exists a strong sentiment that little change will occur.

Movement is a privileged notion. For many reasons, citizens attach meaning to this place, Aamjiwnaang, their home:

> That's why community members want to stay here. It's their home. When I was younger, the land used to be so fresh, and we used to respect the land more and live off the land. Nowadays, with all the talk about pollution back then, maybe they are cleaning it up a little more or trying to hide it with the technology they got now. It's still in people's minds though, I think. You take a car, look how many years it takes to rust if you leave it sitting there ... It's the same way with the land. When I was younger, it was nice and green ... Then they moved in, and it took all these years for it to affect the land and animals. (Denny)

Leaving is not a viable option:

> I would never want to move away from here. This is my home. This is where I was raised. I've lived here my whole life ... So many memories I have. This is my home. This is, right here, a house, that we call our real home. We wouldn't have this place if this world wasn't here. Our Mother Earth. That's our real home. This whole place, this house, is going to be gone if we keep doing the same actions to this world. It is going to be gone someday. (Larry and Sonja)

This is a place to "be" Anishinabek: "Even though we are in the plants, it's the freedom. If you want to blast around, go fishing ... it's not as regulated as in the city ... I feel really close to nature" (Ken). When asked whether it would be viable to move the reserve, one citizen explained, "This is where they are going to lay me to rest, here, 'cause it's my home" (Sam). The environment is a matter of life and death for these citizens.

In lieu of family portraits, funeral cards adorned the mantelpiece of one interview participant. As some suggested, industry "might put food on the table and pay the bills, but it might put you in the ground. That's the pay you get" (Nancy and Bella). Making a living in this community is a perilous affair. A worker noted, "When I got this job, I said, 'I guess I'm sentenced to die' because of the air here" (Lily). Black humour and dark comments are revelatory of death's persistent visceral affront to daily life. As one citizen put it, "I plan on going to our noisy cemetery. That's where I plan on going" (Bob). Another added, "I grew up here, I live here, I'm going to die here" (Nathan). Reserve passersby take note of the community flag's unrelenting half-mast status. One resident said, "If you're not losing someone, you're supporting someone who's going through a loss to cancer all the time" (Lily). When citizens gather together in the reserve's cemetery to pay their respects to the departed and to mourn the loss of their loved ones, ceremonial song, drumming, and tears coincide with the sound and sight of whizzing, vibrating, flaring stacks. The location of the reserve's cemetery, encircled by industrial refineries, further demonstrates that dead or alive the reserve is not a place where one rests peacefully.

In this setting, ecological vitality cannot be separated from cultural vitality. Although "just being here is fine enough" for survival, citizens' loss of a connection to the land constitutes a much deeper disconnect: "When the youth lose that identity, being part of the land ... it takes away from personal growth ... all those areas, land and resources, and way of life that we live. Talk about cultural genocide" (Ned). This notion of "genocide" is not simply about the loss of people – as Canada's colonial history reveals – but also about the loss of a way of life. In the words of another community member, "People have already given up. They've already kind of figured that we've lost it. The habitat is destroyed. It's gone" (DJ). The idea of relocating from this place is difficult to accept given the community's lengthy history and deep attachment to and rooting in this place: "A lot of things tie us into the land, for a long time, since the 1600s. That's a long time just to move" (DJ). To maintain an Anishinabek way of life and sustain their inherent rights, citizens must practise their teachings about fishing, hunting, gathering, and so on.

Although they are indeed concerned about the loss of culture and traditional ties to the land and about the impact of pollution on present and future generations, the reserve is one of the few remaining places where citizens maintain a connection to their way of life, no matter how contaminated. They cope with catastrophe and contamination to maintain cultural ties, teachings, and traditions. Despite acknowledging that the chemical plants make Mother Earth sick, a former Suncor worker and current community member noted:

> When you go up top, you can see how the river bends. It snakes through. When you look at the reserve, you cannot see a house. All the trees are surrounding it. It hugs the reserve. It protects it all. You look over, and you can't see a single house. It's like Mother Nature is just hugging the First Nation like that. You can't see anything. They say the leaves do protect. I do enjoy being here, hiking, sweats, absolutely. (Ken)

Citizens lamented the imminent possibility of relocation: "To survive, our people, that is probably what we will have to do" (Ken). Cultural loss is consistently on the minds of many community members.

It is difficult to dispute that changes to the landscape impact how citizens practise territorial and ceremonial ways. One resident said, "I was sitting here with another committee member. He won't pick the heart medicine" (Frank). The pollution impacts healing practices in this community. According to an elder, "We have four medicines – cedar, sage, sweetgrass, tobacco – which I use from here. I have cedar. We put our tobacco down when we use it. I feel that if you do it in a good way, then it's okay ... but people are afraid to use the cedar because of the pollution" (Kimberly). Ceremonies, too, are not exempt from contamination's impact: "When we go into a sweat, which is a ceremony which we call the womb of Mother Earth, we have steam coming up from the grandfathers [heated rocks] in the sweat. That is going to be the purest air in Sarnia [but] you can still smell the pollution" (Mike). The impact of contamination on culture continues to affect the way of life in this community.

Cultural survival includes the preservation of community, land, and language. Some refuse to use the sacred medicines of the community; few carry on as usual. Language, too, plays a part in the loss of a "traditional," or Anishinabek, way of life: "It's almost like our language died out ... held on a little bit, and it's growing again" (Frank). Elders articulated a dire need for ceremonies to preserve a way of life (Kimberly). Examples are the jingle dress, which is a sacred dance of healing, and the fancy dance, which can be performed for visitors. Such dances are not done for money but for deeper spiritual healing and connection to the four directions. In describing entanglements of community, land, and language, one community member stated, "It's all connected" (Ken). Relationships are formed, maintained, and mediated by song, drum, and dance. Connecting with the North, East, South, and West through acknowledgment of the elements of earth, water, air, and fire, community members attempt to survive and thrive in this place through the preservation of customary and ceremonial ways of life.

Loss of this lifestyle continues to threaten their livelihoods. Citizens expressed concern about not knowing where to turn to remediate this loss: "Don't really know too much about the process of what it would take to get the land back to normal, other than healing itself" (Frank). The surroundings clearly impact citizens' daily realities. They feel that they have lost control. Many feel trapped because of limited options:

> I honestly think it's too late for my generation. Every single day I think about the cancer rate around here. I just think to myself, when is it going to hit me? What type of cancer am I going to get? ... Every day. Maybe that contributes to my anxiety. I do have anxiety. I am a worrisome person. I do worry about my family a lot. I do think about the environment and how it's affecting us. Now that this interview is happening, I'm beginning to wonder now. (Elle)

When asked whether there is "hope" for future generations and what their role might be, one community member lamented, "Will there be a role? That is what I ask. Will there be?" Is there hope for cultural survival? How can community members connect to a "traditional," or Anishinabek, way of life when encircled by this "modern" environment?

Making life better in the present involves thinking differently about human–more-than-human relationships. This entails reimagining citizenship. Rather than existing in an environment where toxic plumes blanket individuals, citizens wish to "be in an environment where culture blankets an individual" (Ned). This kind of cultural preservation and consideration of an individual's rooting in larger environmental processes offers an alternative way of thinking about relationships between humans and their environments – an alternative ontology. Ned's story offers an embodied and embedded way of thinking about citizenship as *ecological citizenship,* illuminating the inherent deep-seated interconnection between human and more-than-human life. Acknowledging the importance of this perspective, a provincial environmental official stated, "The Aboriginal thinking is far better. It is far more consistent with ecological theory and a sophisticated science approach than our general conception, which is set down by the bureaucratic separation, our institutional separations" (Gerry). This advanced ecological thinking – about humans and their relationships to each other and to the more-than-human world – not only offers an alternative way to think about citizenship as ecological citizenship but also provides a framework for addressing reproductive injustice, fusing physical and cultural survival with human and more-than-human life.

This Anishinabek perspective contests an egocentric view of the individual body. Discussing the body and its relationship to the surrounding environment, an elder said,

> I was told one time about a story about a filter that is within the human bodies. That filter is the liver ... I would say that breathing all this air from

> the industries in here, we have to filter that air. A lot if it is toxic air, we have to filter that, so that filter is the liver. It's going through our bodies ... When that filter is damaged or polluted with toxins that come into our body, then it dilutes or blocks any emotions, emotional concerns, that we have within our bodies. We just don't care about ourselves, our community. We show less care about what to do. (Mike)

In contrast to the atomistic stance of the predominant Western biomedical mode of thought, bodily function and emotional capabilities are connected to one's relationship with Mother Earth. As this elder further stated, "Your emotions travel to your heart, from your liver, which emit[s] these emotions. They travel to your heart and brain. When the emotions aren't pure and don't travel to the heart and brain, then you lose the sense of a happy lifestyle. You lose the ability to shed tears about things and acceptance" (Mike). Citizens in this community look on as fellow members pass away. This affects the emotional register: "There was an elder who stopped here one time on a walk. Passing through First Nations territory, she said, 'There's no spirit in Aamjiwnaang.' There's something lacking" (Mike). That reveals a community perspective that pollution has killed the spirits of Aamjiwnaang citizens and the spirits of their land.

Some ceremonial practices take place on the reserve, whereas others occur in a more serene setting with the aim of bringing knowledge back to the community. One practice is the humbling experience of a vision fast, which situates one's human relationship with nature: "You get to understand yourself and see what you appreciate in life. You sit out there and look around and see the trees and plants and animals. You find out how weak and pitiful you really are. You look at those little birds – you can crush it and kill it. A human is just a blanket. That's how you look at yourself as pitiful" (Frank). This ceremonial endeavour serves to remind humans of their place in the world. As one elder suggested, "Let's not be so egotistical to think that it's the only thing the pollution is killing – the birds, trees, have to breathe in just as much as us. They're part of the territory – animals, fishes, and all of life upon the waters and the land" (Mike). Animals, life, land, and humans share this relational connectivity. Confronting the egocentrism of our modern liberal society, the vision fast allows Anishinabek people to "see how the earth could swallow you up and make you disappear. It makes you humble" (Frank). Thus citizens of Aamjiwnaang live in a continuous state of dwelling between "modernity," "progress," "industrial development," and "technological advancement" on the one hand, and the humbling knowledge that as humans we cannot master or own nature, on the other hand. They are but one element among other animate beings in a complex world.

Facing the severity of our circumstances involves rethinking the individualism and egocentrism of our roles in, responsibilities for, and relationships with the "natural," or more-than-human, world. Community members contended that "if you respect Mother Earth," she will "respect you back" (Larry and Sonja). Some citizens said that environment takes on a deeper meaning in this place: "When I say environment, I'm talking about everything – human, animals – [and the] direct impact it has on the land and all those upon it." Furthermore, "we've all got a role. We all have a role and responsibility. We want an environment. It can be ... as an individual, family, community, nation. You want an environment that is going to be safe, healthy, and sustainable" (Nathan). Environmental protection is a shared practice. This connection between people and place highlights an ecological, embodied, yet territorial approach to citizenship. Such an understanding challenges technocratic and institutional models of environmental health policy. It also contends with Western, Eurocentric, liberal subjectivity.

An Indigenous approach to "ecological citizenship" can be understood through the words, actions, and practices of citizens trying to maintain an Anishinabek way of life in Aamjiwnaang. Citizenship, according to many Anishinabek beliefs, takes on multidimensional meaning in relation to a set of social, political, and civic entitlements. Citing an inherent right to the land, one community member said, "When we have a Constitution in place, it will speak about citizenship and the natural laws that we always had" (Ned). He spoke of the Anishinabek people's inherent right to the land and the inexorable tie they maintain to their territory and ways of being: "We do have, as an inherent right, land. That is the reason why we have continued to be here. If we lose that land, that is when the state governments or colonialism really takes effect. We have to have that identity – drums, dances. We have to have those traditions. Ancestors speak about that." These activities, or practices, are essential for cultural survival. Ongoing interaction and engagement are core components of Indigenous citizenship: "You take tools from the environment. You give respect and ask for permission" (Ned). Respect for the earth in the present is rooted in knowledge of the past. For example, the "medicine wheel, circle, continuum of knowledge, passed down for thousands of years," informs an Anishinabek ethic or way of being on the land and in the world today (Ned). This practice, a way of life, prompts residents to think about citizenship as interactive, relational, and placed.

Anishinabek ontology – as a way of being in the world – considers a multiplicity of relationships to be an inherent component of how we relate to ourselves, to each other, and to the environment. This approach takes into consideration the medicine wheel teachings, clan system, and a view of health that focuses on a "way of life." As elders note, this is "not just a governance and governing system but a way of life" (Mike). The residential school legacy sought to extinguish "traditional," or Indigenous, ways of being and of governing the world. In contrast to a hierarchical ordering of humans above nature, from an Anishinabek perspective, responsibilities were bestowed upon individuals by the Creator: "We talk about Nanabozho, who had a relationship with everything. So when you start talking about that relationship between Anishinabek and creation, you start to realize the importance of the mutual respect we have for one another" (Ned). In contrast to a hierarchical model, an Anishinabek approach examines the fluidity between humans and the more-than-human environment: "Environment is Anishinabek [and] Anishinabek is environment. Our passion in life is a clean Mother Earth, a clean environment" (Mike).[4] According to an Anishinabek worldview, respect for Mother Earth constitutes a crucial foundation for ecological citizenship.

To situate oneself and relationships, community members adhere to an Anishinabek view of citizenship that regards "natural law" as including the place of humans among the four elements: earth, water, air, and fire. Moreover, citizenship is corporeal, territorial, and practised. It cannot be separated from consideration of land, treaties, and the environment: "When we start talking about that natural law – for instance, one of the treaties up north talks about the sun: 'As long as the sun shines, and the grass grows, and the water flows' ... And they were encompassing the different ... spheres. You could talk about the 'stratosphere,' or 'biosphere,' or 'lithosphere' ... which is the ground" (Ned). Citizenship from a "traditional" view includes all of that and more: "It's kind of like the medicine wheel, with four directions, winds, grandfathers/mothers, four medicines ... Within that, we talk about the life cycles: child, youth, adult, elder. There are many other teachings [that are] a part of the medicine wheel" (Ned). Rights and responsibilities are inherently attached to the lived practice of caring for and building a *relationship* with the land.

As Ned's interview emphasized, citizens must advocate for both humans and more-than-humans and reimagine (in)animate relations, "for those [other] species, because that was the responsibility that was given to us" (Ned). Nature's resources are to be cared for, nurtured, and respected. According to Ned, "The oak tree provides either shelter, structure, or warmth." Acknowledging the significance of these resources to the community's sense of wellbeing is crucial to community development, identity, and culture. Adverse health outcomes result when this relationship with nature is ruptured:

> For people to be trapped, and to feel unprotected in our environment, either to go swimming, hunting, or to play, you know, it's tough for them to realize the opportunities that we do have, especially when we do have twenty-four hours a day, 365 days of ... pollution of noise, light, air ... and that affects not just us but the land itself. Some animals, all they see is light every day. It's affecting their lifestyles as well. (Ned)

The location and articulation of this community's struggles refocuses our gaze by drawing it away from an autonomous model of self-management, responsibility, and healthcare. It moves beyond a stewardship model of environmental management and toward an intersectional, experiential, place-based understanding of health and well-being. It is this very place, the Aamjiwnaang First Nation's home in the polluted heart of Canada's Chemical Valley, that is at stake in the preservation of the community's vitality. As a matter of physical and cultural survival, it is a matter of environmental reproductive justice.

Conclusion

The lived experiences of Aamjiwnaang citizens trying to come to terms with their environment reveals how making a home in Aamjiwnaang is a bittersweet endeavour, combining a mix of anxiety and attachment. As the voices, stories, and everyday experiences of citizens living in Canada's Chemical Valley depict, the impacts of pollution and their interpretations are multifaceted. On the one hand, daily activities and concerns reveal a disciplined responsibility for coping with and responding to encroaching threats; on the other hand, they bring into focus the deep relational connection that citizens of this First Nation have to their home and territory. An intersectional, affective, place-based focus on situated practices of citizenship presents an alternative way of thinking about *sensing policy* and about citizenship in Canada. In this respect, citizenship encompasses more than a status. It is not something to be attained. It takes place from below. It is embodied and corporeal, situated on the ground, rooted in place.

The experiential dimensions of citizen articulations, actions, reactions, and responses to living within Chemical Valley highlight connections to place and outline various ways that individuals interact with their toxic environment in everyday life. Such actions are heavily imbued with meaning. By revealing the embeddedness of individuals in their environments, an intersectional account of citizen interactions with "place" move us beyond an approach to political science or public policy that focuses solely on "individual responsibility" for the environment. This relational, embodied, or experiential, view of citizenship emphasizes the important role of attachment to the land in one's relations with the spiritual world, which is in stark contrast to a model of citizenship that considers "good citizens" to be individual, property-owning humans set apart from broader socio-political, economic, and environmental forces and processes.

The tie between physical and cultural survival is crucial to reproductive justice. A *sensing policy* framework draws this into focus. This perspective highlights the role of the body as a conduit for knowledge generation and mobilization. As Parr (2010, 1) suggests, "Our bodies are instruments through which we become aware of the world beyond our skin, the archives in which we store that knowledge and the laboratories in which we retool our senses and practices to changing circumstances." Relationships between humans and the more-than-human world are mediated through the body and involve practices and experiences that produce corporeal knowledges. This perspective is crucial to rethinking relationships between humans and their environments and to rethinking citizenship, expertise, and policy. Chapter 6 illustrates how policy arrangements mediate and interpret "truth" claims while privileging some claims over others. This chapter does so by examining the relationships between citizens, public officials, and "experts." In discussing citizen efforts to contest scientific expertise, it highlights how situated bodies of knowledge within this community encounter, confront, and interact with the following discursive fields: *science, scale, lifestyle blame,* and *jurisdictional ambiguity.* The findings in Chapter 6 reveal how large-scale epidemiological surveys fail to account for the specificities of small-scale, placed, ecological knowledges rooted in site-specific locales. Chapter 5 first turns to how this site came to be.

5

Digesting Space
The Geopolitics of Everyday Life

Geopolitical Catastrophe

Jurisdictional ambiguity pertaining to on-reserve environmental health policy became most apparent on May 18, 2004, when Sarnia police located an overturned tractor-trailer containing corroded forty-five-gallon drums of toxic chemicals such as styrene, toluene, and ethylbenzene on and adjacent to the Aamjiwnaang Reserve. Daniel Thomas, a Sarnia resident and "scrap dealer," had been renting a property at 650 Scott Road, across Highway 40 from the reserve's northern edge (see Figure 2 on p. 21). While Thomas was in the process of transferring the barrels from the off-reserve Scott Road site – a numbered property listed under the name Lawrence Brander – to a reserve property at 701 Scott Road, his trailer hitch broke (Poirier 2004a). Barrels tumbled to the ground, one of them exploding and alerting band members. Sarnia police responded to calls from the community about peculiar odours. Some of the chemical barrels were found lying thirty metres away in a brushy, swampy area. Prior to that, the Ministry of Environment (MOE) had inspected the holding site at 650 Scott Road. Although hazardous waste was being stored, it concluded that there was "no offsite impact." This finding did not account for risks associated with the transportation of the barrels.

The following day, the band held an Emergency Control Group meeting with municipal and provincial authorities. Federal representatives were largely absent from the deliberations. On Monday, May 20, two days after the accident, the *Sarnia Observer* ran a cover story illuminating Chief Phil Maness's frustration with his community being a local "toxic dumping ground." Explaining that he had "had enough," he declared a "state of emergency" over the barrels in accordance with the Emergency Management Act (Poirier 2004c). Perturbed by the lack of government enforcement, Maness stated that the band might need to start enforcing its own justice on environmental offenders. His response was fuelled in part by the legacy of concerns over findings from a 1996 study conducted by the University of Windsor that had revealed more than a dozen sites on the reserve contaminated by mercury and heavy metals (Leadley and Haffner 1996). In 2004, researchers worked with Aamjiwnaang community members. Another abandoned property on Scott Road, once the location of Welland Chemical, continued to house toxic chemicals for years following its shutdown in 2000, until its designation as a "brownfield site."[1] Meanwhile, young people from the community have used the site as a location for recreational activities like paintballing.

Following Chief Maness's declaration, federal and provincial authorities began to drum up the political will necessary to weigh in on this divisive issue. In 2004 the provincial minister of environment, Leona Dombrowsky, issued an order for cleanup control and stated, "When I came into work today I said 'we have to get this dealt with as the environment and people in the community are being exposed'" (Bowen 2004b). The order required immediately securing all the barrels, cleaning up all the leaked material, conducting an inventory of the barrels, and categorizing them as industrial product or waste (ibid.).

According to listed property owner Lawrence Brander, with the introduction of a catalyst, material could be converted to a fibreglass resin that would then harden and thus could be sold for profit to be used as a building material like concrete (Bowen 2004a, 2004b). Brander was, apparently, unaware of Thomas's plans to transport the materials across the highway onto reserve land, although in later court proceedings, witness testimony indicated that Brander was to pay Thomas close to $20,000 to dump the waste on First Nations land (Huebl 2005a, 2005b). Scientific experts were called in to clarify the composition of these chemical compounds. According to University of Victoria chemistry professor Reg Mitchell, the mixtures could be understood as solvents, with a little bit of plastic dissolved in them (Bowen 2004a, 2004b). The Sarnia police pledged to investigate possible violations of the Transportation of Dangerous Goods Act and the Highway Traffic Act when the barrels were being moved across the highway, charges indictable as provincial offences.

According to the MOE cleanup control order, Brander and Thomas were to devise a remediation action plan by June 4. Brander was instructed to provide a revised plan, including an inventory of the drums and steps for their removal, which was never submitted (Poirier 2004a). The ministry issued follow-up orders to four parties – Daniel Thomas of London, Campbell Street Industrial Park Limited, Charles Dally of Bright's Grove, and 569006 Ontario Limited, care of Sarnia's Lawrence Brander – each of whom either had possession or ownership of the barrels held at 650 Scott Road. The order gave parties until August 3 to abide by the latest order or else be liable for environmental cleanup costs. If the parties did not meet the August 3 deadline, the ministry would have grounds to proceed with the cleanup at the expense of the parties. As the June 4 deadline came and went, Sarnia's MOE office forwarded the noncompliance report to the ministry's Investigative and Enforcement Branch for a decision on whether to press charges. Finally, London police arrested Thomas while he was attending a court appearance for fraud under $5,000.[2]

Paid jointly by Indian and Northern Affairs Canada and with band funds, an independent environmental remediation company began to clean up the leaking barrels; however, the 650 Scott Road site continued to host some remaining toxic refuse. MOE hired a contractor to remove a total of 669 barrels, containing 25,000 kilograms of surface material (Bowen 2004a, 2004b). An ongoing debate over payment for subsurface contamination ensued, with an estimated cost in the range of $400,000. Finally, in December 2004, under the Environmental Protection Act, Leona Dombrowsky authorized provincial staff to remove and safely dispose of the contaminants from the off-reserve site. However, confusion ensued over jurisdictional responsibility for the on-reserve contamination associated with the accident. When it was time to determine who bore the responsibility for cleaning up the mess, band officials complained that "every time there is a spill, the jurisdiction card is played" (Poirier 2005b). The "point source" for the origin of the barrels remained in dispute. It was unclear whether the barrels were in "provincial" territory, on reserve land, or in federally regulated waterways.

In January 2006 the Aamjiwnaang First Nation Health and Environment Committee, led by Chairman Ron Plain, and the Office of the Environmental Commissioner of Ontario, led by Gord Miller, met to clarify transjurisdictional responsibilities for this murky policy domain. Afterward, on January 26, 2006, citizens of the Aamjiwnaang First Nation invited representatives of all levels of government in Canada – municipal, provincial, and federal – and neighbouring residents of First Nations communities to attend a day-long policy meeting. Notes from the Office of the Environmental Commissioner outlined that words like "jurisdiction" and "border" have very specific meanings for government representatives. Thus the meeting would focus on ways to improve the resolution of environmental issues in the community without challenges to any department's legal authority, jurisdiction, or mandates. In other words, the meeting examined ways that things could be improved given the existing legal and regulatory framework (Office of the Environmental Commissioner of Ontario 2006, 3). Some jurisdictional issues remained beyond the scope of the meeting, such as the Ontario Municipal Board's decisions, annexations, and land sales, as well as the intricacies of responding to contaminant effects, epidemiology, and human health concerns.

The Health and Environment Committee came forward with a long list of agenda items for discussion. These included:

1. Onsite contamination in sediments.
2. Concern over consuming local game and produce from gardens.
3. Chronic health issues.
4. Historical land transfers and decisions of the Ontario Municipal Board.
5. The Scott Road barrel incident.
6. Levels of government and their roles.
7. Frequency and nature of spills and releases.
8. Sirens and the fear of the unknown.
9. Air-quality data and monitoring.
10. Two-way communication.

Each of the ten items was discussed at length. Commissioner Miller noted that the Province of Ontario had previously demonstrated "creative use" of its legislation to ensure public safety. An example was the province's use of emergency evacuation powers for northern communities under forest fire legislation to evacuate Kashechewan residents on the shores of James Bay when their town had a contaminated water problem (Office of the Environmental Commissioner of Ontario 2006, 3). General concerns ranged widely and included the issue that there was no inventory of contaminated sites on and adjacent to the reserve; toxins in Talfourd Creek, which originates in provincial territory and flows through the reserve; accessing funding from the Treasury Board's fund for contamination cleanup (most designated sites are located in Canada's North); plants that began operations prior to the Ministry of Environment's legislative mandate, which originated in 1974; possible contamination of traditional medicines and sweat lodge materials like cedar and stone; accessing up-to-date health records of Aamjiwnaang citizens; a regulatory gap regarding hazardous waste on federally regulated lands such as First Nations territories;[3] emergency response; fear and episodic events such as leaks, spills, and fugitive releases; air-quality monitoring, data, and access; lack of MOE consideration of ambient air quality; and finally, lack of adequate consultation on emerging industrial expansions. These concerns revealed the chronic and cumulative impacts on the community of the toxins spewing from its Chemical Valley neighbours. Each of these points illuminates the reality that in contrast to jurisdictional borders, ecosystems naturally transcend and nuance rigid geopolitical demarcations.

Canada's division of powers makes the remediation of contamination and the safeguarding of environmental health a multifaceted policy domain that is difficult to navigate. In 2007 the Office of the Environmental Commissioner contracted environmental legal firm Ecojustice to produce a legal opinion on "spills to First Nations land." This opinion articulated that the Canadian Environmental Protection Act, 1999 (CEPA) contains significant legal mechanisms to ensure the cleanup of spills both on and off reserves, where provincial legislative regimes are either inapplicable or lacking in efficacy. Tools under the Act are rarely used effectively by the federal government to ensure that First Nation lands are cleaned up (Ecojustice 2007b). The opinion further stated,

> Experience suggests that the federal government is unwilling to apply CEPA to provincial lands despite its ability to do so. Similarly, Ontario appears unwilling to seek avenues to apply provincial regulation on reserve. This situation leaves First Nations in the conundrum that neither level of government will adequately ensure the clean-up of spills on reserve. (Ibid., 3)

This legal formulation leaves First Nations communities with limited avenues for redress. According to Ecojustice, given this "less than ideal scenario," the ultimate solution requires the political will of the Ontario and federal governments to recognize the "inherent self-government of First Nations to manage their environments" (ibid.). "Spills management" should be negotiated nation to nation in order to reconcile legal regimes and thereby ensure protection of First Nations from spills on and off reserve lands. It is further significant to note that Aboriginal laws exist to deal with land and environmental management. Although Indigenous communities and cultures have a diverse range of traditions, many adhere to core principles that value a close relationship with plants, animals, people, spirits, the land, and creation. Indigenous law refers to natural powers and forces that shape human interactions with the more-than-human world (J. Borrows 2002, 2010; LaDuke 1994a, 1994b, 1994c, 1997). This natural, or Indigenous, law has been referred to as "the good life" and "continuous rebirth" (LaDuke 1994c, 128). Despite numerous attempts by the federal government to extinguish Indigenous law, it continues to thrive and coexist with legislative and common law systems (J. Borrows 2002, 2010; Ecojustice 2007b). Finding a way to reconcile these legal systems is mandated by Section 35 of the Constitution Act, 1982.

Moreover, the "duty to consult and accommodate" Aboriginal peoples flows from the Crown's fiduciary duty to seek reconciliation. The other option available to First Nations communities is to pursue litigation themselves in order to ensure the cleanup of spills, which can be difficult given their limited access to resources. As discussed in Chapter 1, citizens of this First Nation were actively pursuing litigation at the time of writing. Such recourse is rare. It assumes that First Nations have the capacity and resources to act against a large corporation and to challenge the government. Since the *policy assemblage* of Indigenous environmental justice remains in limbo, citizens take action themselves.

Whereas physical boundaries are the most visible or evident and may be either demarcated through "natural" means like rivers, lakes, and streams or "built" through means like walls, buildings, and streets, they may also include legal or political arrangements like municipal, provincial, or federal delineations and responsibilities. They also inextricably intersect with identity and belonging. Thus places are defined and differentiated by boundaries, which, like the spaces they demarcate, can be literal, figurative, or metaphorical (Stein 2006). For example, places can be simultaneously literal and figurative, located "downstream" and/or "across the tracks" – both of which are the case in Aamjiwnaang.

Aamjiwnaang First Nation is uniquely situated within Lambton County. Administratively, it falls within the municipal boundaries of the City of Sarnia. According to Sarnia's mayor, Mike Bradley, his is the only city in Ontario that has a Native reserve within its boundaries, thus indicating the importance of a "close working relationship" between the city and Aamjiwnaang (Carruthers 2010). He frequently refers to this unique situation as "one of a kind" in the country, leading to a positive relationship between Indigenous and non-Indigenous Lambton County citizens. How did this "unique" configuration come to be? A turn to the past illuminates the present configurations.[4]

Pre-Confederation Nation Building

Canada's pre-Confederation period was a time of expedited "civilization" and "modernization." The earliest documented explorers included French fur traders and explorers as well as Jesuits (Elford 1982). In 1615 French explorer Samuel de Champlain arrived in Georgian Bay, and waves of explorers and missionaries soon followed his path across the Great Lakes. The seventeenth century encompassed a period of "naming," soon followed by eighteenth-century colonial policies of *terra nullius* and the consequent "claiming" of "empty" space in the name of colonial rule. In 1670 the St. Clair River, which today passes by the Aamjiwnaang First Nation Reserve, was given its name by Father Louis Hennepin. Some of Sarnia's earliest French settlers, preferring British to American rule, came from Michigan after the British surrendered Detroit to the Americans in 1795 (ibid., 141). Several settlers rented land from Indians, which they farmed, exchanging their produce for goods in Detroit.

The eighteenth century witnessed the Seven Years War between France and Britain, by which time the "Chippewas," as they were then known, had established historic ties to France. By 1763, when the Royal Proclamation came into effect, British rule reigned supreme. This period spawned the onset of various treaties, and those who remained loyal to the British were rewarded with land in present-day "Canada." Although treaties were formed, conflict ensued yet again with the War of 1812. In the 1800s the colonial Department of Indian Affairs generically referred to the First Nations communities in Lambton County as "Chippewas," although each group also had a French name. The Walpole Island First Nation was part of the "Chippewas of Chenail Ecarté," the Stony and Kettle Point First Nation was part of the "Chippewas of Rivière Aux Sable," and the Sarnia Reserve was part of the "Chippewas of Rivière St. Clair" (Elford 1982). Alliances shifted with the War of 1812. During this time, "Indians" of the Great Lakes predominantly assisted the British against the Americans, and the British government encouraged their settlement in southwestern Ontario as a form of repayment.

On July 10, 1827, the Treaty of Amherstburg, also known as Treaty 29 or the Huron Tract Purchase, was signed in the Upper Canada Treaties Area. This treaty aimed to set aside lands "reserved" for these Indians. The Ojibwe nation – the Chippewa – ceded land to the Crown with the understanding that it would receive adequate compensation in due course. An area of land named Enniskillen was never formally surrendered and remains the subject of an outstanding land claim to this day.[5] Signed by the Sarnia Band and the British Indian Department, these treaties continue to be a source of consternation today.

Moreover, this period of "civilization" and "modernization" coincided with oil discovery and industrialization. The town of Sarnia soon began to encroach on Chippewa land as offers emerged to acquire land south of current Davis to Clifford Streets. The establishment of a Lands Office gave an Indian Agent the power to sell lots and then reimburse the tribe through the government. By 1857 the "Chippewas" surrendered Stag Island to the Crown. Today, it remains a popular vacation destination among American cottagers. The neighbouring town of Petrolia's discovery of oil in 1848 birthed an oil boom by the 1860s. In this period, one pivotal event led to the reduction and compartmentalization of the Chippewas' territorial base: their separation from Walpole Island. Thereafter, the Department of Indian Affairs referred to the remaining bands of the Huron Tract as the Sarnia Band, with distinct reserves at Sarnia, Kettle Point, and Stony Point.

The discovery and exploitation of oil reserves in Lambton County affected the landscape of the territory and the subsequent formation of the Chippewas' neighbourhood. On March 24, 1871, Dominion Oil purchased twenty-three acres for $4,000 from the reserve government (L.K. Smith and G. Smith 1976). On June 21, 1872, Dominion Oil received these twenty-three acres on the reserve, an area that extends fifty metres along the river south of Indian Creek. Mr. Mackenzie, the Indian Agent, valued this land at $3,345; his superiors later raised the amount to $5,000, and the company's manager said it would have paid $6,000 if pushed (ibid.). On April 5 of that year, the Board of Trade asked the Department of Indian Affairs to sell part of the reserve; on March 7, 1873, new shipyards were proposed on Indian land (ibid.). The mere fact that the reserve has maintained the land base that it holds today is a testament to the perseverance of this Indigenous community in its struggle for survival, although its sustained existence has been continuously under attack due to the acquisitive logic of colonial rule and the colonizer's voracious appetite for capitalist expansion.

From Confederation to Postwar Nation Building

As the Indian Act came into force in 1876, Sarnia Band 45 came into being. Shortly thereafter, both the Kettle and Stony Point First Nations sought separation from the Sarnia Band. During the end of the nineteenth century, the Department of Indian Affairs encouraged reserve subdivisions by mandating that reserve land be comprised of separate lots.[6] These lots were to include "location tickets" for individual families. The goal was to encourage First Nations to adopt an "individualistic lifestyle" and to farm. By "reserving" the bodies of Indigenous people on these marginalized land bases, government policy continued to encourage and foster their sedentary lifestyle, which supported living in one place, farming, and becoming good Christians – that is, becoming "civilized."

Chemical Valley's postwar climate continued to enframe territorial struggles. In 1919 the Dominion Alloy Steel Corporation began to negotiate with band officials for over 900 acres of land, bounded on the east by Scott Road, on the west by Vidal Street, and on the north by Churchill Road all the way to the

Imperial Oil facilities. Dealings culminated in a 1919 surrender of land to the company for the price of $200,000, paving the way for the occupation of this land by Polymer Corporation, Dow Chemical, Imperial Oil, Fibreglass, Cabot Canada, and residential dwellings in the former village of Bluewater. These "negotiations," or "surrenders," made possible the encroachment of heavy industrialization that ensued as part of the "welfare state" that characterized Canada's economy during the First World War.

Canada's war economy impacted the landscape of Chemical Valley by initiating a period of heavy, mass industrialization. As the state enhanced petrochemical and polymer production in the valley, "Indians" who had fought for Canada in the war received the "privilege" of Canadian citizenship and became enfranchised. This also meant giving up any special "Indian" status and the rights that went along with it (Debassige and Pyne 2011, 2). The state's severe grip affected Aamjiwnaang on numerous levels. It was during this time that the City of Sarnia sought to annex the reserve and ensconce it within municipal boundaries.[7]

Controversial land dealings marked the following decades of Chemical Valley's geopolitical becoming. Earmarked for sale, much of Sarnia Band 45's reserve land came into dispute over suspect deals between private investors and the Crown.[8] Demonstrating the separation of authority from the community, lawyer D.B. White of the Sarnia real estate firm D.B. White and Sons Limited handled negotiations and in November 1956 sought backing from New England Industries Limited, which had ties to Wall Street.[9] Dimensional Investments Limited backed a second round of negotiations between band officials and Crown representatives, including a Sarnia law firm acting for D.B. White, while also representing the Sarnia Chippewa Indian Band. It remains unclear the degree to which the First Nations community members themselves had a legitimate voice in these deliberations.

Archival documents from the federal cabinet reveal how negotiations over the sale of reserve land reached Canada's highest seat of executive power. Cabinet decisions in the 1950s demonstrated just how far removed citizens of the Aamjiwnaang First Nation were from these dealings. From deliberations about Interprovincial Pipe Line Company's request for a right-of-way through the reserve in 1953 to high-level discussions about the sale of reserve lands in 1959, this decade reflected the asymmetrical power of the Canadian state, which left a lasting impression on Aamjiwnaang's geopolitical landscape. In particular, leading up to the 1959 land sales, following a series of intensive meetings and talks, the band council gave Crown representatives, acting as the Crown Trust Company of Canada, permission to open negotiations with locatees[10] regarding the purchase of 3,100 acres of reserve land, valued initially at $5.95 million (LAC 1959a).[11] This desirable reserve land represented a "final frontier," as it was the last remaining large portion of land in the rapidly developing downriver industrial area, located alongside Imperial Oil, Polymer, Sun Oil, Canadian Oil, Ethyl Corporation, and a projected site for the DuPont linear polyethylene plant, among others (*Sarnia Observer* 1958). Band members twice rejected offers leading up to the final sale in 1959.

As Cabinet conclusions marked "secret" from March 7, 1959 reveal, the minister of citizenship and immigration recommended the sale of reserve land to Dimensional Investments Ltd. for an increased amount to $6.5 million, after several attempts to negotiate with Sarnia band members (LAC 1959a). Negotiations took place between federal Indian Agent Ward Leroy, acting on behalf of the community, and the Crown Trust Company as it bid to purchase the 3,100 acres. Prior to the 1959 sale, community members had expressed concern about the loss of riverfront land and claimed that the offer was too low. Initially, the band had voted unanimously – by a vote of 68 to 0 – to reject an offer of $5,950,000 for the whole area (LAC 1959a; Lack 1958a, 1958b) (see Figure 4). This deal failed to receive approval from an absolute majority of more than 50 percent of eligible voters; thus the deal was ruled inconclusive, and a request was forwarded to the Honourable Ellen Fairclough, minister of citizenship and immigration, for a second vote (Lack 1958a, 1958b). This second vote of 50 in favour of surrender and 45 against also failed (LAC 1959a). Part of the deal included the construction of a "special Indian village." According to the band solicitor – "Indian lawyer" John McEachran – this was the "last opportunity" for the band to make an offer. Eventually, at a third band meeting a final round of voting took place (ibid.). The price remained the same; however, the initial down payment increased from $750,000 to $1 million (ibid.).

During this third voting period, following a series of heated discussions, the 12:30 a.m. vote, monitored by the Royal Canadian Mounted Police, showed 88 in favour and 37 against the surrender, with 3 spoiled ballots, amounting to 54.6 percent of eligible voters, thus meeting Indian Act requirements (LAC 1959a; Lack 1958a, 1958b). Eighty-four votes in favour were required to make the surrender valid (Lack 1958). Chief Telford Adams was the last to cast his vote. Cabinet documents raise concern about the way in which Crown Trust representatives and Toronto trustees Clark and White handed out $100 to each locatee following the vote (LAC 1959b, 1959c). Cabinet rejected the minister's request for the land sale on March 7, 1959, but approved it by an order-in-council a week later, following an increased land appraisal of $100,000 (LAC 1959a). Cabinet documents conclude: "There was a good deal of agitation in the

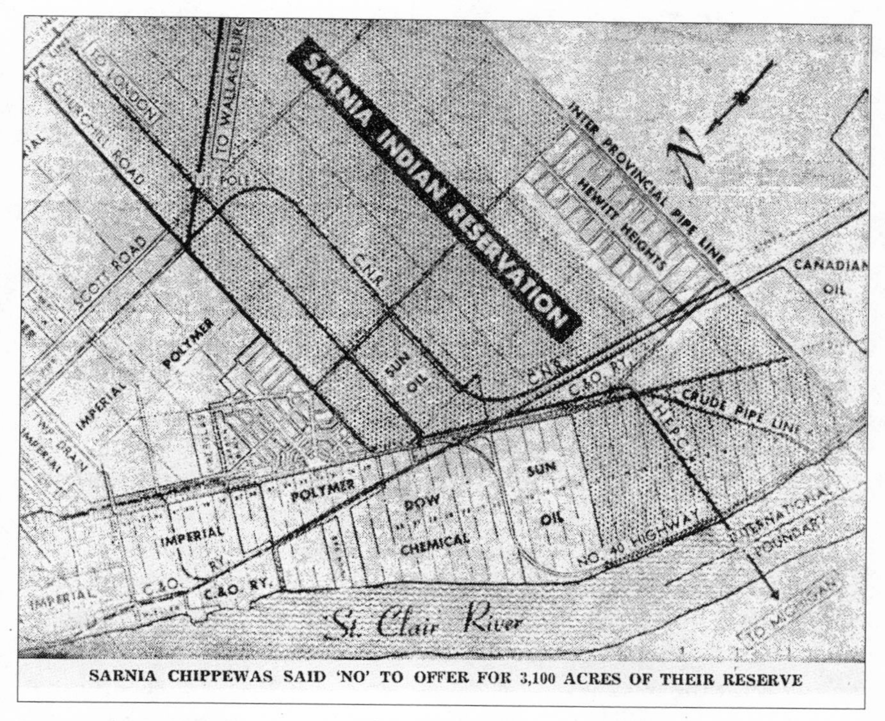

Figure 4 Sarnia Indian Reservation bid, *Sarnia Observer*, 1958

Sarnia district about the sale with a feeling that the Indians were not being fairly treated" (ibid.). A week later, on March 14, 1959, Minister of Citizenship and Immigration Ellen Fairclough recommended the sale (LAC 1959b). Two months later, on May 19, 1959, Cabinet documents noted concerns surfacing in the Ontario election campaign about "bribery" – $100 paid to voting band members – for this land sale (LAC 1959c). These land surrenders remain controversial to this day.[12]

The Cabinet's $6,500,000 deal revealed how state rule was, as now, insepar-able from reserve management, administration, and governance. Initially, the member of Parliament for Sarnia-Lambton West, J.W. Murphy, proudly stated that 3,100 acres of "prime industrial property" would be made available at the price of $6,500,000 (LAC 1959a; Nicholson 1959). In March 1959, touting "long-term development" and the promise of "job-creation," Murphy gleefully added that the Honourable Ellen Fairclough would sign the contract letter right away. Cabinet went into session in the House of Commons East Block at 9:00 a.m. with a day-long agenda ahead. By noon the director of Indian affairs in the Department of Citizenship and Immigration had arrived and summoned the representatives of the principals in the transaction so that they would be on hand to deal with the Cabinet's decision (Nicholson 1959). A second attempt to promote the massive single sale was approved through the negotiations of local agents who had secured the necessary vote of December 20 from the band council and community members for the land surrender.[13] Emerging from this lengthy Cabinet meeting, Prime Minister John Diefenbaker asserted, "The sale of Indian Lands at Sarnia will now go through" (ibid.).[14] Pursuant to the Indian Act, the order-in-council of March 14, 1959, approved the land surrender to Dimensional Investments for $6,500,000 (LAC 1959b). This approval set the stage for spinoff petrochemical industries to enlarge Sarnia's established Chemical Valley.

Several years later, controversy flared up in the House of Commons over the sale of Indian reserve land when Liberal member of Parliament for Toronto Trinity, Paul Hellyer, interrogated the Honourable Ellen Fairclough regarding questionable authority for sale of the land to a company without proof of its financial ability to undertake the transaction.[15] Monies had been held since April 27, 1961, when Fairclough, as minister of immigration and citizenship, had cancelled the agreement between Dimensional Investments and the Indians because the company had failed to meet a deadline for final payment of $4,500,000, despite a thirty-day grace period (*Sarnia Free Press* 1963). Funds held in trust by the federal government finally reached the band in 1963. Chief Adams announced that the Department of Indian Affairs would release partial funds held in trust to approximately 500 band members (ibid.). The band received $1,650,000 of the $2,682,500 paid to the government. According to Chief Adams, as per the Indian Act, these monies were held by the Canadian government, which thought that "Indians would not spend the money wisely" (ibid.). Although Chief Adams lauded the efforts of the member of Parliament for Lambton West, Walter Foy, in getting the monies released, the sale remains an outstanding matter of dispute and raises questions about the inextricable fusion of colonial control and capitalist expansion in Sarnia.

Although formal state-Indigenous relations changed shape in subsequent decades, subtle and informal practices of colonization continued to affect these relationships. Law and policy pertaining to Indigenous citizenship and enfranchisement reconfigured Canada's geopolitical landscape across the country, resulting in local impacts for Aamjiwnaang and its citizens. Dissatisfied with these configurations, citizens increasingly began to mobilize and take action in order to defend their land, culture, and heritage.

Social Mobilization: Canada's Changing Geopolitical Landscape

At the time that the initial industrial negotiations took place, prior to Indian Act amendments in 1951, Indians were not permitted to have their own lawyers (RCAP 1996; UBC 2015). The 1960s marked a turning point with respect to Canada's treatment of Indigenous citizens. It was only in 1960 that Canada's "Indians" received the right to vote. Changes to the Indian Act began to take shape in public discourse and consciousness. Shortly thereafter, a series of social policy movements, actions, and (non)decisions emerged. Inspired by Rachel Carson's book *Silent Spring*, a mainstream environmental movement began to form in Canada and the United States. Moreover, in 1966 the neighbouring industrial community of Bluewater, originally located within the heart of Chemical Valley, was relocated for "health and safety concerns" – as indicated on a present-day plaque marking the site. This period corresponded with expansion of the Lambton Industrial Society and bore witness to an increase in the number of its member companies from three to fourteen, culminating in its status as a nonprofit corporation in 1967.

Strained relations between the City of Sarnia and Aamjiwnaang distinguish this period of social change. Under the leadership of Fred Plain, a "special" joint meeting between the band council and the City of Sarnia was held, where Plain voiced concern that the municipal annexation of the reserve's land had happened without the community's knowledge, making its members unwilling residents of the city's municipal boundaries overnight. Shortly thereafter, the city began a comprehensive study of how to seize the reserve roads. The threatening promise of industrial "development" lurked at the reserve's perimeter. Notably, advice provided to the band council in November 1965 by the planning firm Acres Research and Planning Limited indicated that the economic "potential" of the Sarnia Reserve was dependent on the present and future growth of the petrochemical industry and related services. The report stated, "This location has seen rapid development of a major petrochemical complex since the end of the Second World War; there are eleven major oil, gas and chemical industries in the area" (Acres Research and Planning Ltd. 1965, 6). The report went on, "Regarding "present land use': except for a few small garden plots and orchards, the land is not used in a productive capacity. It is used as residential land for the homes of the Band members. Even this utilizes only a portion of the total acreage" (ibid., 7). The 1965 report to the Chippewas of the Sarnia Band explained why this place was so desirable for industrial development:

(i) The gas and oil pipelines from Canada's western oil fields pass through the United States south of Lake Superior and cross back into Canada at this point
(ii) The St. Clair River provides process and cooling water of the desired quality and temperature in large quantities
(iii) Economical transportation by water is provided by the St. Lawrence Seaway system using the St. Clair River
(iv) Industries are dependent one upon the other for sources of materials so that a complex of industries creates an attraction for other industries of the same type
(v) Sarnia is close enough to serve the major Canadian market lying around Toronto and is also favourably located to the US market for certain products used in agricultural production
(vi) The salt beds lying between 1,500 and 2,700 feet below the surface represent the greatest depth of salt deposition in Southern Ontario and are a source of chemicals for the industry. Caverns hollowed out in the beds provide economical storage for liquids and gasses. (Ibid., 5–6)

It further highlighted the "special *nature* of reserve lands." The unique features accounting for this "special nature" included its political status in the Canadian Confederation, policy arrangements, and scenic qualities. These "special" relations preceded Confederation; as per the 1763 Royal Proclamation, only the British Crown was empowered to negotiate with Indians for land settlement. In 1827 the Crown and Chippewa bands signed the first treaty to set aside a 6,160-acre reserve. The report noted that "reserve land is set apart for the use and benefit of a Band," that the majority of "Band electors" must agree to releasing any part of the reserve for use by a non-Indian, and that all "dealings must be done with Crown sanction, which must accept final responsibility for the equity of the deal" (ibid., 9, emphasis added).

Moreover, the report noted the unique properties of the reserve's "natural parkland," specifically advising that this natural area should remain located along Talfourd Creek to keep it "open as a drainage way" that could serve as a buffer approximately 120 metres wide and that no building should be erected within 60 metres of the line between industrial and residential uses (Acres Research and Planning Ltd. 1965, 26). These points reveal competing views of land use: on the one hand, the land is to be a source of "development," and on the other hand, it is to be a collective resource for the entire band's use. These points particularly pertain to land transactions, as reserve lands are not available on the "open market" without prior review under the auspices of the Indian Act.

The following decade continued to reveal the persistence of industrial advancement on reserve land. In 1977 the *Sarnia Observer* reported that Polysar sought a right-of-way from the adjacent "Indians" to run an overhead pipe bridge across the reserve (*Sarnia Observer* 1977). This strip, 20 metres wide, crossed Tashmoo Avenue, extending onto land "owned" by the Department of Indian Affairs, not the City of Sarnia. Under the leadership of Chief Ray Rogers, the First Nation citizens and Polysar representatives remained at an impasse. Shortly thereafter, another parcel of land to the west of Tashmoo Avenue and north of LaSalle Line came into dispute.

Past policies regarding Indian enfranchisement have led to the formation of territorial donut holes on First Nation reserves. One contested tract came before the Ontario Supreme Court in a case involving citizens of Aamjiwnaang and Shell Canada Limited. This case, regarding 200 acres of land west of Tashmoo and north of LaSalle, had resulted from an appeal of a past decision by the Ministry of Indian and Northern Affairs, which did not support the band's claim and would not front any costs for the band's legal battle (Pattenaude 1978). Industrial development officer Wilson Plain questioned the title of the land, which had been transformed into private property during the 1920s when band members Francis Wilson Jacobs, a former chief, and his son Henry Wilson Jacobs had become enfranchised – that is, "citizens" and thus no longer "Indians" – so that they could buy property allocated to them by the band. These men took out mortgages and then bought the land from the band at $8 an acre, for a total of $1,600 (ibid.). Plain questioned their title to the property, as a government proclamation was never issued before the land was mortgaged, thus leading to the question of whether they truly "owned" the land subsequent to enfranchisement.

According to Plain's claim, the non-issuance of a proclamation had been an oversight, thus rendering land transactions after 1926 illegal. The contention here centres on the fact that clear title to the land was never certified. Plain sent the minister of Indian and northern affairs, Hugh Faulkner, a letter noting this concern. The ministry responded, "In our opinion, Henry and Francis Jacobs held the land in fee simple and were under no special restrictions regarding its use or disposal" (Pattenaude 1978). In 1931 Sarnia had begun taxing the land when the Lambton Loan and Investment Company had foreclosed under the power of sale after holding the mortgage for five years. A public auction for the land soon followed. Priced at fifty dollars an acre, the land drew no offers, nor did the band, unaware the land was "theirs," place a bid or claim it outright (ibid.). Lambton Loan and Investment held the property under power of sale until 1944, when it was purchased for $8,000 by Russell Hewitt of Sarnia, who intended to develop the land for residential use. This land, valued at approximately $1 million, was annexed by the City of Sarnia in 1951. Shell Canada, located south of the disputed property, was eagerly waiting to purchase the tract of farmland for future expansion, prompting a legal battle.[16]

The fall of 1978 continued to witness struggles between the band, corporations, and government officials. Yet again industrial development officer Wilson Plain argued that the Ministry of Indian Affairs had failed to adhere to its responsibilities for reserve land and citizens. He argued that the ministry had given land to Imperial Oil in 1947, contravening federal statutes at the time (Stevenson 1978). The disputed land, which comprised five acres at the south end of Christina Street off of Clifford Street, within the boundaries of Imperial Oil, had been sold without band consultation. Plain argued that this sale was contrary to Section 51 of the Indian Act, which stated that "no release or surrender of a reserve or portion of a reserve shall be valid or binding unless assented to by a majority of the electors" (ibid.).[17] According to Plain's claim, the Department of Indian Affairs had acted negligently. The band was not entitled to independent legal representation at the time of the land sale, which occurred prior to the reversal of this stipulation by the Indian Act amendments of 1951. Consequently, concerns over the federal government's breach of "trust" loomed large.

Conclusion

Situated in one of the densest petrochemical and manufacturing complexes in Canada, the Aamjiwnaang reserve's social and geopolitical location is embroiled within a jurisdictional assemblage. As this chapter has discussed, local, national, and international developers continued to set their sights on this territory, culminating in the aforementioned attempts to "dispose" of the reserve by New England Industries and Dimensional Investments. A geopolitical orientation moves us beyond conventional interpretations of state boundaries, authority, and rule to reveal the inner workings of power relations in particular locales. At the same time, state power is inherently connected to the social, political, and economic formation of such sites. Aamjiwnaang's ongoing and jurisdictional concerns often take place in a regulatory gap pertaining to responsibility for environmental health catastrophes in large part due to Canada's constitutional division of powers. Although there appears to be a lack of authority, responsibility, and direction for the policy field of Indigenous environmental justice in Canada, the state's shadow lingers.

6

Seeking Reproductive Justice
Situated Bodies of Knowledge

The impact of pollution on the reproductive body in Aamjiwnaang makes it a focal point in the struggle for justice within Lambton County. In addition to locating the community's disproportionate burden of toxic exposure, reproductive justice entails a consideration of the multifaceted ways that contamination affects this community's ability to reproduce future generations. Discussing reproductive justice, the US grassroots organization SisterSong (2013) states, "The right to have children, not have children, and to parent the children we have in safe and healthy environments is based on the human right to make personal decisions about one's life, and the obligation of government and society to ensure that the conditions are suitable for implementing one's decisions." Moreover, as noted by Hoover and colleagues (2012), the politics of reproduction uniquely affect Indigenous communities; thus an *environmental reproductive justice* framework must support policies to ensure that a community's reproductive capabilities are not inhibited by environmental contamination, which compromises a community's ability to reproduce cultural knowledge. In this way, reproductive justice fuses health and environment policy, coupled with a need to protect culture and knowledge. A reproductive justice framework for policy analysis acknowledges that individuals must have the right and ability to reproduce in culturally appropriate ways: "For many Indigenous communities to reproduce culturally informed citizens requires a clean environment" (ibid., 1648). Examining both structural and discursive dimensions of public policy affecting citizens of the Aamjiwnaang First Nation requires an assessment of the politicization of reproductive health knowledge involved in shaping and constraining struggles for recognition within a deliberative public health process, the Lambton Community Health Study.

Fleshing Out Reproductive Environmental Justice

Experiential concerns propel citizen claims for environmental reproductive injustice in Aamjiwnaang. In this way, bodies act as knowledge generators. As an embodied or corporeal "body of knowledge," experiential knowledge challenges the notion of the epistemic neutrality of biomedical expertise (Orsini and Smith 2010, 53). Examining the body in this way enables new categories of meaning and discourse about situated and lived experience to come to the fore. Moreover, bodies constitute "messy data" with which to advance claims and articulate injury (Epstein 1996). Bodily experience forms the foundation from which citizens declare they have been harmed. Lived or felt experience thus constitutes the "expertise," or grounds, upon which corporeal claims are both consciously and unconsciously enacted and articulated by citizens seeking policy change. As previously discussed, examples of this include biomonitoring, body-mapping, and bucket brigades. Through these techniques, communities are called to take action themselves, with their bodies on the line, in order to gather knowledge about pollution exposures affecting their everyday life. Expressions of these techniques may range from protests to the production of rap music. Such expressions simultaneously generate knowledge and move people both to take action and to speak out about ongoing injustices.

In response to continued concerns about the Aamjiwnaang First Nation's ability to reproduce, a team of researchers used a community-based participatory research model to assess the sex ratio for live births on the Aamjiwnaang reserve (see Appendix 1). This assessment emerged out of a broader community-based investigation undertaken by citizens of the Aamjiwnaang First Nation in collaboration with the Occupational Health Clinic for Ontario Workers – Sarnia (OHCOW), as well as with scientific consultants, professionals, and students from a wide range of disciplines (Mackenzie, Lockridge, and Keith 2005).[1] The exploration encompassed quantitative measurements, including soil, sediment, wildlife, fish, and air sampling, along with a door-to-door health survey and interviews. It also included body-mapping exercises.

As Chapter 4 depicted, subsequent to gathering health data, community members hung body maps on the walls of a gymnasium and placed coloured stickers on the maps to indicate and visualize ailments experienced in the community. Body-mapping of 411 individuals between 2004 and 2005 revealed that

26 percent of adults experienced high blood pressure, 26 percent of adults and 9 percent of children experienced chronic headaches, 23 percent of children aged five to sixteen had learning and behavioural problems, 27 percent of children experienced skin rashes, and 39 percent of women had experienced a miscarriage or stillbirth (Ecojustice 2007a; Scott 2008). Statistics collected by Aamjiwnaang band member and community activist Ada Lockridge and her team indicated that one in four Aamjiwnaang children had a behavioural or learning disability and that four in ten women on the reserve had had at least one miscarriage or stillbirth (Ecojustice 2007a). Results further indicated that 40 percent of band members required an inhaler and that about 17 percent percent of adults and 22 percent of children had asthma (nearly three times the national rate). In comparison, the Lambton County asthma rate sits at approximately 8.2 percent (ibid.). Results from the community health survey were published in the Ecojustice report *Exposing Canada's Chemical Valley* (2007). They were not published elsewhere.

The esteemed journal *Environmental Health Perspectives (EHP)* published Aamjiwnaang's controversial sex ratio data in 2005 (Mackenzie, Lockridge, and Keith 2005). For the study period 1984–2003, the number of live births, and their sex, was determined using the data on births that had been self-reported by band members to the Department of Indian and Northern Affairs, now Aboriginal Affairs and Northern Development Canada. Between 1984 and 1992, findings revealed a relatively stable birth ratio, whereas the period between 1993 and 2003 showed a rapid decline in the percentage of live male births (ibid.).[2] Linear regression as a research methodology was deployed to examine the trend in the proportion of live male births over time. This method drew from data sets of statistical units, with the goal of being potentially "predictive" or "forecasting."[3] Although the study's findings remained contentious, they spawned widespread media attention.

The "birth dearth" findings began to make waves. Leading up to and following the *EHP* publication, news headlines about living in a place "Where the boys aren't" put this small community under the media's microscope (De Guerre 2008; Mittelstaedt 2004, 2005). News stories claimed that males were an "endangered species" and that it would perhaps be only a matter of time before what was happening in Aamjiwnaang happened in other communities across the world (Mittelstaedt 2004, 2005). A 2009 feature in *Men's Health* magazine expressed fear about this community's "lost boys" (Petersen 2009). Although these stories lamented the loss of male babies, stories pertaining to the lived experiences of difficult pregnancies and births among community members continue to be invisible.

Scientists and members of the Aamjiwnaang community contend that hormone-mimicking pollutants known as endocrine disruptors could be to blame for the skewed birth patterns, due to the interference of synthetic organic chemicals with natural hormones. According to the Canadian Broadcasting Corporation's documentary *The Disappearing Male*, written and directed by Marc De Guerre (2008), these endocrine disruptors can interfere with hormones that determine the sex of a baby. Consequently, many individuals living in Aamjiwnaang are concerned not only about each birth but also about the future viability of their community.

Moreover, the maternal body in this scenario is deemed particularly vulnerable to toxins as a carrier for the community's children. Toxins are generally stored in fat. During pregnancy and lactation, women's fat is metabolized and exposes fetuses and newborns at vulnerable stages of development to these chemicals (A. Smith 2005). Toxic endocrine disruptors mimic natural hormone production, disrupting reproduction and fetal development. The ways that the maternal body is hailed in the media as "vulnerable to environmental contaminants" reveals some of the gendered dimensions of reproductive health. Popular and media reports suggest that the maternal body is especially susceptible to these hormone-mimicking, endocrine-disrupting chemicals, nicknamed "gender-benders," which infiltrate the body and affect the reproduction of future generations (De Guerre 2008; Scott 2009). Despite all the media that concentrated on the "lost boys," a gendered analysis of the Indigenous body was missing from the analysis. Indigenous perspectives of gender must also be taken into consideration when looking at discourse around the Aamjiwnaang First Nation's reproductive health.[4] Expectant mothers are commonly hailed as the first line of defence against toxins in the environment, which have the potential to harm future generations. Consequently, the maternal – reproductive – body is constructed as a "site of contamination" in material and discursive ways (Scott 2009). Women have become gatekeepers, demarcating the boundary between some "environment out there" and some "body inside."

Bodies at this juncture are made "vulnerable," affected physically by pollution exposures, in addition to gendered framing. "Vulnerability" discourse shifts the burden of responsibility for managing health toward pregnant mothers, who are assumed to be individually responsible for their well-being. This approach is based on an incomplete picture of the broader discursive and structural factors that shape and constrain access to reproductive health and justice. Words and seemingly inclusive and deliberative processes alike have the potential to reproduce colonial power relations by the act of discrediting or delegitimizing bodily claims.[5]

Although the human health effects of environmental contamination due to toxins in the environment are largely unknown, scientists investigating local wildlife populations in the Great Lakes have documented the problem of "gender-bending" chemicals, which are the result of an unknown mixture of toxic chemicals in the air, soil, and water (Kavanagh et al. 2004; Weisskopf et al. 2003).[6] Scientists use sex ratio as a sharp indicator of exposure to chemicals disrupting the endocrine system and reproductive health.[7] According to Marc Weisskopf (Weisskopf et al. 2003), a research associate at the Harvard School of Public Health, there are a lot of unknowns. In Lake St. Clair, about 50 kilometres from the Aamjiwnaang Reserve, fish have been discovered with both male and female gonads. The condition, known as intersex,[8] is caused when a young fish that is genetically male is exposed to chemicals such as atrazine, a herbicide found in some fertilizers, which causes female gonads to develop by acting like the hormone estrogen (Kavanagh et al. 2004; Weisskopf et al. 2003). Research has also identified increased reproductive abnormalities for women who consume the fish. Weisskopf's findings suggest that maternal exposure to polychlorinated biphenyls may alter the sex ratio of offspring (Mackenzie, Lockridge, and Keith 2005). The phenomenon has been documented all over the southern Great Lakes, not just in fish but in birds and amphibians as well (ibid.). Whereas the science has revealed the impact of toxins on wildlife, the human impacts remain unknown. Aamjiwnaang citizens live with such unknowns daily.

Following the *EHP*'s publication of the birth ratio study, civil servants scrambled to grasp the ever-growing concern about the "girl baby boom" in Canada's Chemical Valley (Miner 2005; Mittelstaedt 2005; Poirier 2005a; Spears 2005). Health Canada correspondence from the time shows that questions about this community led to confusion within the ranks of government. Federal officials scrambled to find out who was in charge.[9] The data, composition, and methodology of the study itself remained matters of continued debate, and the study's credibility was criticized inside and outside the community.

Shortly after publication of the *EHP* study, local politicians met with Health Canada representatives at Lambton County headquarters in Wyoming, Ontario, at the request of the voluntary, industry-led Sarnia-Lambton Environmental Association to discuss the formation of a community-based health study that would focus on the county as a whole. Following a July 2006 request from the Office of the Lambton County Warden, Health Canada pledged support, subject to the provision of local leadership.[10] At the same time, the Lambton County Health Unit produced its own reproductive health report. That report's findings concluded that sex ratios in Lambton County did not differ from Ontario rates

(LCHS 2007). The health unit considered the small number of births recorded on the reserve during the same time frame to be unrepresentative and too small to determine conclusively whether there were any abnormal health harms and patterns. Aaamjiwnaang's data were thus considered statistically insignificant due to the overall low number of reported births. Health Canada soon began discussions with municipal authorities, industry, and county representatives, widening the scope and scale of reproductive health concerns away from Aamjiwnaang to generate a broader data pool. Shortly thereafter, the Lambton Community Health Study, a participatory project that included intensive civic engagement, came into being.

Encountering Expert Knowledge: The Lambton Community Health Study

Deliberative health studies are not neutral. They actively (re)produce discursive regimes, which shape and constrain citizen action. There is a wide and vast literature discussing the "deliberative turn" and the promise of the public arena for reasonable communication, interaction, and governance (Dryzek 2000; Fischer 2003, 2007, 2009; Fischer and Forester 1993; Fischer and Hajer 1999). As Hobson (2013, 64) suggests, these processes continue to be "embroiled" within governmentality as an advanced liberal form of rule and rely on responsibilized citizen action with limited state intervention. Institutional processes like the Lambton Community Health Study (LCHS) are mechanisms that reproduce discourses and knowledges, which some actors may appropriate and internalize in their mobilization for justice through formal and informal avenues.

In 2008 the LCHS established its board membership and mandate to examine the relationship between industrial activity and human health. The study drew funds from the Province of Ontario and the Sarnia-Lambton Environmental Association, as well as the Chamber of Commerce. The federal government pledged in-kind support. The board's formalization comprised a diverse group of stakeholders, including municipalities, First Nations, business, labour, industry, occupational health representatives, victims of occupational illness, and county public health officials (LCHS 2011). The board determined that the health study would contain three distinct phases: phase 1 would involve establishing a community-based governance structure and identifying a board of directors to oversee the project; phase 2 would include a comprehensive literature review, community engagement (i.e., a phone and online survey as well as townhall meetings), the development of research questions, and a call for study proposals; and phase 3 would be for the undertaking of identified studies, the communication of results to Lambton County residents, and the identification of next steps (ibid.). Phases 1 and 2 were completed early in 2011, yet at the time of writing, phase 3 – actually carrying out a systematic and scientific health study – remained subject to funding.[11] From the beginning, many questions emerged about whether the LCHS process adequately represented the Aamjiwnaang First Nation's unique reproductive health concerns.

Health policy development takes place within the rubric of government decisions or nondecisions. Thus encounters with the healthcare system operate in politically charged environments. By examining the meanings embedded within health policy discourse – namely the spoken and unspoken language of various documents, terms of reference, and media statements, among others – we glimpse how social power and disparities are produced, contested, and resisted in a particular domain. An interpretive analysis of such text, language, and communication calls underlying assumptions into question. When citizens are brought "into" a conversation about health and, in this case, about the recognition of reproductive health concerns, a paradox of engagement becomes apparent: citizens are expected to adopt the terms of dialogue or debate, which may not necessarily provide a context for empowerment and the recognition of particular claims. In this situation, the claims of citizens participating in the health study's deliberative process have become marginalized. How this outcome has occurred is highlighted by focusing on four distinct yet interrelated discursive fields: *science, scale, lifestyle blame,* and *jurisdictional ambiguity* (see Table 2).

Science

Canada's public health regime places a high degree of importance on large-scale, population-based epidemiological knowledge. "Truths" in this model often assume the neutrality of science. As Orsini and Smith (2010, 47) observe, privileging scientific knowledge and expertise as resources external to the mobilization of actors separates knowledge from the lived experiences of those mobilizing for change. As a result, knowledge becomes an instrumentalized object. Expertise as such functions as a resource external to the movement. Actors become parcelled off from scientific knowledge and expertise, which are more readily accessed by state authorities. Consequently, the state has resources to reaffirm existing policies and assumptions. "External expertise" thus forms a hierarchical triangle, with "scientific" authority disseminating knowledge from the top to the citizenry below as they vie for recognition and justice.

Communities have a complicated relationship with experts – governments, scientists, and academics. These authority figures constitute a kind of "necessary evil" to be engaged with as communities seek redress. Several community

Table 2
Encountering knowledge

Theme	Pseudonym	Role	Interview location
Science	Daniel	Policy official	Ottawa
	Edward	Policy official	Aamjiwnaang
	Gerry	Policy official	Toronto
Scale	Claire	Policy official	Sarnia
	Daniel	Policy official	Ottawa
	Dawn	Policy official	Sarnia
	Elliott	Policy official	Sarnia
	Glen	Policy official	Sarnia
	Kier	Policy official	Sarnia
Lifestyle blame	Billy	Community member	Aamjiwnaang
	Dawn	Policy official	Sarnia
	Elliott	Policy official	Sarnia
	Glen	Policy official	Sarnia
	Heidi	Community member	Aamjiwnaang
	John	Policy official	Sarnia
	Lloyd	Policy official	Sarnia
	Mike	Community member	Aamjiwnaang
	Ned	Community member	Aamjiwnaang
	Sally	Community member	Sarnia
	Tina	Policy official	Aamjiwnaang
Jurisdictional ambiguity	Claire	Policy official	Sarnia
	Cora	Policy official	Sarnia
	Ethan	Policy official	Sarnia
	Glen	Policy official	Sarnia
	Henry	Policy official	Sarnia
	Kier	Policy official	Sarnia
	Lloyd	Policy official	Sarnia
	Oliver	Policy official	Sarnia
	Tina	Policy official	Aamjiwnaang
	Steve	Policy official	Sarnia

members contended that governments bear the responsibility for tightening up laws and policies to create healthier peoples and environments in Aamjiwnaang: "The best thing you can do is get the government to tighten up their regulations to make it more stringent" (Edward). Health Canada, which maintains a fiduciary responsibility for First Nations health, has approached Aamjiwnaang on several occasions to offer guidance and to help the community better understand the relationship between their health and environment.

Public health processes reveal contested divisions between scientific and community-based knowledges. According to one public official, scientists are frequently asked by communities to confirm data: "the scientists say, 'Here is the data,'" and the resulting difficulty is that sometimes the data does not confirm or deny specific health concerns (Daniel). Consequently, tensions come to the fore between knowledge carriers. As is the case in both Aamjiwnaang and Lambton County, "access to specialized expertise free of charge to help communities develop proposals has been difficult" (Daniel). In an attempt to correct, or plug, this gap, Health Canada has developed the First Nations Environment Health Innovation Network to provide access to researchers from affected communities.

Tensions between on-the-ground experts and "fly-in" expertise have deep historical roots in past practices where academics would appear in communities and tell Indigenous people what to do. As a result, scientific research carries an unsettling legacy. According to one federal official's observations, there exists a legacy of skepticism on both sides between "scientific" and "traditional" knowledges; thus today there remain philosophical differences "between community-based ontology and scientific method" (Daniel). This was most clearly illuminated by the controversy surrounding the publication of the *EHP* birth ratio study.

If a community voices concern with the reproductive health and biological makeup of its citizens, there is a policy protocol in place to generate scientific findings. From one official's perspective,

> The study was offered to the community. The director of this division at that time asked me to go to the community and meet with the chief and council and do a biomonitoring study, so we actually look at the levels of contaminants in human tissues, blood, and hair, and examine the birth ratio for every year in relation to that, as well as examine the birth outcomes. (Daniel)

The community considered this proposal in 2004 and refused it. This was one year prior to the publication of the *EHP* study. The self-reported administrative data indicated a gender imbalance. However, the data did not account for where people lived, which to the federal government was the minimum requirement for assessing health impacts. "You have to link exposure in the particular geographic location" to be able to look at particular outcomes (Daniel). Health Canada began to conduct a follow-up assessment of community exposure; yet it never received support from the chief and council, "so that was it" (Daniel).

The proposed assessment would have comprised a Public Health Surveillance Project to address public health concerns at a particular emergent data point. Such refusals have left officials perplexed:

> Fundamentally, research well done decreases the amount of political power that can be applied. Until you have research, then the decisions are value-based; you can claim whatever you want. When you have the research, then the knowledge you have limits your ability to achieve results. When you have resistance to research, sometimes it is because of the power of knowledge. In this particular case, it may not be convenient, but that is speculation. (Daniel)

Reasons for the study's rejection stemmed from community concerns about control over the process. Why a revised study with amended community-based protocols in place has not emerged remains an issue for future discussion.

Generating credible data continues be a central issue for citizens of Aamjiwnaang and Lambton County. As a county official noted, "Any epidemiological study, it's about 95 percent argument about methodology and 5 percent about the results" (Glen). The Lambton County Health Unit is responsible for public health. In this capacity, staff conduct risk factor surveillance and gather health statistics and health data through national and regional surveys to conduct reporting and evaluation. Staff with expertise in epidemiological studies collect and analyze public health data for chronic and infectious disease, in addition to conducting programs aimed at health surveillance and health promotion.

The work of the LCHS falls upon overburdened county staff. As a local policy maker noted, there was an expectation early on that "expertise" would be led by external authorities, not by county staff. During the board's development, skilled facilitators came forward to construct a model based on a Sudbury health study, yet there were considerable differences between the two places: whereas "Sudbury was funded by industry on the direct order of the Ministry of Environment, we don't have such a situation here" (Glen). The Ministry of Environment does not have an active role in the LCHS but attends board meetings as an observer. As a result, "there's certainly been no great enthusiasm to fund this since then." Moreover, as this official continued, "Frankly, I have tried to be careful not to involve our resources – I mean public health resources – in this study. I wanted it to be an independent study" (Glen). Thus the county maintains a concern that its resources are limited in the face of competing priorities. The LCHS has the potential to be an overwhelming project beyond the staff's capacity.

Scale

County programs are based on "evidence" and seek to ensure the effectiveness of service delivery. The LCHS falls within the research responsibilities of the public health unit's staff, and "environmental health" has increasingly been at the "forefront of the types of research that we want to do around here" (Dawn). Following the release of the birth ratio study in Aamjiwnaang, the Lambton County Health Unit determined the need to hire an environmental health specialist. One of the first projects this specialist led included an examination of the available data on reproductive health countywide to move beyond the small-area geographical analysis (LCHS 2007). The county health unit monitors data related to population health statistics to the best of its abilities by drawing on available data sources. These "data sources" for the Aboriginal study, according to one official view, were "questionable" because "we couldn't replicate" the findings (Glen). Lambton County's study did not show the same statistics countywide as were apparent in Aamjiwnaang.

The scope and scale of this study are relevant. Results of the birth ratio study were disputed within Aamjiwnaang, Lambton County, and the federal government. A public official cautioned, "Read the *EHP* article very carefully. StatsCan did an internal analysis on the basis of postal code. They haven't seen the same picture that was shown in the article" (Daniel). Clearly, the data are contested. "The specific dataset – the best we could figure out – the dataset was an administrative dataset of children who were born to band members. However, this includes those people who live in Aamjiwnaang as well as those who don't. In fact, for those who don't, we don't necessarily have information on where they live" (Daniel). Consequently, nothing according to this official could be definitive or conclusive. The results were merely speculative. Board members noted that to achieve the goal of obtaining substantive government support for a health study of this scope, having reliable and scientifically sound data was important. One local policy maker maintained the position that the health unit would not fund a geocode (as opposed to postal code) study to delve further into Aamjiwnaang's reproductive, respiratory, and cancer-related concerns because, in terms of epidemiology, the sample size would be too small. In consolation, he noted that they would be welcome to attend educational events (Glen). The epidemiological model itself, hailing the importance of large-size samples to the creation of generalizable results, discredits localized communities with smaller-scale concerns.

According to another board member, a good health study would need to be "meaningful, scientifically valid, and [be] accepted by the public" (Elliott). Epidemiological expertise is considered to be a crucial component of the board's work. As one local policy official noted, "We just wanted to make sure that this wasn't a problem on a wider scale that we should be doing something about" (Dawn). Answering the question of whether there exists a skewed birth ratio in Aamjiwnaang requires considering many variables from an epidemiological perspective: "It's one of those things we'll continue to track. It's unfortunate that it always falls back on data ... Is it really an issue? With a small population ... was it an anomaly?" (Dawn). The issue of sample size, in addition to "lifestyle factors" like smoking, diet, and drinking, colours the findings by limiting the scope of Aamjiwnaang's health concerns. With a measure of sex ratio, the larger the sample, the more stable the findings. Although the Ontario and Lambton birth rates remain relatively constant, fear of the "unknown" too remains constant with respect to Aamjiwnaang's unique reproductive health concerns.

Population size reappears as a statistical caveat for situated concern. Regarding the data, some board members brushed off the existing statistics: "When you look at the data, we aren't far off other populations." This board member further noted that rather than focusing on small data, "you have to look at a broader scale" (Claire). This requirement raises significant questions about small-scale population data generated by communities like Aamjiwnaang. Although Aamjiwnaang's population may be too small to produce statistically sound results, its geographic location is a recurring theme within the board's deliberations. Noting that "some pockets of the community are more concerned" about their health, one board member said, "Obviously, the closer you live to it [Chemical Valley] the more concern there is." He continued, "That's a concern that I don't hear from anyone else ... That study was reviewed by people from McMaster, and they said the sample size is far too small to make any conclusions, but if you look at Lambton County as a whole, you don't get those numbers." Consequently, he concluded, there is "too small of a sample size to really make concrete assumptions or whatever, findings" (Kier). Regarding cancer, cardiovascular illness, and respiratory concerns, there is some consensus that these issues have raised alarm bells across the county.

Official responses to the birth ratio study suggested a need for more "reliable data," while noting that "Aamjiwnaang is concerned" and that although there might be a need to look at "smaller areas within the community," major differences were not prevalent at present across the county (Claire). With respect to the unique health concerns in Aamjiwnaang, the community's sample size renders the local population vulnerable to being eclipsed by large-scale studies. As stated by an LCHS board member, "The problem I have with the First Nations is the population, the N factor, the sample size, is not big enough" (Elliott). It seems that under this paradigm, such a small population cannot generate credible statistical results.

Board officials outlined the need for larger sample sizes in order to make generalizable findings. The official response maintained that everyone needs to be included, "not just a specific little population" (Claire). This requires broader citizen engagement. Although citizens were able to voice their concerns during five town hall meetings in the fall of 2010, one of which took place on the reserve at Aamjiwnaang's health centre, the need for a countywide, large-scale study continued to carry weight in the board's deliberations regarding how to generate valid data and concrete results. To correct the disputed data, as well as the contested biomarkers coming out of Aamjiwnaang, one official noted the importance of longitudinal studies like the Ontario Health Study, which would "encourage as many citizens to participate as possible" and provide more information about citizens and their health (Claire). This voluntary Ontario-wide study generates data based on a much larger population base, drawing on standard epidemiological scientific principles.

The doubt over credibility of Aamjiwnaang's 2005 birth ratio study continues to linger and silently informs the board's deliberations. Moreover, concern with the "image" of Sarnia as a negative place – due to the legacy of asbestos exposure, mesothelioma, and a reputation as Canada's "cancer capital" – continuously prompts board officials to rebrand Lambton County as a desirable, healthy, and flourishing place to work and live. Striking the balance between citizens' health and economic prosperity is a constant juggling act in Lambton County, and tension between these poles plays out within the LCHS board structure. Considered to be the "lifeblood of the community," the chemical refineries are needed to sustain a healthy economy (Glen). Thus a significant factor motivating the board to complete the study is a desire to "clear the air" in order to reverse Sarnia's negative public image, stemming largely from media coverage regarding mesothelioma in Sarnia and a skewed birth ratio in Aamjiwnaang.

Several questioned whether the birth ratio is a "community concern or more of an Aamjiwnaang concern" (Elliott). The contested data appeared in a 2008 *Chatelaine* issue, which noted even the chief's acknowledgment that much of the population resides off the reserve, thus making data difficult to track (Giese 2008). The same article illuminated the frequency with which individuals assume responsibility for environmental health in order to hold their industrial neighbours to account.

By the end of 2011, the board had gathered data from the town hall meetings and from online and phone surveys and was unsure of where to turn next –

hence the potential partnership with the Ontario Health Study or possibly Cancer Care Ontario. This led to calls for external expertise: "I don't have my expertise in these types of studies. We need a team that says to the board, 'Here are your options,' and helps the board move forward" (Dawn). In fact, county officials noted that further work on the study would be beyond the scope of their capacity: "Now it's up to higher levels of government to provide higher levels of expertise" (John). The quality of expertise is presumed to be located at a different level or scale of government, external to the board and Aamjiwnaang.

Lifestyle Blame

In 2004 Health Canada approached the Aamjiwnaang Health and Environment Committee to conduct a biomonitoring study, but the community declined. Individuals perceived the model of the study to be overly technocratic and top-down, wherein government researchers would maintain authority over the process, conduct random body sampling, and provide the overall direction of the project. From the perspective of members sitting on the committee, the individuals who approached them were not sensitive to on-the-ground concerns: "You can't just randomly ask people, 'Oh, we need your blood and urine,' and if they said 'no,' they would assume there was no interest ... We had done a fish and wildlife study. You need the fats and organs to test properly for chemicals ... We were suspicious [they would] destroy samples ... It's hard to believe or trust the government ... but it's always been that way for First Nations people" (Sally). Several community members expressed concern that during a conference call public servants had stated that it was "no wonder" citizens were sick since their smoking and drinking were surely to blame. From the view of these officials, lifestyle transpired as a major caveat (Heidi; Sally).[12] Shortly thereafter, Aamjiwnaang refused the biomonitoring study.

Some in Aamjiwnaang believe that when the community raised concerns about the birth ratio issue, Health Canada hired experts to refute the data and tried to blame the outcomes on "lifestyle and everything else." "Instead of being helpers, they are always trying to come into the other side by denying that things are happening instead of being supportive. They don't want to let the public know and be held responsible" (Tina). The recurring discourse of "lifestyle blame" offends and serves as a roadblock for systemic change. As observations from town hall and board meetings highlight, in addition to arising in interviews, the "lifestyle" language appears in the epidemiological framing of the LCHS operations, questionnaires, public forums, and discourse. For instance, in response to the launch of a Charter challenge by two individuals from the Aamjiwnaang First Nation, discussed in Chapter 1, board member Dean

Edwardson, who is also the director of the industry-led Sarnia-Lambton Environmental Association, told the *Sarnia Observer,* "The cumulative effects of pollution are hard to establish, given local weather patterns, *resident lifestyles* and other factors. It's hard to predict the impact the legal challenge will have on local industry" (Jeffords 2010, emphasis added). This discourse shifts the emphasis away from the systemic and structural conditions that shape and constrain citizen health, and it places blame upon the shoulders of individual citizens.

Findings based on official interviews within the county further illuminate this quandary: "The other issue, whether you like it or not, you have to look at genetics and lifestyle. A lot of our health issues are directly related to what we do, red wine ... etcetera" (Elliott). In this respect, individuals in Aamjiwnaang continuously come up against the language of "lifestyle factors" and the notion that they should be more personally responsible for their health and well-being. Skepticism about the reproductive, respiratory, and cancer health concerns coming from Aamjiwnaang appeared at the town hall meeting held on the reserve, in previous studies, in media accounts, and at the board level.

Blaming "lifestyle factors" for Aamjiwnaang's health issues was a recurring theme during phase 2 of the LCHS. Citing these factors, particularly tobacco use, one official noted that certain actions could impede the credibility of the birth ratio study's findings (Glen). This perspective is an essential component of biomedical epidemiological studies: "We do that automatically because we are public health. It's part of health promotion. We wouldn't want to be part of a study that didn't account for that stuff" (Dawn). The next step, actually carrying out the study, may be best aligned with an approach that employs small-area analysis to further narrow the data so that specific clusters can be examined.

Addressing "lifestyle factors" falls under the rubric of "health promotion," a key feature of county programming. Under this framework, county staff play an active role in the LCHS. Aware of the limitations of a pure biomedical model, which focuses on individual choice and lifestyle behaviours, the Lambton County Health Unit sought to move toward an approach to public policy that considers the "social determinants of health" and "creates environments where people can be healthy" (Lloyd). The county staff's duties include providing accurate data on health status in a timely and accurate fashion. Noting that "the Aamjiwnaang birth ratio study was a watershed report or moment," staff discussed the importance of working collaboratively with multiple stakeholders of equal standing (Lloyd). Thus environmental health concerns involve multiple stakeholders, advocates, science, and governments. Consequently, "when we are doing something like this, it's fragile. If we don't have all the stakeholders around the table, we have a risk of being unsuccessful" (Lloyd). Although the LCHS has not been an easy process, many officials argue that it is an essential one.

Casting individuals as responsible for the care and management of the body follows a lengthy Canadian history of biological regulation, surveillance, and self-discipline. As one interview participant observed, "'Indians' were always numbered off. My dad's number was 687. Everyone is still numbered by the government ... You're numbered ... and then reserves are numbered. Of this reserve, I'm 809. I'm the 809th Indian born on this reserve" (Billy).[13] It has always been simple for the government to compartmentalize Indian citizens as bodies rendered calculable and categorizable.[14] Consequently, the community feels that the government has a duty of care for the treatment of its citizens, who face the results of government decisions on a daily basis: "I think they should be doing a lot more because they put the plants here ... They took the land away from us to build the darn things. Why do they get to sell the land? We should be compensated" (Billy). There is only so much self-care that Indian bodies sequestered to this place can practise.

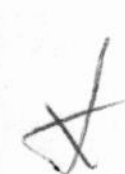

Moreover, experiential, "traditional," Anishinabek knowledge continuously confronts scientific knowledge or expertise in the ongoing struggle for environmental health and reproductive justice. That policy makers request "traditional knowledge" when conducting environmental assessments incited one community member to state, "It's up to us to talk about traditional knowledge. It's up to us ... There are two points of view. There is traditional knowledge and scientific knowledge" (Ned). Often, these worldviews are at odds. Ongoing LCHS proceedings make this clear. In response to the recurring theme that poor "lifestyle choices" are the key reason for the adverse health outcomes in Aamjiwnaang, one elder spoke out: "This isn't rocket science ... You don't need all these reasons as to, for instance, 'lifestyle,' to know that there is something wrong here ... It's the cumulative effects of what's happening here. If cumulative emissions are of concern, are these the causes of cancer-related occurrences within people around here?" (Mike). The official and predominant discourse of "lifestyle blame" continues to trouble the community. Furthermore, attributing "responsibility" for environmental health outcomes is further complicated when scaling from individual behaviours outward to the government's conduct in this policy arena.

Jurisdictional Ambiguity

Although the LCHS has representatives from both Aamjiwnaang and Lambton County, financial responsibility for the creation of this kind of study remains in limbo. There is a sense within the board's membership that "change is not going to come from Aamjiwnaang or Sarnia. It's got to come from provincial or federal" governments (Steve). Frequently, Lambton County's representatives on the LCHS look to the federal government – Health Canada – to intervene.

Early stages of the board's formation prior to 2008 have been characterized as a battleground. The "real battle" occurred during the first few months when the board "didn't want Aamjiwnaang or OHCOW involved" given their particular stakeholder positions (Oliver). From this city official's perspective, "health Canada started this [and] then ran for the hills after a few meetings when it was believed that they would be the funder and driver of the process." This prompted him to ask, "Is Health Canada an oxymoron? Are they designed to protect the status quo? They've been defenders of the status quo in a fairly bureaucratic organization." The former executive director of OHCOW left Sarnia and the study early in 2008. At that time, the city ceased attending LCHS meetings: "It just didn't feel like a valuable use of time" (Oliver). Aamjiwnaang's position also remained ambiguous regarding its continued role in the study.

Municipal officials lacked clarity on the chief and council's mandate for the health study. There existed "differing opinions between [the] chief and council and [the] Health and Environment Committee"; moreover, the chief rarely – if at all – attended health study meetings (Oliver). As this city official added, "Communities can't afford these studies – millions of dollars," and finding information is difficult. Noting liability issues as a rationale for federal governmental inaction, he argued that Canada takes pride in the denial of such controversial information. Communities thus find themselves caught within the jurisdictional cracks of Canadian federalism.

External validation appears within the ongoing discourse of the LCHS board. Health Canada and the federal government become the "go-to guy," maintaining authority to validate citizens' health concerns (Cora). Health Canada's scientific experts provide "clout" for citizens in Lambton County concerned with seeking recognition of their ongoing health concerns. Although Health Canada offered $100,000 of in-kind expertise, board members continued to be perplexed about the tangible services that would be paid for with this magic sum (Cora). This confusion illuminates the opaque and ad hoc approach to determining jurisdictional responsibility.

Such jurisdictional ambiguity poses a significant challenge for First Nations citizens. As one official discussed, "The way things are divided up in Canada, historically, rightly or wrongly, or whatever, you do have this, um, 'division of labour.' Those people in Aamjiwnaang are all residents of Ontario, so the province isn't washing their hands of them" (Glen). This official raised the question of whether Aamjiwnaang could use its special status – as a federal responsibility

– to leverage funds. He continued, "When we are talking to the feds, I don't think they're much interested beyond the boundaries of the reserve ... but if something goes into the waterways ... In terms of the way they are set up, it's a Native community, a band, opposed to the County of Lambton ... Joint funding would be a hopeful thing to see happen." Hope for jurisdictional clarity constantly dwells on the horizon.

Some local policy makers consider Health Canada to be an appropriate and objective regulator. There is thus a sentiment that Health Canada has a duty to protect Canadians' health:

> I also think that they need to realize that they are not working for the companies. They are here to protect the health of Canadians. That's where they get confused. They're protectionists. If they get information, they think, "Oh, they can't let it out." They put all kind[s] of stops in the way ... And then finally when they have all the experts come, the scientists say there is an issue, HC [Health Canada] had to finally say there was an issue. (Tina)

Both the LCHS board and community members within Aamjiwnaang have expressed a desire for more proactive relationships between local and federal governments.

As health unit staff report to the county and are guided by political needs, counties hold a unique political position within Canada's jurisdictional fabric. They are ultimately accountable to political decision makers (Lloyd). In reference to going forward with the LCHS, this county official articulated the importance of "a facilitated process that is transparent, led by a neutral facilitator that has the skill and political insight and the care to lead that process in a way that leaves everyone feeling valued and listened to." Bridging diverse authorities, stakeholders, and interests is simultaneously an opportunity and a challenge for county staff.

Although it was the federal government that initially approached both Aamjiwnaang and Lambton County officials – in 2004 and 2005 respectively – once the health study began to be formalized, funding for its actual completion at the county level was not agreed upon. As noted, Health Canada pledged $100,000 of in-kind scientific support, but it had yet to provide any real dollars. Moreover, funding for the LCHS arose jointly through the industry-led Sarnia-Lambton Environmental Association and the Chamber of Commerce. The provincial government kicked in $50,000 for a scientific literature review – phase 2 of the study – and as these pages go to press, funders have yet to materialize for phase 3: actually conducting a health study.

Some board members are of the view that there is a need for specialized, external expertise and that provincial and federal environment departments should play a larger role. Specifically, they maintain that provincial and federal environmental departments "should be responsible for coming up with some money" (Claire). This board member went on to state, "I'm surprised when the Ministry for Environment put statutes in place but don't tie it back to human health. They should put forward funding to address that piece." Although the provincial Ministry of Environment sent observers to meetings, it did not provide any financial support. She highlighted the importance of securing specific funding from multiple levels of government, as the community appeared to be "falling between the governments and the cracks." In her view, there existed a need to "make them realize how important this is in the community ... Then a documentary happens, a *Men's Health* article ... [that] points to all the reasons to do the study." Moreover, she maintained the view that the community needs "to make sure that we send this info off to the governments. This is the impression of our community that's been given to others."

According to another board member, "Canadians have all benefited from the success of industry. If there's going to be a better understanding of the benefits of industry, all Canadians should share in the cost" (Henry). There is a feeling within the board that multiple levels of government, corporations, and citizens alike share responsibility for moving the study along. For many, the study did not move along fast enough. Concerned with the slow pace of the study, this board member called for more government engagement: "Typical [of] government organization, it's creeping along. We're waiting for someone else to shape our destiny because they have funding. We don't. It's moving way too slow for how people wish it were moving." Study inputs from senior levels of government serve to pacify concerns about the study's impartiality, or bias. Although a role for the Ministry of Environment has been identified, this board member maintained a strong feeling that it "doesn't seem like HC will do more than provide in-kind support. That's been great so far"; however, "going forward ... then the federal government needs to chip in" and work with MOE, as "both are setting regulations. Both are working hand in hand." Although Health Canada was provided with a provincially funded literature review as well as reports from town hall facilitators Phil Brown and Associates, no concrete plan was put in place to synthesize the results and provide the board with funding or with direction on where to take the study next.

Health Canada's role in the LCHS received mixed reviews from county and city officials. It was upon the request of the Sarnia-Lambton Environmental Association that it pulled together a series of meetings during the formation of the board's governance structure in 2005. Since then, its role has waned. Although Health Canada was instrumental during the study's early stages, according to a board official, "once we got started ... the relationship hasn't been there" (Kier). Subsequent to the "fact finding" that took place in phase 2 – including online and phone surveys, town hall meetings, and a literature review – Health Canada's input "was really quite minimal." This board member further noted, "They've told us that they're willing to give us $100,000 [of] in-kind support for phase 2." This $100,000 of in-kind support continues to be defined on a discretionary, ad hoc basis.

As a result, the board requested another face-to-face meeting. Slightly frustrated, this prompted an official to state, "There's been some communication at the staff level, but this emailing [and] letter writing back and forth is getting onerous. We need to have a face-to-face and lay it out on the table" (Kier). From this perspective, there is a need for government expertise to push the study forward. This official noted that since "the province has given some actual dollars for the literature review, we paid a consultant [to move into the next phase]. That's what we're looking to Health Canada for. We need some guidance." This guidance is crucial to conducting a study of the empirical data and gaining some solid answers. With the lack of governmental support, the LCHS board turned to university partnerships, the Ontario Health Study, and Cancer Care Ontario for direction. Citing the high cost of specialized scientific expertise, officials noted that harnessing in-kind support from the county was a challenge, as duties were placed on staff members in addition to their regular responsibilities. Although the county's Department of Community Health Services continues to change and grow, it does not have the resources to fund a large-scale county-wide health study. As a result, board officials look to Health Canada and to consultants for help:

> I think it's gotta be with Health Canada. We just don't have the expertise. At some point ... I mean the thought of an outside consultant ... but that's gonna take some big bucks. If Health Canada has the expertise, then why don't they just do it? Rather than bringing in ... I would rather see them do it ... in my mind they have nothing to gain or lose from this project. They should have the ability to be fairly independent and unbiased. I think they definitely would have the expertise. I think Health Canada is probably the independent unbiased voice that should be leading something like this. (Kier)

In 2011 the board sent correspondence to Health Canada seeking clarity on the details of $100,000 of in-kind support. In the interim, the LCHS remained at a standstill, awaiting clarification on what Health Canada could offer. During this period, board officials made contact with the Ontario Health Study to determine whether it would be possible to merge some of the local concerns with the provincial study. Although this board official noted frustration that "this thing's moving at a snail's pace," there exists a sense of optimism that Health Canada will provide some expertise and guidance on determining the scope and methodology for the study as it moves into phase 3. He added,

> It's just going to come down to one day we are going to hear from HC, "Yes, we'll help you" [or] "No, we won't." I think we've put forward a good case, but at the end of the day, it's the federal government that has the resources to do this kind of thing. They are either going to have to step forward or get out of the room. If they get out of the room, it's a done deal.

Jurisdictional ambiguity permeates concerns both on and off the reserve.

As one municipal policy maker noted, in consideration of the twin issues of environment and health, the reserve constitutes a kind of regulatory black hole: "That area – really, we have an understanding most of the time that we can go on and assess the odour, but I have no authority, under the EPA [Environmental Protection Act], to do anything out there. I'm a normal citizen on that property" (Ethan). He said that environmental management in Aamjiwnaang requires policy imagination: "If you draw a box, and the source is outside the box – the Province of Ontario – I can deal with the source, but inside the box, I really can't do anything. I'd have to call INAC [Indian and Northern Affairs Canada] or EC [Environment Canada] to deal with the problem." He explained that officials must receive permission to conduct environmental monitoring on a First Nations reserve: "We still ask the chief for permission to come on the property. They are a government; we deal with them as a government. We respect that line. We have to. If I'm caught telling somebody to do something and I have no authority I could be liable. My employer won't back it because I'm not in my area." Consequently, he added, authorities "regulate outside that box as much as we can." For some "outside-the-box" nuisances, such as the "necessary evil" of noxious industrial flaring, little can be done. Evidently, there exists a certain kind of discomfort about how to provide ethical and external expertise.

This policy black hole complicates everyday life when health concerns appear on the landscape of a First Nations community. According to a City of Sarnia official, "This country is constitutionally designed to fail" (Oliver). This situation leaves the community in limbo. It is all too simple for the federal government to cite provincial responsibility for healthcare in the country. Moreover, as this official continued, "when you throw First Nations in, you can deny responsibility." Initial concerns arising from Aamjiwnaang were considered to be advantageous to Sarnia in light of Health Canada's fiduciary responsibility for First Nations health policy. This official noted Sarnia's unique position as one of the few Canadian municipalities "with a reserve within its boundaries"; however, he was equally quick to point out that the reserve is not part of the city's constituency. Thus municipal officials would not necessarily be the most obvious site of political advocacy on behalf of Aamjiwnaang.

In this context, there are numerous concerned citizens fighting for the attention of regulatory authorities: the Aamjiwnaang First Nation, union members, OHCOW, and the not-for-profit organization Victims of Chemical Valley, established by widows of former plant workers concerned with the impact of asbestos-related mesothelioma. All of these bodies seek recognition for health concerns at the county, provincial, and federal levels of government. Consequently, limited responses prompted the emergence of new partnerships.

Engaging Knowledge: On the Promises and Perils of Partnerships

Another form of knowledge mobilization emerges when movements directly instrumentalize knowledge and expertise. From a paradigm of engaged knowledge, in contrast to a hierarchical triangle of authority where scientific expertise is placed high above citizen demands, citizens mobilize themselves within the parameters and language of science. Within Aamjiwnaang, this instrumentalization of knowledge and expertise at the community level takes place through partnerships and interactions with governments and researchers. This framework of knowledge engagement fuses expertise and agents within the movement. As a result, the emergent policy process employs shared language. This vernacular may form through the use of techniques such as citizen engagement and other forms of citizen juries or focus groups to legitimate the "expert" knowledge on which policy is based (Orsini and Smith 2010, 47). Science and scientific terms are used directly by citizens themselves seeking to reshape policy development. To defuse antagonistic contestation, citizens are consulted and engaged. Citizens are invited "into" the policy process through the formation of boards, broad-based consultations with stakeholders, partnerships, collaborative initiatives, and community-based research. This may affect the ways that policy makers present research as increasingly sensitive to community concerns (ibid.). In short, the penetration of scientific expertise into the movement itself disrupts the traditional break between "science" and "civil

Table 3
Engaging knowledge

Theme	Pseudonym	Role	Interview location
Community expertise	Charlotte	Community member	Aamjiwnaang
	Sally	Community member	Sarnia
	Sam	Community member	Aamjiwnaang
	Sonny	Community member	Aamjiwnaang
	Tina	Policy official	Aamjiwnaang
Consultation	Brenda	Policy official	Sarnia
	Charlotte	Community member	Aamjiwnaang
	Ethan	Policy official	Sarnia
	Gerry	Policy official	Toronto
	Mike	Community member	Aamjiwnaang
	Molly	Policy official	Sarnia
	Nathan	Community member	Aamjiwnaang
	Tina	Policy official	Aamjiwnaang
	Walter	Community member	Aamjiwnaang
Partnerships	Brenda	Policy official	Sarnia
	Cora	Policy official	Sarnia
	Gerry	Policy official	Toronto
	Sally	Community member	Sarnia
	Steve	Community member	Sarnia
	Tina	Policy official	Aamjiwnaang
	Wanda	Policy official	Ottawa

society," calling for a more active and mobilized citizenry. The mobilization of "engaged knowledge" can be assessed in three ways: through community expertise, government consultation, and partnerships (see Table 3).

Community Expertise

Officials in Aamjiwnaang interact with multiple layers of governance, from the community and municipality to the province and state. In 2002 the Aamjiwnaang First Nation's Health and Environment Committee formed a direct response to Suncor's plans to establish the largest ethanol plant in Canada. The plant was eventually located on the other side of the reserve, and in 2007 the committee created the position of environmental officer to support the development of community expertise. The creation of this position arose amid the post-Ipperwash political climate in Ontario, a time when the province established the Ministry of Aboriginal Affairs and began seeking more involvement with First Nations communities. This led to some improvements in the working relationships between Aamjiwnaang and provincial authorities on environmental issues. With respect to the federal government – which maintains a fiduciary responsibility for Aboriginal peoples in Canada – department staff mentioned that a federal environmental officer had visited the reserve only three times within the past five years for the purpose of surveying fuel tanks. In addition to these rare visits, the staff reported some contact with officials from the Department of Fisheries and Oceans regarding contamination of Talfourd Creek (Tina). Prior to the Ipperwash Inquiry and the subsequent formation of the Ministry of Aboriginal Affairs, provincial officers charged with responding to and addressing environmental issues in Lambton County had refrained from monitoring the reserve.

Similar to the Ministry of Environment's provincial officers, who are governed by the Environmental Protection Act, Aamjiwnaang's environmental officer provides the community with capacity and expertise while serving as a recorder of ongoing concerns. This employee has thus assumed the position of a kind of "watchdog from within" charged with monitoring ongoing environmental issues in Chemical Valley, while also ensuring more comprehensive consultative arrangements. Moreover, the existence of the environmental officer's position conveys Aamjiwnaang's environmental stance to industries and government. Pertinent issues articulated to provincial and federal authorities have included "concerns regarding contaminants, the St. Clair River, and the airshed" (Tina). Much of the environmental officer's work entails managing relationships between a diversity of citizen interests in Aamjiwnaang and at the stakeholder level – including industry and governmental authorities.

Environmental staff members are largely charged with disseminating important information about ongoing projects to the community. This includes the use of newsletters, website maintenance, and developing effective notification processes when new industrial developments take place. Moreover, staff have sought to "develop a procedure for the certificate of approval process, the notification process," given that "the EBR [Environmental Bill of Rights] system does not work for Aamjiwnaang. This is the part where we require accommodation" (Tina). Due to the volume of ongoing changes, developments, and concerns, the community has hired full-time staff to monitor the Environmental Registry. Even so, given the pace of events within and around the community, they cannot be purely devoted to monitoring activities. The Environmental Bill of Rights requires that anyone the ministry deals with must post a request for a certificate of approval. In place since 1993, the Environmental Registry is hosted on a website, searchable by territory or company. It contains "public notices" about all environmental matters proposed by government ministries covered by the Environmental Bill of Rights: "The public notices may contain information about proposed new laws, regulations, policies and programs or about proposals to change or eliminate existing ones" (MOE 2012a). Obtaining details about each development requires further investigation. From the perspective of Aamjiwnaang staff, there is not enough information to determine the scope and scale of actual impacts. The postings are "really difficult to get through"; moreover, as indicated by a series of unreturned phone calls, so too is it difficult to get through to MOE officials when community concerns arise (Tina). This system does not work for an oversaturated community whose members cannot expect the limited staff of Aamjiwnaang's Environment Department to continuously monitor and investigate each posting to the Environmental Registry.

When Aamjiwnaang's Health and Environment Committee (HEC) formed in 2002, it undertook a variety of practices to raise the community's voices and residents' awareness: "I think the HEC was as active as circumstances would allow. We were paying attention to the issue of an ethanol plant; that was our focus. In the meantime, there was a plant that was going to be added on by Suncor – the Genesis project" (Sonny). Community members were frustrated about the so-called "good neighbour" policies espoused by plant representatives. One said of the proposed ethanol plant, "The goal there was to install facilities to carry out the desulphurization of diesel fuel." It was to cost "something like $800 million," and "the council never got any notice, even though the ministry – the legislation – required it" (Sonny). While community members were busy organizing to protest this plant, they did not realize that plans were concurrently underway to expand elsewhere: "We were busy addressing ethanol, location, and everything, and we didn't get a chance. There was no opportunity to ask about the Genesis project. Of course, they didn't offer, even though they posted it on the EBR. They posted, but again as 'good neighbours,' they should have [offered to talk]" (Sonny). As community members rallied to protest the ethanol plant, they did not have time to monitor the Environmental Registry, where they would have learned about the establishment of the Genesis plant. Consequently, they felt that their voices fell on deaf ears and were ignored by their industrial "good neighbours" yet again.

Community mobilization is not free of charge. In addition to working with scientific experts, community members pick up the tab for their air samples. This is a costly practice at "$15 per bag. Then to ship it off is another $30, then to get it tested ... $500 ... just the raw data. Then someone has to look up the standards" (Sally). When asked what recourse community members would like to see, this respondent said, "Stricter fines, standards." Another stated, "I would like to see those guys pay us compensation. I know it's not going to bring back people who are gone, but maybe it will smarten them up" (Sam). Many of the chemicals used by the plants continue to be unregulated in Canada; yet citizens live here with their bodies exposed. Within the community, there is a limited understanding of where to begin cleaning up the long-term, accumulated pollution burden: "There's no support ... Whenever somebody wants to do something, we're told 'no' ... There is grant money, for just that purpose, to clean the waters. I just found one. I'm trying to do a little bit of everything right now. One of my main objectives when I started my co-op was to find grant money, and I looked at the environment, and there's money for that, cleaning up the waterways" (Charlotte). Finding grant money is one obstacle. Political will is another. Generating community momentum and capacity is an ongoing challenge for communities seeking change.

Consultation

According to Supreme Court of Canada jurisprudence, there is a constitutional requirement for governments to consult and accommodate Aboriginal peoples when projects impact their lands or resources.[15] Specifically, this pertains to their Aboriginal right and title to the land. Many of these requests under the duty to consult and accommodate are presented to Aamjiwnaang staff.[16] There are various grants and funds they can access as "capacity-building for consultation" (Tina). As this policy official explained, Aamjiwnaang's Environment Department successfully secured funding for two people to focus on developing community capacity and "to handle these issues instead of paying consultants and different people who come in." With respect to consultation, industry representatives must come to the communities as more than "good neighbours" or "good corporate citizens."

Councillors and community members who have participated on the Health and Environment Committee for two-year terms have been left wanting when it comes to industry consultation. The committee meets bimonthly, frequently with industry, government, and academic representatives. "Being on council you hear a lot about what they are doing and stuff like that ... Sure they started having meetings and coming here and showing them what they are doing and what they are making" (Sam). This community member gave industry's community "consultation" a mixed review:

> They try to make us at ease ... They do samples. They come along here. I say, "Have you guys been doing samples here?" ... "Oh yeah, we come, once a week or month" ... On a hot day, or rainy day, or I don't know, they come at a certain time ... If they can close the beaches up there somewhere, there's gotta be the same thing coming down here.

The Ministry of Environment has a discretionary working relationship with the Aamjiwnaang First Nation that, based on a "nonstandard procedure," allows MOE staff to enter its territory and monitor environmental contamination, despite MOE's limited mandate to formally regulate on-reserve concerns.

Over time, governmental and industrial authorities have changed the ways that they interact with First Nations communities. Regarding the ministry's certificate of approval (COA) permitting new industrial developments and impacts on Aboriginal peoples, one policy official said, "The Government has put most of the companies on notice that all [applicants for] COAs have to consult with First Nations" (Tina). In Aamjiwnaang community officials successfully leveraged funding from multiple scales of government to secure an industry-standard air-monitoring system at their health centre. The above official explained that in collaboration with government officials, community staff "developed a protocol for information and how it should be done appropriately." A large part of the work of the Environment Department's staff includes sharing information between governments, industries, and scientists, as well as "community outreach," which includes, she said, "trying to provide information and get as much information to the community as possible." Furthermore, the department collaborates with governmental and scientific experts to understand environmental degradation in the community.

The consultation protocol in Aamjiwnaang entails various stages of engagement. Initial contact is made through the chief, who then puts items of correspondence into a "consultation file": "Every Monday the consultation worker collects them and makes a briefing note." The consultation worker then replies with the community's position, which depends on the scale and magnitude of the initiative (Tina). If Aamjiwnaang requests "full consultation," this requires special meetings with the chief and council, community open houses, technical reporting, impact-benefit agreements, and compensation for peer-reviewed consultation. The above official further explained that the community may then ask for "accommodation" under the guidance of the chief and council as well as Aamjiwnaang's Economic Development Department, which may come in the form of scholarships, business opportunities, or employment. Environment staff have files on many, but not all, of the companies that work with Aamjiwnaang. Most of the companies have personnel who liaise with community members, which enables Aamjiwnaang staff to address and articulate requirements. The above official noted that several plants abide by a "good neighbour" policy, which requires community outreach and engagement. Evidently, part of the environmental staff's role in Aamjiwnaang involves liaising both with companies and with government officials.

There is a strong sentiment in the community that consultation is not enough to satisfy citizen unrest: "They just come and say 'hello.'" Consequently, "There are a number of issues that are going on, the challenge with human rights ... and I hope they're successful in that – to build a foundation for environmental concerns ... I really hope it enables us to develop policies" (Nathan).

Community consultation is an activity that consumes much of the Environment Department's time and involves multilevel stakeholder negotiations. According to one employee,

> I'm dealing with a lot of items that come into the office, for when people have dealings with our community. Federal court, the Crown, has to have "meaningful consultation for projects regarding Aboriginal peoples and their territories." They have to consult with the First Nations. It means ... because there is a reserve here, Kettle Point, Walpole, the Crown has to consult. (Walter)

Some members questioned the legitimacy of any "consultative" engagement by the adjacent facilities. One said, "I don't think there is ... unless they do it behind everybody's back ... There's something new on Plank Road that wasn't there last year. You're just driving around, and they appear ... and we are pretty much surrounded. It was only the northwest and Shell were here, and now its on the southeast and pretty much all around the reserve; now there's Praxair and all kinds of things coming up" (Charlotte).

The politics of consultation became apparent during the Health and Environment Committee's involvement in a series of meetings with public officials from MOE in Toronto for the 419 Initiative. This MOE-led regulatory initiative seeks to address community concerns around cumulative impacts. Community experience has come into tension with the Open for Business initiative undertaken by the Province of Ontario.[17] Although MOE continues to have a quasi "open-door" policy for environmental and public health stakeholders interested in meeting to discuss regulatory amendments, it is not always feasible for Aamjiwnaang representatives to attend the deliberations, which predominantly take place three hours away from Sarnia in Toronto. According to one committee member: "I get information on my emails about what's happening ... I guess I still get considered a stakeholder, but I think because of the budget that we have in Health and Environment, they can only send representatives that are picked from the committee. I'd have to go on my own. I don't have the funds. I'm interested and I'd like to. If I could afford to, I would" (Mike).

Although many community members, officials, and employees continue to work with and engage in government-sanctioned policy processes – from the 419 Initiative to the LCHS – those involved also demonstrate a kind of "consultation fatigue": "It doesn't take no year-long study on statistics and data to know there is something wrong here. My statistics on human interactions with what is happening around here is all I need to know that there is something wrong around here. The deaths that are happening on Aamjiwnaang are 80 percent, if not better, cancer-related deaths" (Mike). This statistic reflects the severity and significance of ongoing health concerns experienced in Aamjiwnaang.

Stating that investigating the persistent health concerns of the community was not "rocket science," one community member criticized the government's linear approach:

> What I am really disturbed with is that the form of studies that the government – the approaches that they are making – are all based on a linear governmental approach. You know, they have in their linear government the MOE, the MOE Health, and when you say you have a health-related incident that might have to do with the environment, they say, "No, it's one or the other. If you wanna talk about health, let's have a health meeting. If you wanna talk about the environment, let's have an environment meeting." (Mike)

He explained that this linear approach contends with one that is networked, or circular:

> Everything was interrelated as to cause and effects and solutions ... If there was an environmental issue, somewhere down the line, we knew there would be a health issue. Same for the health ... even with the social aspect of the government, which could've been children playing outside with social activities. So that social activity is a health-related incident, which probably tied in with an environmental concern.

This circular approach appears in experiential knowledge claims regarding health and the environment. It contrasts with a technocratic model, which tends to split health off from the environment: "I mentioned this to our environmental people in meetings sometimes. They sometimes say, 'We are talking about environmental issues, not health.' And I mentioned the linear and circular approaches, so at the next meeting they had a couple of health representatives there, which was a good step forward. It hasn't happened too often" (Mike). Organizing and mobilizing citizens for change continue to be challenges due to external antagonisms with encroaching industry and due to the community's administrative structure itself. Although some citizens cited the importance of fusing "health" and "environmental" concerns, workers and citizens concerned with these two policy domains did not always have a clear understanding of their respective portfolios: The community "separates health and environment too ... Health Committee meets once a month," whereas the combined Health and Environment Committee meets bimonthly (Diane). Although this community organizes to engage with and protect the health and environment of its citizens, even citizens themselves are confused about the manner in which their concerns are addressed.

Moreover, a linear, segregated approach to environmental health policy trickles down from the federal, provincial, and municipal authorities. As a result, it affects the administrative composition of some First Nations communities themselves:

> They have a similar government situation there. It's very– their structure is very much the same as federal and provincial guidelines and structure. That is sad for me to observe that within our community. We talk about [it] within our chiefs' meetings, that I used to attend with my father, and we talked about getting back into the clan system, circular government. It's still being discussed within our systems. (Mike)

It is often within the pre-existing institutional frameworks that communities are incited to make claims and seek regulatory redress for their ongoing concerns.

Community engagement is an active part of policy making at all scales of government. As stated, consultation with Indigenous communities is a constitutional requirement in Canada. A policy official with MOE's Aboriginal Affairs Branch noted the importance of "consulting early and often" (Molly). "Deep consultations" are a continuing theme in Aamjiwnaang in connection with a proposed Shell refinery, the ongoing environmental assessment process, and the changes to Regulation 419. Citizens in this community are consulted on an ongoing basis and are invited to participate in various meetings, open houses, and workshops. As the above policy official noted, providing guidance to community members on technical matters is a challenge and requires specific expertise: "Communities want to be independent, but they may not have experts on hand. Communities want to know what their rights are and all the volumes of information and putting the two aspects together." Developing community "capacity" – technical expertise – is thus a challenge.

This policy official highlighted how the post-Ipperwash provincial context may be more conducive to systemic change in light of the provincial Ministry of Aboriginal Affairs' "new relationship with Aboriginal people," implemented by the Ministry of Environment (Molly). Although the ministry is still working on consultation success stories, officials see opportunities for community empowerment and engagement in beautifying Aamjiwnaang's environment. With respect to Talfourd Creek, this official said, "They probably need to do something positive for the creek, empower people, that there are things they can do. There is funding for that ... There isn't funding to devastate a creek by dredging it." There are opportunities for action within the institutional realm of public policy making and within communities themselves whose members mobilize for change.

Over time, new "nonstandard" or unconventional policy partnerships have emerged between officials and communities. One concrete example is the on-reserve air-monitoring system. More broadly, an overall attempt to work through nonstandard "relationship building" has improved the way that Aamjiwnaang interacts with adjacent regulators. Noting that "building trust is very difficult," one MOE official praised the work of the Health and Environment Committee: "We have to treat this as a personal relationship rather than a government-to-government. I think that would help" (Ethan). He cited the development of "a nonstandard response procedure" that can be implemented "any time of day" as demonstrative of MOE's "level of commitment as an organization."

Enhanced relationship building becomes important for citizen participation when communities face transjurisdictional policy issues. One of the central concerns pertaining to community capacity is the lack of public policy expertise located within Sarnia. According to a local MOE official, there are no "policy folks" in a department with twelve environmental officers (Brenda). All certificates of approval are completed in Toronto. When an accident, spill, or release occurs, "first responders" can be companies, citizens, or MOE officials. As noted, there is a "nonstandard procedure" in place for calls coming from Aamjiwnaang. The above official explained, "If somebody calls from Aamjiwnaang, they get a response right away." Consequently, when dealing with Aamjiwnaang, MOE staff usually go and check out the scene no matter what, whether for specific odour complaints or a visible release.

According to a provincial policy maker, the reserve is, in a sense, a "black hole" for policy making when it comes to on-reserve environmental health (Gerry). As mentioned, the establishment of an air monitor on the reserve involved all levels of government in collaboration. According to this policy official, although the legislative composition of Canada's constitutional fabric may seem to produce this kind of "black hole," enabling a policy assemblage, it doesn't mean that meaningful partnerships and arrangements cannot take place through an ad hoc, special, or "nonstandard" approach: "We build our institutions with our own problems. It is an artificial problem." In his view, communities at the front lines of environmental hazards are well placed to address this problem.

Partnerships

To assist with the numerous responsibilities assumed by Aamjiwnaang's Environment Department, partnerships with researchers, scientists, and academics have developed. Over the community's years of activism, various researchers and "experts" have sought, and been sought after, to liaise on various initiatives. Part of the Environment Department's role is to "guide them through the systems and processes" (Tina). The department thus connects experts to the community's administrative processes by various means, including meetings with the Health and Environment Committee and with the chief and council. One initiative included a partnership with biologist and former International Joint Commission scientist Michael Gilbertson. As the above official explained, the community wanted to have a better understanding of its birth patterns and thus attempted to collaboratively "set up a mapping survey of where the births have happened on the reserve to correlate where possibly some of the miscarriages are happening. Were there more boys born in a certain area of the reserve? Trying to figure out where skewing is happening, and correlating, over time, looking at some of the wind data and some of the chemicals that were in the area." These types of partnerships constitute one mechanism for the community to address its concerns.

Some citizens joined forces with government authorities and citizen groups and sought scientific expertise to raise awareness and voice concern. A few community members cited participation and involvement with the organization Victims of Chemical Valley, initially formed by widows of plant workers who had predominantly been sick with mesothelioma. In addition to involvement with groups like these, Aamjiwnaang citizens and officials conducted birth ratio, biomonitoring, and body-mapping studies, blockades, and bucket brigades. In each of these forums, community members partnered with scientific experts to lobby for change: "We got Gilbertson to interpret the Windsor study, birth ratio study ... [but we] had to keep quiet until it was published" (Sally). This community member explained that Gilbertson was but one expert approached:

"We had talked to Health Canada. They wanted to do random blood, hair, urine sampling ... That didn't sound right to us. We didn't like that, so the OHCOW folks said we could do a self-reporting one. They had done body-mapping and a health survey, and Walkerton folks as well, to see what was happening." When the initial Health Canada study was "offered" to Aamjiwnaang (and rejected), community members instead opted to partner with the Occupational Health Clinic for Ontario Workers – Sarnia to conduct their own door-to-door participatory health study, the results of which included large body-size maps with corresponding colour-coded stickers on relevant body parts indicating the community's ailments.

The mobilization of citizens comes in many forms. Whereas some work within the existing administrative alignments, others contest the system from the outside. According to one community member, successful movements require advocates not only outside but also inside the community – like Ada Lockridge, who sits on numerous boards and committees, including Victims of Chemical Valley:

> We don't need more Adas. We couldn't handle more Adas. We need people to support Ada. We need people like you, who can stand up, who have the credentials, the papers behind them, to say what she is saying is accurate, to qualify everything she says. We need other people there who are better at empowering groups of people. Ada is good with a certain group of people. (Steve)

From his perspective, there are times when mobilizing and accessing scientific expertise can be advantageous to the movement.

During the public consultation phase of the Lambton Community Health Study, one of five town hall meetings took place on the reserve, and two Aamjiwnaang citizens participated in the phone survey. It is unknown how many participated in the online survey. As interest in this study faltered, Aamjiwnaang looked elsewhere for meaningful partnerships to paint a more accurate picture of their environmental health concerns. The community pursued other community health possibilities, from partnering with the University of Michigan in its biomonitoring study to participating in the Assembly of First Nations biomonitoring study. As the LCHS moves forward in partnership with the province-wide Ontario Health Study, there is a strong feeling in Aamjiwnaang that "there's no sense sitting around for another four years for the government [to decide] what they need to do" (Tina). Although the University of Michigan biomonitoring study may not provide community members with the answers they are looking for, it is one attempt to gain some knowledge. Several times, the chief and council have been advised by the Environment Department to pull out of the LCHS, but there has been no official decision about the community's ongoing involvement, and staff members continue to attend monthly board meetings.

The role that citizens should play in developing scientific expertise is a matter of debate for the LCHS board. Within the LCHS governance structure, there is a "technical committee" with specialized biomedical expertise that plays a role in overseeing the process (Cora). This voluntary process – whether citizen engagement in Aamjiwnaang, in-kind services offered by Health Canada and Lambton County, or the continued meetings of the LCHS board – demonstrates citizen action with limited redress. As a voluntary process, this model assumes that individuals have the time, resources, and capacity to change their environment. The above board member noted, "We are a committee not a board," and she asked, "What role do citizens play in environmental stewardship?" In contrast to a top-down hierarchical model of public health governance, this kind of citizenship engagement draws on grassroots expertise to manage environmental health concerns; yet it does not necessarily lead to substantive, structural redress.

As Chapter 3 discussed, Health Canada has a fiduciary responsibility for on-reserve environmental health. One of the core tenets of Health Canada's mandate in this policy field is to support community-researcher partnerships. The First Nations and Inuit Health Branch (FNIHB) is responsible for programs such as the First Nations Environmental Contaminants Program and the First Nations Food Nutrition and Environment Study, which is a partnership among the University of British Columbia, the University of Northern British Columbia, and the Assembly of First Nations. As conducting surveillance of more than 600 communities would be onerous, this model requests that communities tell policy makers what their concerns are.

Federal officials – environmental health officers (EHOs) – establish relationships with communities as advisers and develop federal-community partnerships. EHOs may not have all the expertise required, as specific environmental knowledge is needed, so communities are encouraged to partner with researchers. The role of the federal government in specific environmental cleanup projects or health studies is neither seamless nor immediately apparent. Although the FNIHB can fund specific research, the onus is on communities themselves to request federal support for health studies: "There is no program outside of the Environmental Contaminants Program" (Wanda). This policy official explained that, with community consent, EHOs visit communities to conduct preliminary assessments, bringing expertise with them: "We are talking about this as a collaborative initiative." With respect to environmental health projects, she said, a regional director "couldn't provide individual compensation. All you can do is fund a study, awareness workshops, more support from EHO, more research, go to community meetings, fund a full-time employee if there is a significant concern in the community." With respect to on-reserve environmental health, the paradigm of federal public health partnerships is such that collaboration and engaged expertise require active interaction between communities, policy makers, scientists, and citizens.

Provincial regulators vie for community-legislator partnerships. There is a need for jurisdictional clarity pertaining to responsibility for a community-based health study involving Indigenous people's environmental health. Although responsibility for "funding a health study is directly [with] the federal government, as is contamination of wildlife [since] those are clearly federal," there are other issues that warrant multilevel partnerships: "On the air monitor, everyone agreed, and somehow the money came around. It starts with people cooperating and everyone recognizing there is a problem and then talking about it" (Gerry).

Jurisdictional clarity requires a better understanding of Canada's public health system. Medical officers of health are provincially funded and quasi-municipal, and they have "no natural linkages with the federal"; consequently, "it's tough for municipalities to be helpful or initiate anything" (Gerry). Local health units in the county are partially funded by the province and municipalities. There is a provincial as well as a federal medical officer of health responsible for Aboriginal people on reserves. As the above policy official said, one of the biggest challenges is the "lack of communication between the two." Provincial medical officers are in charge but have no access to on-reserve data.

All levels of government play a role in on-reserve environmental health, albeit in a piecemeal fashion. MOE began to seek a more active relationship with citizens of Aamjiwnaang as of 2004. Since that time, it has become more involved on the reserve: "We have done fish, clam, sediment, water quality [tests] for a number of years" (Brenda). As noted, MOE also put in an air-monitoring station – with federal collaboration – and is now stepping into the "black hole" of on-reserve environmental health issues. This policy official said that MOE actively seeks to "cross the line": "We don't make that line anymore, saying it's just the feds. The feds are not here, so we are stepping in and trying to do the right thing and be responsive." Although more could always be done, with limited resources large-scale activity is difficult, and health issues are outside the scope of MOE's immediate mandate.

As they carry on, committed to living life "as usual" while trying to ignore the impending threats to their home and habitat, both Aamjiwnaang's employees and its citizens develop technical capacity through their responses to and efforts to mitigate environmental health concerns. Such actions by staff include participating in the LCHS, attending Regulation 419 meetings, conducting surveys of traditional plants, providing comments on and being involved in archaeological digs, organizing and participating in various workshops and symposia, responding to and partnering with companies such as Imperial, Suncor, and Shell, informing the community about ongoing projects, identifying spots for remediation, and essentially "trying to develop relationships with different companies and government" (Tina). Effective communication between technical experts and community members constitutes a large portion of the Environment Department's continued work.

Conclusion

There are several reasons ongoing struggles for reproductive justice have been discredited or eclipsed throughout this public deliberative process. These reasons arise from issues associated with the representation of this community's concerns vis-à-vis the larger interests of Lambton County as citizens encounter the discursive fields of *science, scale, lifestyle blame,* and *jurisdictional ambiguity*. Regarding science, the biomedical power and authority embedded within the language of science, epidemiology, and statistical significance overlooks and discredits Aamjiwnaang's situated, experiential claims. There appears to be a presumption at the county level that the 2005 birth ratio study was not statistically sound and is thus not representative of the county's generalizable concerns. As mentioned, Lambton County's Department of Community Health Services analyzed sex ratios for the entire county and individual townships "in order to determine if sex ratios differed from provincial ratios and if communities adjacent to the reserve and local industry were differentially affected" (LCHS 2011, 17). The results of the study revealed "no trends towards a declining sex ratio, i.e. fewer male births, in Lambton County or its individual townships between 1981 and 2001" (ibid.). The report concluded that data on sex ratios in Lambton County did not differ greatly from the data for Ontario as a whole. This study did not look at Aamjiwnaang's distinct data, an undertaking that is crucial to *sensing policy.*

In this paradigm, scientific, epidemiological, and biomedical principles are cast as legitimate, apolitical, technical, and "true." Such privileging of this technocratic model posits a "body of knowledge" wherein expertise is external from the experiential, corporeal knowledge derived from the bodies of those mobilizing for justice. This approach conflicts with a corporeal account, which situates bodies as knowledge generators and emphasizes connectivity. For example, one interview participant from Aamjiwnaang indicated that public servants often cite scientific discourse in public policy processes to classify human life as separate from inanimate life and forget that "we are all tied into one, every human, animal, tree. We are all one. We can't survive without us either" (Tracy).

Regarding scale, the Lambton Community Health Study seeks to understand the health concerns of the county as a whole, which encompasses eleven municipalities. This is in stark contrast to the Aamjiwnaang First Nation health study, which began in 2005. Given the impact of long-term cumulative effects as well as the community's geopolitical location encircled by industry, it is unclear how this history and unique situation would be represented and accounted for at the county level. As Scott (2008) discusses, casting too wide a net has the potential to dilute pollution's effects on human health. The body burden is disproportionately distributed across Lambton County, where Aamjiwnaang is acutely impacted.

Regarding lifestyle blame, public discourse at the board and county levels repeatedly raised the issue of individual behaviours to explain the community's adverse health outcomes. Lifestyle language about risk factors during pregnancy and throughout the reproductive process appeared in public statements, media accounts, and interview data. During Lambton County's town hall meetings, residents said that they were frankly tired of hearing the discourse of "lifestyle blame" in explanations of reproductive harm that alluded to smoking and drinking habits among residents (LCHS 2011). This individualizing framework of public healthcare posits the individual body as distinct from its surroundings and fails to recognize the integrated, placed relationship between health and the environment.

Regarding jurisdictional ambiguity, the issues of funding, resource distribution, and fiduciary responsibility for on-reserve environmental health have led to a power imbalance within the representation of Aamjiwnaang's reproductive health concerns. This problem signals the importance of multilayered analysis. Funding for the health study is provided by a combination of the provincial government and industry (LCHS 2011). Funds pledged by the Province of Ontario early in 2010 covered the completion of a literature review. Prior to 2010 the only real dollars came from stakeholders in the business community, the Chamber of Commerce, and the Sarnia-Lambton Environmental Association, although both Lambton County and Health Canada contributed in-kind services in staff time and technical and scientific expertise (LCHS 2014). According to Ben Martin, assistant to local Member of Parliament Pat Davidson, Health Canada's in-kind services are valued at $100,000, higher than the $50,000 awarded by the province (Morden 2010). As of 2015, the Lambton Community Health Study board announced its intention to seek funds for a multi-million-dollar partnership with environmental toxicologist Dr. Laurie Chan (LCHS 2015). Should it go ahead, the results of this study will surely advance awareness about environmental health concerns in Aamjiwnaang and Lambton County.

When citizens enter the deliberative sphere, they both encounter and create discursive fields of knowledge. These knowledges are bound up within the discursive fields of "science" and "expertise." At the same time, upon entry into these participatory processes, citizens interact with institutional knowledges and enter a "complex field of contingent governance" (Hobson 2013, 63). These encounters with knowledges that are internal and external to the community emerge as citizens form partnerships with governments and researchers. Such processes are highly charged with political meaning and reveal multiple ways of interacting with science and expertise. Chapter 7 advocates for the advancement of *environmental reproductive justice*. To do so, it turns toward some creative avenues for reconceptualizing the theory and practice of collaborative community research.

7

Shelter-in-Place?
Immune No More and Idle No More

Walking Together, Moving Forward

During his keynote address to the 2015 Congress of the Humanities and Social Sciences in Ottawa, Canada's capital city, Justice Murray Sinclair – one of three commissioners of Canada's Truth and Reconciliation Commission – invited audience members to recall the spirit of Idle No More and commit to an ongoing individual and collective movement for truth, reconciliation, and justice.[1] He asked the audience to bear witness to the truths about our dark history, manifested through the systematic discrimination against Indigenous peoples enabled by Canada's residential school policies, in order to move toward a brighter future. By raising our hands in agreement, all present articulated a physical, emotional, and spiritual commitment to honouring our treaty relationships and to sharing responsibility for the creation of a more just society. Although the commission's mandate came to a close in June 2015 with the production of a final report outlining ninety-four "calls to action," Justice Sinclair did not evoke closure but instead extended a dialogical invitation to all Canadians to collaboratively build a decolonial future. The day following his remarks, on May 31, 2015, residential school survivors and Canadian citizens from a diverse range of backgrounds marched together to honour this commitment. By doing so, citizens engaged in and embarked upon an ongoing process of reconciliation. Such actions are the expression of continuous resistance to political violence and a personal and political commitment to being "idle no more."

To move forward, we need to understand how we got to this place. In the fall and winter of 2012–13, a widespread Idle No More movement, spurred through Twitter and Facebook, emerged as a loosely knit protest against omnibus bills C-38 and C-45 that included blockades, rallies, and flash-mobs. As noted by the University of Winnipeg's director for Indigenous inclusion, Wab Kinew (2012), Idle No More is "not just an Indian thing"; it is about engaging youth, finding meaning, claiming rights, protecting the environment, and upholding democracy. Four Saskatchewan-based women, frustrated with the lack of consultation about sweeping legislative changes affecting federally protected waterways, natural resources, and Indigenous rights, pledged to be "idle no more" (Coulthard 2014, 160). Although no sole leader emerged with a concrete list of demands on behalf of the movement, the considerable momentum across the country and beyond demonstrated the loud, chaotic, beautiful, and messy features of democracy. Consequently, details about the lived realities experienced by many Indigenous communities across the country exploded into the public arena.

Like Idle No More in some respects, Chief Theresa Spence's high-profile hunger strike reveals the contemporary biopolitical stakes for Indigenous peoples in Canada. The hunger strike took place because she could no longer be idle; her body could no longer be immune to the persistent corporeal practices of Canadian colonialism. On December 11, 2012, as a form of protest, Chief Spence commenced a hunger strike, undergoing considerable physical, mental, and emotional duress to raise awareness about the dire straits facing Indigenous communities across Canada and to demand a discussion about mutual respect, treaty rights, and relations (Coulthard 2014).[2] A year prior, her home community of Attawapiskat declared a "state of emergency" due to poor housing conditions (Asch 2014, 150). On Victoria Island, an Algonquin territory in the shadow of Parliament Hill, she subsisted on tea and broth for forty-four days to seek recognition of a nation-to-nation relationship between Indigenous peoples and the Crown.[3] Her body became a symbol of sacrifice, a mirror of the bare life experienced by the communities she represented, and a powerful site of resistance. As noted by Alice Klein (2013), this act "crashes against the unconscious non-Indigenous Canadian certainties and political calculations. It demands that we recall instead the actual history of our country and how it still lives in the unrelentingly colonized amongst us." Frustrated with the constant need to fight for physical and cultural survival due to the past and present manifestations of Canada's colonial legacy, Chief Spence put her body on the line – a fine line between bare and political life (see the discussion of this concept on p. 27) – as a physical and symbolic gesture for Canada, and the world, to see. Thrust into the spotlight of Canada's body politic, her body became visible and highly charged with biopolitical meaning.

This was not the first time that Indigenous people mobilized their bodies to draw attention to their lived experiences, and as the 5,000 supporters of truth and reconciliation demonstrated in Ottawa on May 31, 2015, it will not, and must not, be the last.[4] Numerous Indigenous communities across Canada and the world live in a constant state of insecurity due to their perpetual corporeal exposure to contamination. The Aamjiwnaang First Nation is one such community. Here, individuals reside in a risky environment, where uncertainty reframes the conditions for one's life, being, and citizenship. Although transborder exposure to environmental harm is indicative of a globalized, deterritorialized threat, examining community practices of resistance prompts a different kind of thinking about citizenship and reterritorializes our focus. With respect to Aamjiwnaang in particular, and Anishinabek thought in general, "place" is a core feature of Indigenous citizenship, which challenges biopower's insidious and sometimes explicit hold on Indigenous life. Although the everyday experiences of Indigenous citizens underscore biopolitical concerns, their activities demonstrate how citizenship is relational: it is simultaneously embodied, rooted, and territorial. These practices propel us to think differently about policy, mobilization, belonging, and justice.

The idea of being "idle no more" strongly resonates in Aamjiwnaang. Solidarity with Spence's hunger strike included actions such as fasting, demonstrating, and blocking the Canadian National Railway line leading into Chemical Valley (Wright 2013). According to blockade spokesperson Ron Plain, local leaders wanted to grab Ottawa's attention. On December 21, 2012, the railway responded with a court injunction that called for the blockade's removal; however, the protesters remained in place a full week longer.[5] Imperial Oil and Nova Chemicals, among other facilities nearby, claimed that the blockade had led to reduced production in the area (ibid.). Finally, in mid-January, Justice John Desotti ordered that the blockade be cleared. Although injunctions were issued, Sarnia police remained hesitant to make arrests for fear of inciting violence. As citizens of this community blocked the railway line with their bodies and camped out in tents in the dead of winter, their mobilization caused neighbouring industry to sit back and await a more peaceful solution. Citizens of all ages began to take action, demonstrating this community's agency.

The staff and children of the Aamjiwnaang Binoojiinyag Kino Maagewgamgoons Daycare took to the streets on January 16, 2013, to demand the right to a cleaner environment for the community's young. Framing their action as an Idle No More demonstration, these concerned citizens, frustrated with the incessant spills, leaks, and accidents, demanded answers from their industrial neighbours. The long-term health impacts of such spills and accidental releases are unknown. This action is but one form of activism among a lengthy history of many others, from fasting and rail blockades to biomonitoring studies, bucket brigades, door-to-door health surveys, and body-mapping. In the midst of life's opacity here, what becomes clear, as Bargu (2011) suggests, is the "theoretical register" and prominence of the body as a conduit for agency. As such, the body makes a statement on life itself as both a stage and a key actor. Like Chief Spence's hunger strike, these acts illuminate how life, reduced to bare life, may not be worth living without recognition of a radically different kind of politics. All Canadians bear the responsibility for recognizing, respecting, and creating space for these radical actions. Chief Spence's action demanded recognition of equitable treaty relationships and a profound acknowledgment that we are national partners sharing the vast territories that make up present-day Canada. In Aamjiwnaang and Attawapiskat, we see how the body is powerful and regenerative. This illuminates Grosz's (1994, 120) assertion that it is a "force to be reckoned with." In the context of the hunger strike and everyday existence in Aamjiwnaang, life itself is both an object and a subject of political action. Thus bodies are crucial conduits and agents for social change in ongoing struggles for justice.

Justice

As an alternative approach to linear, technocratic, positivist policy, *sensing policy* is oriented toward justice and thus underscores the diversity of experiences, voices, and knowledges across sites of difference. Consistent with intersectionality-based policy analysis (IBPA) in theory, method, and practice, a consideration of resistance and resilience is crucial to the reframing of environmental justice and the advancement of reproductive justice, which considers policy to be a kind of "political action" (Hankivsky 2012, 18; Orsini and Smith 2007). Much like IBPA, *sensing policy* is a transformative approach that highlights inherent inequities in our political institutions and discourses while making space for diverse, situated discourses and knowledges to intervene in the policy-making process. This reframing of policy is crucial to achieving more equitable Indigenous environmental justice in Canada. Ensuring environmental reproductive justice in Aamjiwnaang is just one of the many challenges facing Indigenous peoples in Canada.

An interpretive and intersectional view of struggles for environmental reproductive justice must couple citizen action or behaviour with the structural configurations of injustice to work toward substantive change in the deliberative and discursive realms of political life. Although a focus on the body and corporeal experience takes primacy in my analysis, which is conventionally associated with the private realm, commitment to justice would be incomplete without consideration of the public arena and the relations between the two. For this reason, a *sensing policy* framework of analysis requires a *multilayered* approach to understanding the policy assemblage that constrains equitable advances in Indigenous environmental justice. As Kymlicka (2001, 143) states, "There are many aspects of economic, social and environmental policy that can only be effectively dealt with at the federal level. Too much decentralization of power may result, not in the empowering of communities, but simply in leaving everyone powerless in the face of global economic and political trends." This problem highlights how decentralization does not necessarily reconcile claims for justice. Devolution in this regard redistributes the regulatory burden downward to communities. What becomes evident, Kymlicka (ibid., 151) observes, is that we need to reconceptualize justice so that it is sensitive to the needs of, but is not offloaded to, communities. Thus we must think critically in equal measure about discursive and distributive justice when struggles for the recognition of environmental reproductive injustices emerge.

An ongoing commitment to respecting diverse expressions of justice is central to *sensing policy*. Schlosberg (2013) explains that "environmental justice" is a discursive term that entails more than the distribution of "bad" social ills, as it is also about the language, rhetoric, meanings, and processes that shape, constrain, and enable citizen opportunities for policy change. As Chapter 6 highlighted with respect to the Lambton Community Health Study, there are procedural dimensions that affect environmental reproductive justice. Although outside the formal arena of institutional politics, this health study's deliberative structure has revealed some of the challenges to equitable democratic participation. These deliberations bring into focus some of the ways that procedures are "complex ensembles of practices," both structural and discursive (Mouffe 2005a, 68). Chapter 6 discussed how marginalization occurs in the decision-making process as citizens struggle for recognition of their corporeal concerns while trying to confront an elite model of scientific expertise and knowledge. *Sensing policy* suggests that achieving reproductive justice requires a collaborative and experiential approach to public health and to environmental policy and planning. It also accounts for Aamjiwnaang's unique cultural place, health, knowledge, and experience in public deliberations.[6] This approach entails creating policy that makes space for *lived experience, situated bodies of knowledge,* and *geopolitical location* through *multilayered analysis*. Thus working toward social change in pursuit of justice requires retooling the deliberative sphere to create space for and integrate diverse ways of knowing, aligned with Hall and colleagues' (2013) conception of "knowledge democracy." Such an approach cultivates the deliberative conditions necessary to hear and listen to diverse voices. Doing so requires attention to the discursive, distributive, and procedural dimensions of justice.

An experiential, affective, place-based approach to public policy is crucial to substantively addressing environmental reproductive justice. This understanding is consistent with an "environmental reproductive justice" orientation (Hoover et al. 2012). As stated in Chapter 1, this place-based emphasis extends environmental reproductive justice discourse to communities and "to the human relationship with the non-human world" (Schlosberg 2013, 38). To do so, accounting for corporeal and ecological claims is a necessary component of deliberative justice. Moreover, as Gabrielson and Parady (2010, 379) note, linking citizenship to environmental reproductive justice cannot be "body blind"; our deliberative processes require an intersectional consideration of the axes of race, class, gender, and place. Green theory, green governmentality, and Canadian citizenship studies have conventionally been "body blind." As Adkin (2009, 5) notes, much of this scholarship to date focuses on the rational, "normative," or "procedural" dimensions of the cultivation of active ecological citizens. Consistent with her call for a critical citizenship theory that integrates social justice and ecological reform, the task of working toward a more equitable society in pursuit of reproductive justice involves not only consideration of the corporeal experiences of biopolitical engagement in the private realm but also an interrogation and reconfiguration of the discursive and structural features of our democracy. Aligned with Gabrielson and Parady (2010, 387), advancing an approach to *sensing policy* shares the goal of working toward a "fleshier democracy." A fleshier democracy requires a focus on the body – as bodies enact citizenship – and also locates bodies within larger power assemblages. This conception corresponds to Adkin's (2009, xii) turn away from a discursive emphasis on "sustainable development" and toward "ecological democracy." To achieve justice, it is not enough to examine autonomous practices of citizen action.

Achieving environmental reproductive justice requires new thinking about citizenship. Drawing on the work of feminist theorist Elizabeth Grosz, Gabrielson and Parady (2010, 380) accentuate the ways that bodies counter rationality and "naturalist" accounts of politics; they are socially and culturally inscribed and embody difference. Western, liberal philosophy has tended to regard the body as something with passions and appetites to be tamed and controlled. By bringing the body forward and making corporeality a prominent feature of politics, we can begin to retool citizenship and policy toward socially just ends. Furthermore, by centring on the agency of bodies and by countering predominant accounts of how "rational" citizens should manage "responsible lifestyle practices," we can contemplate a more relational, practised, embedded, and embodied approach to citizenship that counters a rational, liberal, Eurocentric worldview.

We must recall that the vibrant human body is connected to a nonpassive world. Bodies are resilient. They move, regenerate, and reproduce. As Gabrielson and Parady (2010, 381, 387) suggest, corporeal citizenship forces us to reimagine individualist accounts of civic duty and to quash such instrumentalization of the body and environment with a more embodied account. Rather than separating citizens from their environments as instrumental stewards to care "for" the environment, a corporeal and further ecological approach locates individuals as embedded within their more-than-human environments. Counter to classic, modern, and liberal accounts of citizenship, an ecological approach to citizenship does not position human life as superior to the more-than-human world. Human subjectivity, through an ecological lens, begins from an embedded rather than hierarchical account of human–more-than-human relationships.

Environmental and reproductive injustices in Aamjiwnaang reveal some of the ways that bodies are sites of harm. Human bodies are porous, vulnerable, and susceptible to toxic encroachment. Situating a concern with biopolitical subjectivity in the context of current struggles for environmental reproductive justice highlights harm and the possibilities for agency. In addition to being vulnerable sites, bodies also intersect with cultural, social, political, and environmental forces. Such an intersectional approach to understanding the body opens up possibilities for justice claims within a framework of a radically different conception of citizenship and policy, which may lead to a more socially and environmentally just account of democracy.

A more inclusive, democratic conception of citizenship and policy accounts for corporeality and place. Such an ontological shift troubles human-nature, mind-body, and individual-environment dualisms to situate bodies within socially constructed human and nonhuman contexts. Counter to much of green theory, green governmentality, and liberal state theory, an ecological account of citizenship, as Gabrielson and Parady (2010, 387) explain, "recognizes the centrality of the environment to human subjectivity by acknowledging the variety of places that bodies inhabit and the diversity of human relations with the natural world." This ecological account of human subjectivity takes into consideration that claims for corporeal recognition are entangled with questions of social justice and attempts to flesh out a more socially just form of belonging – of citizenship – in our modern democratic society.

On the Contours of Modern Democracy

Struggles for environmental reproductive justice uncover implications for democratic politics. As Adkin (2009) attests, examining these struggles points toward new directions regarding the potential to democratize and decolonize ecological knowledge in Canada. Examining policy and citizenship through an intersectional and interpretive lens makes space within theories of environmental justice for reproductive justice, a process that requires a close evaluation of the discourses, practices, and structural constraints shaping political action. The aims of ecological citizens cannot be achieved without radical transformation of the existing liberal, democratic norms and institutions.

A fleshier democracy makes space for ecological citizens and cultivates the conditions for meaningful citizen participation. The claims of ecological citizens demand a more complex articulation of corporeal and environmental concerns in order to work toward justice and participatory democracy. Rather than attempting to "reconcile" or "solve" persistent and pervasive injustices, we can draw inspiration from Mouffe's (2005b, 5) account of the inherent pluralist features of contemporary politics to guide us in our ongoing quest for democratic justice. Mouffe's notion of modern democracy commits to an anti-essentialist lens yet advocates for a positive consideration of difference as a kind of pluralism that questions ideal notions of unanimity and homogeneity. Difference is thus a celebrated feature of anti-essentialist democracy. This radical orientation to democracy aims to create multilogical space for dialogue rather than to impose discursive uniformity in pursuit of reconciliation.[7]

To envisage democratic politics from an anti-essentialist perspective, it must be recognized that no one form of political life maintains a privileged foundational position over another. This treatment of democracy fundamentally challenges the subtle violences implicit within the "rationality" or "neutrality" assumed by objective liberal philosophy. Mouffe (2005a, 29) contends with the "dangerous utopia" of moral and political philosopher John Rawls's universalizing liberal theory, which pertains to how one might establish peaceful coexistence as a matter of reconciliation. She critiques the Rawlsian paradigm of justice – which assumes that individuals can begin from an "original position" of equality and that principles of justice can be selected behind a "veil of ignorance" – for its presupposition of value-neutral procedural democracy. Mouffe (ibid., 23) contests the objective of achieving "consensus on political fundamentals," which is at odds with a contextual, pluralistic society, sequesters dissent from public life, and conceals alternative forms and visions of political agency. Rawls's concern with political justice requires fair terms of social cooperation between free and equal citizens by underscoring "reasonable pluralism." As Mouffe (ibid.) draws out, any claim to "reasonable pluralism" overemphasizes a deliberative democratic life that seeks to erase difference, an impossible and violent feat. Such an account assumes that citizens appropriate the terms set by a rational, liberal approach. It also distinguishes between "reasonable" and "unreasonable" citizens.

In contrast to an approach that begins from a vision of a well-ordered society, from an original position behind a veil of ignorance, a "fleshier democracy" aligns with Mouffe's approach to endorse a democracy of difference. Mouffe's vision of a radical and plural democracy acknowledges the value of diverse ways of knowing, which has considerable implications for the deliberative arena. These pluralisms must be brought to the fore and made visible. Noting that "consensus" is a conceptual impossibility, Mouffe (2005a, 33) argues that this does not put the democratic ideal in jeopardy but instead "protects pluralist democracy against any attempts at closure." The Lambton Community Health Study (LCHS) is an example of liberalism's blind spots, demonstrating the limitations of rational participatory democracy for situated knowledge.

Since its inception, the LCHS has moved away from the difference-based, fleshier dimensions of Aamjiwnaang's corporeal concerns and has continued to seek "closure" by opening up the community's suffered injustices to the broader scale of the county and subsequently the province. The discursive act of scaling-out eclipses the specificities of political life, reveals the exclusive edges of citizenship, and polices the political grammars of possibility for reframing environmental justice. In doing so, it forecloses avenues for site-specific environmental reproductive justice. In occluding the distinct place-based corporeal articulations of harm or injury, this participatory process has failed to account for Aamjiwnaang's experiential and consequently subjugated knowledges. Rather than trying to "erase the traces of power and exclusion," as the LCHS sought to do with its widening of the scale, a fleshier democratic politics brings these injustices to the fore in order "to make them visible so that they can enter the terrain of contestation" (Mouffe 2005a, 33–34). Making visible and distinctly accounting for environmental reproductive injustices in this participatory and deliberative health study would offer a much more transformative and socially just approach to addressing Aamjiwnaang's embodied, corporeal, and ecological concerns.

Finally, a fleshier democracy reconfigures the boundaries of citizenship. Several contemporary political theorists contend that "in an age of globalization" citizenship cannot be confined to the boundaries of a nation-state and must be "transnational" (Mouffe 2005a, 37).[8] Whether or not the "nation-state" *should* be the key arbiter of citizenship claims is not the focus here. Instead, *sensing policy* turns our attention to the particular places where citizenship is embodied and enacted. With respect to the lived experiences and articulations of residents in Aamjiwnaang, citizenship cannot be deterritorialized. Attempts to achieve reproductive justice must contend with liberal, rational accounts of deliberative democracy to make space for a messier, fleshier, more corporeal version of policy and citizenship that counters the liberal primacy of mind over matter and that brings a multiplicity of voices, bodies, and experiences to the fore.

Sensing Policy: Toward Environmental Reproductive Justice

The persistent struggles in Aamjiwnaang prompt a new, affective, place-based, intersectional, and relational way of thinking about citizenship and policy. This approach to *sensing policy* is an *affective framework for analysis* and is critical to developing new policy strategies for environmental reproductive justice. Inspired by Michel Foucault's notion of governmentality, the discussion of power and government extends beyond the formal, institutional, hierarchical realm of politics to examine broader citizen encounters with ensembles of power. In contrast to focusing on "government" solely as a hierarchical, centralized institution or set of institutions and groups, a governmentality approach hones in on political analysis as an examination of the outcomes of thoughts and practices that shape assumptions about what government is and about how, by whom, and for what purposes it should be exercised (Murray 2007). In this view, language, speech, and communication carry and transmit power relations. Consequently, the freedom, agency, and mobility of actors is constrained by the material and discursive contexts in which citizens are embedded. In Aamjiwnaang, citizen agency and individual responsibility for the mitigation of health and environmental risks are at once bound up with uneven power relations; yet they simultaneously reveal a radical form of belonging. For this reason, any solution or gesture toward "justice" requires a focus on the structural and discursive constraints impeding agency rather than a critique that calls for citizens to change their individual behaviour. Making changes only to citizen action leaves the unjust policy and procedural configurations intact.

Going from a discursive analysis of texts to engaging with community members opens up some possibilities for thinking differently about political organization, values, and beliefs. The aim of cultivating the conditions for dialogue between a Eurocentric, Enlightenment-refined approach to citizenship and an Anishinabek approach to justice is to revisit and articulate a different way of understanding political life. As numerous conversations with community members revealed, despite the modern manoeuvre of separating "humans" from "nature," more-than-human elements are central to human existence. The ontological portrayal of an animate view of the earth and more-than-human world was most clearly articulated by elders and traditional knowledge carriers of the Aamjiwnaang First Nation. This approach comes into direct tension with a possessive, positivist, atomistic, rational, liberal ontology. Theoretically, methodologically, and empirically, *sensing policy* acknowledges the power of citizen storytelling as a kind of truth telling. Thus it sheds light on diverse voices and worldviews as a means to challenge any strict separation or possessive relationship between human and more-than-human life. This orientation to policy making aims to create space for other ways of thinking about the constitution of political life itself.

Multilayered Analysis

As discussed, policies take shape across levels of government, scaled from the global to the intimate. These policies include those of Aamjiwnaang, the City of Sarnia, Lambton County, the Province of Ontario, and the Government of Canada. Each policy layer entails laws and regulations pertaining to the management of Indigenous lands and bodies. Moreover, it is undeniable that the situation of Chemical Valley is embedded within transnational capitalist systems of production. Thus a comprehensive analysis of power requires an examination of policy impacts on everything from global capital to daily lived experiences.

Chapters 3 through 6 exposed the *multiple layers* of Canada's legislative and policy arrangements for on-reserve environmental health, demonstrating a policy failure for Indigenous environmental reproductive justice. The *policy assemblage* of these configurations includes citizenship, health, and environmental policies, each of which distinctly impacts Indigenous citizens vis-à-vis Canadians at large. Notably, Indigenous peoples in Canada are regulated by the Indian Act, Canada's primary means of defining what it means to be an "Indian." As Chapter 3 explained, Canada has always regulated, governed, and monitored the "bodies" of Indian citizens. This coupling of population-based and bodily governance as a form of biopower impacts Indigenous peoples Canada-wide and within local communities such as Aamjiwnaang.

Biological management continues to be a part of state-making practices in Canada. By examining Canada's constitutional design, this book exposes some challenges that our jurisdictional matrix poses for Indigenous communities concerned with on-reserve environmental health. Chapters 3 and 5 advanced the argument that this biopolitical *policy assemblage* shapes and constrains an emergent field of Indigenous environmental justice, thus presenting a "wicked policy" problem that decision makers struggle to address (Kreuter et al. 2004). Administratively, there exists a lack of clarity about Canada's jurisdictional composition and responsibility for Indigenous health and, further, for environmental health. As a result, services are often poorly defined. There is overall confusion about the requirements and responsibilities for adequate federal funding. Whereas for most Canadian citizens the provision of healthcare services is a provincial responsibility, for people on reserves, even in areas that fall under provincial jurisdiction, these services are provided by the federal government.

These constitutional configurations produce public policy gaps, illuminating a messy and dense assemblage. Consequently, citizens confronting this *policy assemblage* become embroiled in this field of relations and assume the burden of ongoing corporeal and ecological concerns. As the interviews revealed, citizens and policy makers interpreted the problem, expertise, and appropriate solutions differently. Uncovering and discussing the apparent policy configurations of on-reserve environmental health as a *policy assemblage* twins environmental and reproductive justice to achieve more substantive place-based public policy developments that account for citizens' lived experiences and experiential knowledge. Normatively and empirically, the intention here is to speak to policy gaps in order to make this policy issue less vacuous, contribute to a broader, more robust conversation about environmental reproductive justice in Canada, and think rigorously about the theory and practice of Indigenous environmental justice.

Lived Experience

Sensing policy centres knowledge in stories and *lived experience*. It supports Anishinabek approaches to research that centre "stories" through a range of traditional and contemporary narrative forms, including song, dance, and drumming (Doerfler, Sinclair, and Stark 2013). Emphasizing citizens' grounded, local expressions brings discursive and experiential dimensions of policy and citizenship into view. Doing so creates space for constructing news ways of thinking about citizenship and justice that contend with rationalist accounts of biological and environmental citizens as stewards of their bodies and land. To conceptually, methodologically, and practically move from environmental to reproductive justice, the analysis intervenes in status quo, liberal accounts of justice by emphasizing the conception of "place." Thus the theoretical orientation in this book aims to confront biopolitics, liberal individualism, subjectivity, and Eurocentric citizenship by situating the emergence of citizen practices and struggles for justice "on the ground" and in relation to place.

Indigenous citizens' ongoing struggles for environmental reproductive justice are simultaneously struggles over knowledge and power. Specifically, Chapter 4 highlighted citizens' embodied, emotional, felt, lived experiences through grounded narratives pertaining to community views about living perpetually on alert in a "sacrifice zone" (Lerner 2010). As a matter of reproductive justice, findings revealed the multifaceted ways that citizens must mobilize for change to protect both *physical* and *cultural* survival. As a result, citizens have become active, responsible environmental stewards of their land and life, while expressing an ontological *relationship* to their home, place, and cultural survival that is radically different from the one offered by a Western model.

Going beyond textual analysis, this study moved into the field to examine the experiential dimensions of Canada's *policy assemblage* through *lived experiences* and *situated bodies of knowledge* in the ongoing struggles for environmental reproductive justice in Canada's Chemical Valley. This turn toward the empirical site of Aamjiwnaang is as vital as the theoretical insights gained through more academic fields. Such a turn is crucial to developing an in-depth, community-based understanding of the everyday realities confronting citizens of the Aamjiwnaang First Nation. Linking an interpretive study of policy with an account of political ethnography draws attention to lived experience and engages with this *geopolitical location*. A *sensing policy* approach argues for a form of policy making that goes beyond tokenism in engagement with diverse groups to account for the diversity of lived experiences.

Geopolitical Location

As a site imbued with meaning, Aamjiwnaang's *geopolitical location* represents a unique place whose character is shaped by the daily activities of the local citizenry. Aligned with critical Indigenous scholarship and geopolitical thought, it is a core assertion of *sensing policy* that an emphasis on "place" paves the way for a more localized and situated understanding of public policy concerns on the ground (Alfred and Corntassel 2005; Coulthard 2014; Cresswell 2004; Ingold 2000, 2011; L. Simpson 2011; Thornton 2008; Tuan 1975). Deepening environmental justice policy through an affective approach to reproductive justice extends beyond atomistic models of public policy that frame individuals as "at fault" or to blame for their adverse health outcomes.

Moreover, an affective framework is necessary for effective policy making on environmental justice. Linking individual practice with "place" as an analytical category to address ongoing and persistent environmental and reproductive health concerns on a First Nations reserve provides an alternative way to think through the emergence of reproductive injustices in Canada and may open the door to more robust forms of place-based policy on public and environmental health.

Given the ongoing and unanswered questions about the impact of pollution exposure on reproductive health, we need to take reproductive justice more seriously in Canada. Building on experiential bodies of knowledge, including interview findings, media accounts, and grassroots, participatory involvement in the community, in addition to relevant literature, the theory of reproductive justice developed here brings a lived, experiential, and affective approach to "place" into policy. Moreover, an empirical and qualitative investigation of the situated concerns expressed by citizens of the Aamjiwnaang First Nation draws on voices in the field to challenge and contend with the predominant Eurocentric, Western notions of citizenship in Canada – in theory and practice – that discursively and structurally centre on the rational individual, who is considered to be distinct from location, situation, or environment. This investigation is one of justice from below. It is an examination of practices of citizenship that are experienced and expressed by individuals situated within relations of power. As this research takes place on and adjacent to an Anishinabek First Nations reserve, this book aims to make space for an Anishinabek approach to justice in order to radically rethink the meaning and ontology of citizenship, policy, and justice.

By constructing an approach to citizenship and policy informed by Anishinabek thought and lived experience, this book is a concrete attempt to share stories and knowledge about citizens' ongoing struggles as they confront an opaque, political problem – an ad hoc, discretionary, murky *policy assemblage* – in their work to create better avenues for addressing reproductive and environmental justice concerns in Canada. In doing so, it connects citizens' lived experience with broader contexts of current and historical geopolitical power. This requires a kind of "relational ethics," or a kind of relational citizenship, if we are to reframe how we think about encounters between the human and more-than-human (Rutherford 2011, 197). Such relationality aligns with a radical democratic approach to difference (Mouffe 2005b). This intersectional approach to the relations between human and more-than-human life gives meaning to the manifestation of complex power dynamics and furthermore draws into focus the extent of past and present policy impacts. A relational approach prompts us to recognize the "multiple actors, both human and non-human[,] that form our bodies, ourselves and our world," as well as to move beyond biopolitical subjectivity and spaces of green governmentality (Rutherford 2011, 203). It also presents a starting place for thinking differently about the policy assemblage of Indigenous environmental justice, reproductive justice, and citizenship.

Situated Bodies of Knowledge

To examine people, knowledge, and power in a personal and intimate setting, it is crucial to foster the conditions for meaningful relationships and in-depth, qualitative research with policy makers and community members. This approach situates political analysis beyond purely institutional parameters. That is not to say that power relations operate "outside" these parameters – indeed, such an escape is neither possible nor desirable – but this approach does stretch the limits of such parameters, revealing that grounded fields demand careful attention. As an ethnographic engagement of this terrain reveals, the state is but one site of governance to be taken up by political inquiry. Seeking to decentre political science's grip on the state as a primary axiom of analysis, an examination of multiple modalities of power, authority, and rule moves away from the state and into the field – literally and figuratively – to investigate the discursive and structural power relations that shape and constrain citizen action in a specific geopolitical locale.

Chapter 5 expanded a discussion of the systemic constraints that impact avenues for justice. The contested terrain of environmental reproductive justice reveals the disputed conditions for action, knowledge, and power. These disputes are corporeal, discursive, and structural. Discursively, an analysis of reproduction and the politics of reproductive justice highlights both Foucault's (1994a, 244) discussion of the genesis of the state and the ways that power today operates through productive forces, the "reproduction of relations of production," and the ways that citizens become governmentalized. As bodies mobilize, they generate and regenerate forceful meaning.

Chapter 6 shifted this study's lens from the community's experiences to the institutional public arena by focusing on encounters within the ongoing LCHS. This chapter illuminated contending *situated bodies of knowledge* – experiential, external, and engaged – to assess how Aamjiwnaang's embodied concerns became eclipsed by this countywide study due to the politics of science, scale, lifestyle blame, and jurisdictional ambiguity. Moreover, Chapter 6 discussed the difficulties citizens face when they mobilize engaged knowledge through resource- and time-intensive processes such as consultation and partnerships yet see limited systemic and regulatory change.

The occlusion of Aamjiwnaang's unique concerns raises important questions about the role that local knowledge should play in deliberative processes. There is often a lack of clarity about who or what constitutes expertise. Further, ideas about "evidence" or "science" underscore the "primacy of rationality" (Adkin 2009, 306). As LCHS deliberations demonstrated, scientific and epidemiological data provide only partial knowledge and present an incomplete picture of the reproductive concerns of Aamjiwnaang citizens in relation to their neighbours. There is thus a need for deliberative processes to creatively integrate alternative forms of iterative and nonlinear knowledge.

Decolonizing Environmental Justice

By making visible the ways that existing power relations shape policy processes and citizen struggles, and by creating space for diverse ways of knowing, *sensing policy* advocates for a decolonizing approach to policy making. A decolonizing lens draws into focus intersecting and inequitable forces of power. Working toward more just social policies requires acknowledging and celebrating diverse forms of life. In addition to drawing attention to experiential knowledge, the inclusion and discussion of Anishinabek thought through interviews with local knowledge carriers foregrounds an alternative way of conceptualizing human–more-than-human relationships as a matter of environmental reproductive justice. It requires thinking about our responsibilities to the more-than-human world and the intersection between physical and cultural survival. Equally, such recognition of responsibilities also entails creating conditions for thoughtful encounters between "humans and non-humans as participants in this dance" (Rutherford 2011, 201). This is only a starting point for decolonizing the current policy assemblage of Indigenous environmental justice. As Martineau (2014) notes, decolonization in theory, practice, and method entails "Indigenous ontological understandings of land and landscape." Such place-based understandings do not refer to a romantic precontact period; rather, they rely on embodied, grounded normativity (Coulthard 2014; L. Simpson 2011). Thus they offer some suggestions for political theorists and policy makers interested in engaging with the ontological and epistemological foundations for how we construct relationships with ourselves, each other, and environments.

Policy solutions to ongoing toxic exposure must be rooted in community and cultural practices. A *sensing policy* approach to environmental justice thus involves an examination of citizens' lived experiences and a focus on situated knowledge to achieve reproductive justice. As Hoover and colleagues (2012, 1648) discuss, future intersectional research requires "collaborative partnerships among researchers, health care providers, and community members ... to determine the impact of environmental contamination on community members' health and to develop necessary remediation, preventative measures, and protective policy interventions." Following suit, a *sensing policy* approach aligns with intersectionality and critical policy scholarship committed to a decolonizing research methodology (Fridkin 2012, 121; Hankivsky 2012; Orsini and Smith 2007) in order to ask crucial questions such as:

1. What kinds of policy problems are being framed and what assumptions underlie them?
2. How are policies framed and how has this framing changed over time?
3. In what ways do policies and policy processes represent, define, and portray knowledges structurally and discursively?
4. How do structural and discursive configurations enable or disable certain communities' access to policy making?
5. What are some avenues for the enhanced representation and inclusion of diverse voices and epistemologies in policy?

Moreover, research comparing the policy-making contexts that affect environmental justice in Canada and other countries will advance thinking in this field. In contrast to the US context, which has a robust policy framework for environmental justice, there is no formal overarching framework for environmental justice in the country. Overall, Canadian scholarship on environmental reproductive justice has been limited in theory and practice. An examination of the evolution, experience, and articulation of corporeal and environmental harms in Aamjiwnaang highlights, responds to, and addresses a prevalent scholarly and policy gap in pursuit of creating more substantive policies on environmental reproductive justice at all levels of government, from the micro to macro scale. This undertaking requires affective, experiential, embodied, and place-based policy making that brings situated, community experience at the micro level into conversation with the broader systemic meso and macro social, political, economic, legal, and environmental forces shaping ongoing struggles. This place-focused, *sensing policy* approach is important for "low-level geography" or for communities with a "small sample size."

In the Canadian context, there is a dearth of reproductive justice policy and scholarship. Reproductive justice in theory, method, and practice must connect lived experience to broader systemic political processes, including the institutional, discursive, and symbolic. It must interrogate a specific population's ability to reproduce future generations. Quoting tar sands activist Melina Laboucan-Massimo, Naomi Klein (2014) interrogates the intersectional logics of violence that powerfully mark Indigenous life: "Violence against Mother Earth is violence against women," as Indigenous women are at the forefront of Indigenous resurgence. When the capacity to physically reproduce is compromised, the viability of the entire community's cultural survival is at stake. "Slow violence" – physical and cultural – zaps community strength (ibid.; Nixon 2011). But as widespread, creative, regenerative movements like Idle No More are thrust into view, the story does not end here.

Local expertise and ways of knowing frequently emerge within struggles for environmental reproductive justice in dynamic and nonlinear ways. As with many forms of social mobilization, contending bodies of knowledge play out differently at various stages of a movement's activity. Interviews with citizens and stakeholders involved in the public policy process shaping Aamjiwnaang's reproductive and environmental justice concerns revealed how these concerns fell along a continuum of diverse bodies of knowledge. There is much more work to be done in order to account for the alternative forms of knowledge, science, and expertise that are rooted in the distinct practices of daily life. Arts-based approaches offer an avenue to access and generate new forms of knowledge in order to address injustice, while working toward a more socially just, deliberative, and participatory democracy.

How can policy officials make sense of the dynamic features of Indigenous environmental justice? Doing so requires rethinking how knowledge becomes recognized, understood, and communicated. A pressing concern in advancing intersectionality-based policy analysis is the need to develop explicit, clear, and user-friendly methods for translating theory into practice so that it may be used by decision makers and policy makers rather than being used merely to deconstruct policy or language (Fridkin 2012, 128; Hankivsky 2012, 20). How can we think about the vibrant modes in which expressions of Indigenous environmental justice transpire? As a transformative approach committed to justice, not only does this framework require a *multilayered analysis* that accounts for *lived experience, geopolitical location,* and *situated bodies of knowledge,* but it also requires attention to five key principles of creative engagement: *reflexivity, relationships, reciprocity, respect,* and *resurgence.*

Creative Engagement

Policy making is an art and a craft. As new policy puzzles emerge, those responsible for making critical decisions must find new ways to engage diverse forms of knowledge. Storytelling is a way of doing so. Stories are rich sites of knowledge. They include meanings, activities, and articulations expressed and enacted by those situated in the field of these relations. Stories are place-based. They are not a "formal authorized kind of transmissible knowledge beyond contexts outside those of practical application"; on the contrary, they are "based in feeling, consisting in the skills, sensitivities and orientations that have developed through long experience of conducting one's life in a particular environment" (Ingold 2000, 29). Stories shed light on an array of vantage points, revealing the range of practices, activities, worldviews, and knowledges generated within communities based on emotions, intuition, and perception. Such experiential knowledge is not inferior to reason but is crucial to justice, substantive policy, and a fleshier democracy.

A fleshy democracy requires innovative thinking about the meaning and practice of citizenship. Enacting citizenship is a creative, practice-based action. It is a form of "feeling citizenship" (A. Simpson 2003, 10). The experiences of communities facing reproductive and environmental degradation challenge conventional understandings of citizenship. We must think about citizenship as more than a rule or status. It is an enacted practice, not simply a "category" for citizens to receive or a passive object for citizens to attain. As Tully (2008b) discusses, a creative approach to justice moves away from thinking about citizenship in terms of the granting of civil, political, or social rights and toward an examination of citizenship as a set of ongoing practices and responsibilities in relation to one's livelihood and environment. The approach to citizenship advanced here moves beyond a conventional status-based approach, and thus beyond thinking about the inclusion or exclusion of citizens in society, by examining the ongoing activities and engagements that citizens enact, experience, and feel in their daily lives.

Reflexivity

Community-engaged scholarship requires a careful examination of identity and an awareness about our own positionalities and privileges. It is important that researchers think critically about the values, perspectives, and biases that they bring to the research setting. When a researcher approaches a community to conduct a study, he or she must acknowledge the diverse forms of knowledge that exist in the community and adopt a position of learning. This stance requires a considerable degree of humility and a commitment to ongoing dialogue and personal transformation. It often entails multiple layers of accountability to keep one's privileged vantage point in check.

A reflexive and interpretive lens draws into focus what is both visible and obscured in our society. It investigates which techniques enable certain forms of power to emerge while marginalizing others. Scholarship committed to engaged and empirically grounded research using a *sensing policy* approach acknowledges the multiplicity of views that citizens hold about "the world" of their experiences. This approach seeks to witness,[9] hear, document, and render visible microscopic and marginalized aspects of our societies that are inexorably linked to broader socio-political forces outside the purview of mainstream society.

With the intention of contributing to policy making that is rooted in place-based and experiential approaches to reproductive justice, reflexive analysis stands apart from formal, or conventional, models of social science inquiry to generate theoretical findings about ongoing injustices through engagement with the messy contextuality of life experience while acknowledging that our shared futures are embroiled within existing struggles for environmental reproductive justice. This "messiness" stems from the fact that politics emerge through assemblages and extend beyond the realm of institutions to include government's apparatuses and administration as well as citizenship, revealing how power relations are formed through the extension of the state's tentacles into the spaces, intimacies, and micro practices of everyday life. This view rejects the notion that "government" is coterminous with formal or official institutions of power, known as "the state"; rather, "government" encompasses a multitude of processes and practices inside and outside the state that shape individuals and communities toward desired ends.

An intersectional and interpretive investigation of these issues is informed by a desire to present findings about citizen struggles for knowledge, science, and expertise that will contribute to a shared creation of spaces for concrete policy change that recognizes alternative ways of thinking, being, and articulation. This intention aligns with a commitment to justice and inspires a larger objective of enhancing substantive deliberative dialogue about environmental reproductive justice. Overall, the interpretive approach, paired with a commitment to community engagement as a decolonizing methodology, seeks concrete social change. For those committed to social action and political mobilization, the most appropriate way to conceptualize and engage with participatory research is as a passionate supporter, without trying to guide, steer, or dominate activism within a community mobilizing for change.

Relationships

When researchers enter these relational fields, the task of building, maintaining, and sustaining relationships – from witnessing injustice to listening to stories and walking or paddling together – is an important part of this community-engaged methodology. Aligned with the principles of the Two Row Wampum and Canada's ongoing responsibilities as treaty peoples, a commitment to relationships is as crucial to decolonizing Canadian politics as it is to research methodology (Keefer 2014; Kovach 2009; L.T. Smith 1999). Relationship building before, during, and after is central to the project's ethics, engagement, and long-term success. An approach to data collection that infuses interpretive analysis with a commitment to decolonizing methodology incorporates a collaborative, participatory, and community-engaged model. Conducting an engaged, participatory study connects research with ongoing practice by sharing knowledge and authority about the study's design, development, and results with the community and by inviting their involvement in all stages of the process.

Sensing policy, as an affective framework for analyzing environmental reproductive justice, hones in on macro and micro scales to grasp the multidimensional complexity of such policy issues. In McGregor's (2009) words, an appropriate approach to environmental justice must include the concept of "all our relations" and the understanding that relationships based on environmental justice are "not limited to relations between people but consist of those among all beings of creation." In an Indigenous context, environmental (in)justice entails a concern with human–more-than-human relations, in addition to both physical and cultural survival.

Citizens in Aamjiwnaang and the surrounding area interpret the relationship between oneself and environment in many ways, which expose contesting subjectivities. At times, experiential community concerns come into tension with scientific knowledge. Many of these tensions centre on different philosophies of human-nature, body-environment, and self-earth relations (J. Borrows 2010; Doerfler, Sinclair, and Stark 2013; Johnston 2005). These tensions highlight ontologically contested notions of how humans relate to their selves, lands, and environments and problematize the meaning of citizenship itself. Citizenship, as a relational practice, is inseparable from identity. Relational ecological citizenship intersects with Indigeneity, place-based belonging, and what it means to "be" an Indigenous person. This radically troubles liberal approaches to citizen subjectivity, which portray citizen subjects as distinct from, and masters over, the inanimate nonhuman world.

Identity is central to being in place for many Indigenous communities across the country. As Indigenous scholar Nick Claxton stated before a National Energy

Board hearing on November 28, 2014, in Victoria, British Columbia, when describing his local environment, reefnet-fishing practices, and ways of life in Coast Salish territory, "Those islands are our relatives ... That really reflects our connection to this place as very deep. Our word for islands, *tetaces,* [means] relatives of the deep. They're our relatives" (NEB 2014, 11565). In his oral testimony, Claxton continued to articulate the significance of the local ecosystem, including the islands, fishing, and ceremonies, as the backbone of Coast Salish society. He noted the responsibilities of his community to the salmon and to future generations. This is exemplary of an intersectional and relational approach to ecological citizenship and place-based belonging.

Similarly, according to Alfred and Corntassel (2005, 597), being Indigenous is characterized by a "place-based existence." Cultural survival in a settler-colonial world stems from heritage rooted in attachment to land. Leanne Simpson (2012) articulates this deep-rooted connection: "I stand up anytime our nation's land base is threatened because everything we have of meaning comes from the land – our political systems, our intellectual systems, our health care, food security, language and our spiritual sustenance and our moral fortitude." Maintaining an inherent connection to land is central to being Indigenous and is the crux of Indigeneity. The spirit of Indigenous nationhood and Indigeneity entails a connection to a distinct existence, to each other, and to territories, communities, ceremonies, languages, and histories (Alfred and Corntassel 2005, 599). Continuing to practice a connection to place thus presents a starting point for cultural resurgence in the face of encroaching colonialism and subjugation, as well as toxic exposure. Sustaining this connectivity is an inherent feature of a conception of ecological citizenship that is radically different from environmental citizenship and liberal subjectivity.

Reciprocity

Examining environmental and reproductive (in)justice requires methodological innovation. As Chapters 4 and 6 discussed, lived or felt experience frequently constitutes the knowledge and expertise shaping corporeal claims articulated by citizens seeking policy change. Communities take action themselves, with their bodies on the line, to gather knowledge about perceived problems affecting their daily lives. The manner in which these claims are articulated differs from the conventional scientific model and may occur through a forum that is more artistic, emotive, and feeling.

The task of accessing, interpreting, and examining situated knowledges requires creative thinking about how to conduct research on environmental reproductive justice. In my experience as a participatory researcher, connecting with Aamjiwnaang citizens of all ages flowed from my passion for artistic forms of expression. My initial introduction to the community through a youth PhotoVoice project paved the way for engagement with young people and enabled me to gain an understanding of their concerns (Flicker et al. 2008; Scott and Smith 2012). Subsequently, young members of the Aamjiwnaang Green Teens presented their images – photographs, paintings, collages, and sketches – all of which were revelatory of their situated and ongoing concerns about the impact of pollution on their way of life. Music, particularly rap, also provided a form of expression through which these young people could speak out about their lived experiences. Thus future trajectories for research on environmental reproductive (in)justice will benefit from integrating arts-based research methodologies to access and share the voices of young people and those who may not be comfortable with traditional qualitative research methods like focus groups and interviews. Such opportunities enable researchers to connect with community members on a profound, shared emotional level, creating intersubjective knowledge exchange.

Moreover, visuality presents an intellectual and theoretical challenge to dominant discourses when words fall short. That which is seen – visible – can lead to social awareness, critique, and change. Exploring "art" is a way to upset or contend with dominant narratives and discourses. It can counter the "hit and run" approach to ethnographic research.[10] By participating in a youth-driven documentary film project in the final stages of my immersion, I engaged in an interactive process that countered Western models of knowledge, which often privilege monolithic models of visualization, representation, and aestheticization. As knowledge production involves "abstraction, interpretation and representation" (Campbell 2007, 379), artistic media offer a potential avenue for resistance.

The inclusion of multimedia in research sources is "democratic" insofar as it can "weaken the role of the specialized producer or *auteur* by using procedures based on chance, or mechanical techniques which anyone can learn, and by being corporate or collaborative" (Sontag 1997, 149). Film has power, striking an emotional chord and eliciting an affective response. It fleshes out bodies of knowledge when words fall short; it nets chaos and challenges dominant discourses and stereotypes. It can be subversive and give presence to absence. Through creative means like photography, film, and music, communities can vocalize and destabilize dominant discursive paradigms. This ability suggests possibilities for resistance to biopower and injustice through interactive, intersubjective, and emergent aesthetics.

Respect

Despite the continuous presence of contemporary colonialism, Indigenous communities demonstrate ongoing resistance and resilience. Emphasizing ongoing injustices does not go far enough to achieve justice. Instead, we must respect Indigenous experiences, knowledges, and stories. Examining adverse health outcomes and indicators can pathologize individuals and communities. This effect is especially problematic in colonial contexts. Thus moving from a "deficit" model of health toward an assets-based approach is crucial to centring the strength, resistance, and innovation of Indigenous peoples as they search for self-determination (Loppie and Marsden 2014, 1). Creative, strengths-based methodologies of engagement can promote optimal health outcomes from the ground up, while highlighting diverse knowledges in pursuit of decolonizing research.

In light of the ongoing practices in Aamjiwnaang, where citizens are drawn into governmental processes like participating in health studies, reporting concerns to a Spills Action Centre, and following shelter-in-place protocols, the links between participatory democracy and social justice come to the fore. Such processes reveal how citizens mobilize and struggle for knowledge, science, and expertise to mitigate their corporeal and ecological concerns. The treatment of these concerns in administrative and deliberative processes illuminates the boundaries of Canadian democracy and highlights relationships between institutional configurations of power assemblages and lived experiences on the ground.

Citizenship is thus an analytical concept that extends beyond a narrow focus on the role of the state and its extension into the citizenry. In contrast to thinking about citizens in terms of a category of meaning imposed from above, the approach to ecological citizenship and reproductive justice advanced here builds up from community experience. As an affective, place-based ontology of citizenship, it focuses on the feelings, attachments, sentiments, and aspirations spoken and enacted by citizens who express concerns regarding their bodies and environments.

Citizenship, understood here as ecological citizenship, is place-specific. It pertains to an interconnected relationship between the human and more-than-human worlds. In the documentary *Force of Nature*, scientist and environmental activist David Suzuki states, "When you destroy the air, you destroy us" (Gunnarsson 2010). This eloquently captures how many citizens of Aamjiwnaang ascribe meaning to their ways of living with the more-than-human world. It speaks to the ways that the conditions shaping how one lives have much to do with how individuals act and with how they respond to and feel about their environments and consequently about themselves. Individuals relate to and are impacted by their environments. As Tully (2008a) argues, individuals are embedded in larger relationships and habitats, for which they are responsible. The more-than-human world is essential to one's being. One cannot be separated from this world as a managerial steward. Many Indigenous elders explain that the identities of their people are related to the places where they live and "that the creator has placed them here with the responsibility to care for life in all its harmonious diversity" (ibid., 250). Thus the responsibility to care for all ecologically interrelated forms of life is timeless when one looks back to the wisdom of ancestors and seven generations forward to the future. Tully (ibid.) continues, "This unshakeable sense of responsibility to the source and network of life is at the core of Indigenous identity." This is coupled with an individual's sense of his or her place in relation to nature. It is not a "stewardship" mode of care but an ontological practice. It is a way of life and, ultimately, a way of being.

In Newtonian-Cartesian fashion, a Western, Eurocentric, liberal worldview of ecological citizenship treats land as distinct from human action and regards it as needing management and care by individuals cultivating the environment as responsible stewards. In radical contrast, Indigenous worldviews tend to articulate a relational, embodied, and *storied* connection to place, land, and the environment (Alfred 2009; Alfred and Corntassel 2005; J. Borrows 2002, 2010; Bryan 2000; Doerfler, Sinclair, and Stark 2013; McGregor and Plain 2013). As Alfred and Corntassel (2005, 609) explain, Indigenous peoples understand that all entities of "nature" – plants, animals, stones, trees, mountains, rivers, lakes, and a host of others – represent "embodied" relationships that are to be honoured. "Land is life" (ibid., 613). This dynamic and interconnected respect for land, as "Mother Earth," is a central tenet of Anishinabek ontology, which considers the earth to be an animate living being, where everything has a heartbeat. We are all related.

Resurgence

Widespread movements, from healing walks and studies on traditional plant use to flash-mob powwows, demonstrate multiple forms of resistance. As expressions of cultural resurgence, music, song, dance, and drumming enable communities to speak out. At the same time, resistance in order to protect cultural resurgence also emerges through standing one's ground, physical and cultural survival, and being alive in the face of environmental injustice. Confronting ongoing forces of colonization is an act of resistance itself. In various ways, art can be both "medicine" and a "survival tool"; it is a sign of identity, place, and presence (France Trépanier, cited in Flicker et al. 2014, 17). Art propels people, raises awareness, and builds community. It "provides space for meaning-making, for the negotiation of identity, and for the expression of counter-hegemonic political realities" (ibid., 29). The artistic medium takes on particular resonance in Indigenous communities, many of which have long-standing practices of oral traditions and ceremonies to pass on cultural knowledge. From drumming to dancing, actions are important means of storytelling about particular places and identities. These affective practices have deep roots in resistance. Amendments to the Indian Act in 1884 banned the potlatch and, with it, cultural expression and the right to sing, dance, and gather (ibid., 17). Thus, in reclaiming these creative arts – through gathering together, singing, and dancing – each process becomes an inherent act of resistance. Citizens' bodies become physical and cultural conduits for social change. For many Indigenous peoples who are confronting cultural erasure, art has the potential to aid in transformation by showcasing both how things are and how they could be otherwise.

The time is certainly ripe for thinking about new forms of research that imagine alternative possibilities for environmental reproductive justice. Given that Indigenous youth are one of the fastest-growing populations today, strengths-based approaches that rely on the "talents and energies" of Indigenous youth are central to developing new forms of decolonizing knowledge that emphasize research as resistance (Flicker et al. 2014, 16). In the protection and promotion of Indigenous culture and expression, valuing and respecting youth voices through the processes and products of collaborative art making can open up possibilities for democratizing knowledge, revitalization, and healing. As Flicker and colleagues (ibid., 25) draw into focus through collaborative, arts-based, participatory research, contemporary and traditional art – from carving to hip-hop and graffiti – has the power and potential to "promote dialogue and transmit important messages." It can help others to see culture through an accessible medium, while challenging stereotypes and promoting a dynamic sense of Indigenous identity, or Indigeneity. Art can also speak truth to policy. In this intersubjective, multilogical, and poetic vein – and with the aim of contributing to an ongoing conversation about Indigenous environmental justice – I close a chapter with images of the community and with words from its citizens.

Our Home
Mother Earth

Each night I look up to the Moon and Stars
And thank the Creator they yet have no scars
Not like the Earth, our home and Mother
She is being abused almost beyond repair
On sunny days I trace the sun through the haze
Who freely sends to us heat and light each day
Elders told me wildlife ran unafraid and free
Pictures of extinct ones now are just a memory
Once all the forests bloomed fresh, green leaves
Where today now stand skeletons of trees
Fishing and swimming will be a thing of before
As we see dead fish lying on polluted shores
Flowing water is known to be the veins of Earth
When her arteries stop flowing so will all of birth
At one time the water was clear, pure, and free
Today we buy it cleaned and bottled as a luxury
The Old Ones say, once we could breathe fresh air
Inhale the air these days, there is danger here
Nature is life, without it there is no humanity
People won't see living with all creates harmony
Many beautiful cultures all live on this world
All have a tremendous heritage, they feel so proud
We could share our good traits and precious values
Keeping our spiritual beliefs and sacred traditions
People would all smile, laugh, and live in peace
They then would see how much they are truly blessed
As I speak to the Creator with my daily prayer
Giving my respect and thanks for life here
One day I vision all people to open their hearts
To respect and live as one with Mother Earth
~ To you, your children, and their children

Keith Rogers, Aamjiwnaang First Nation

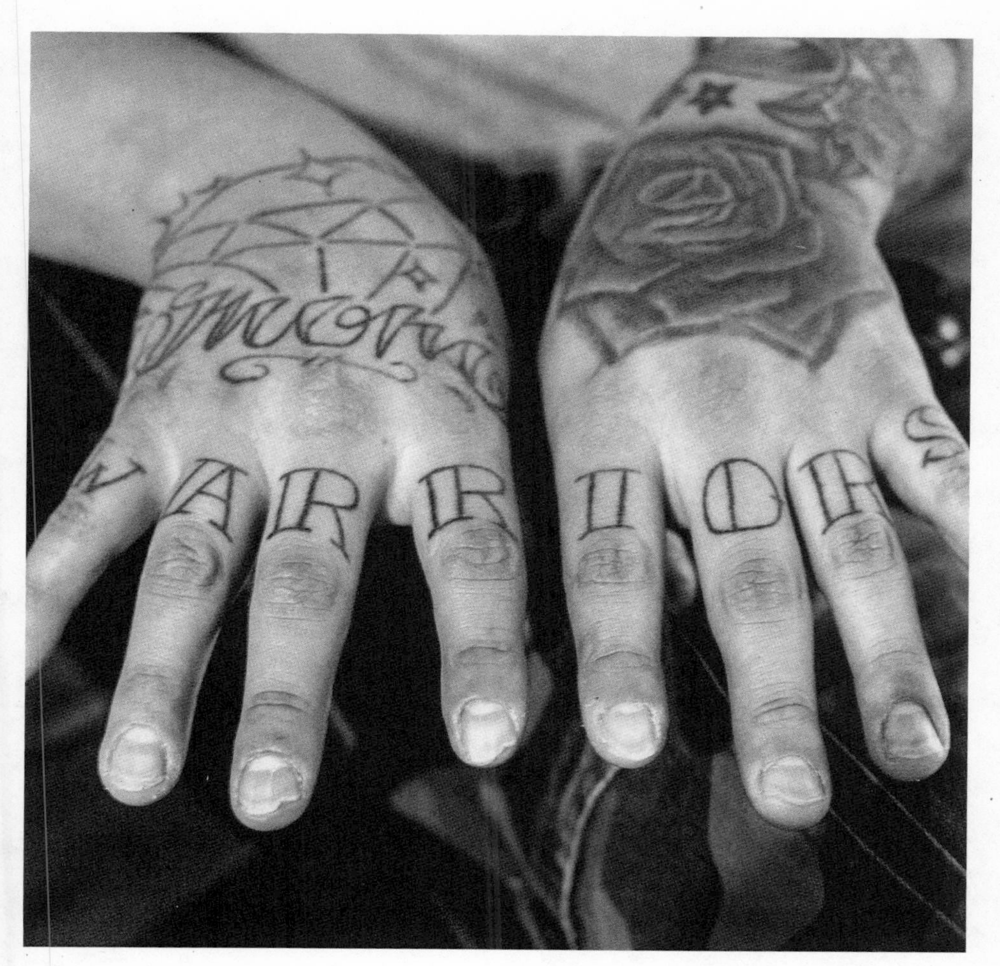

14

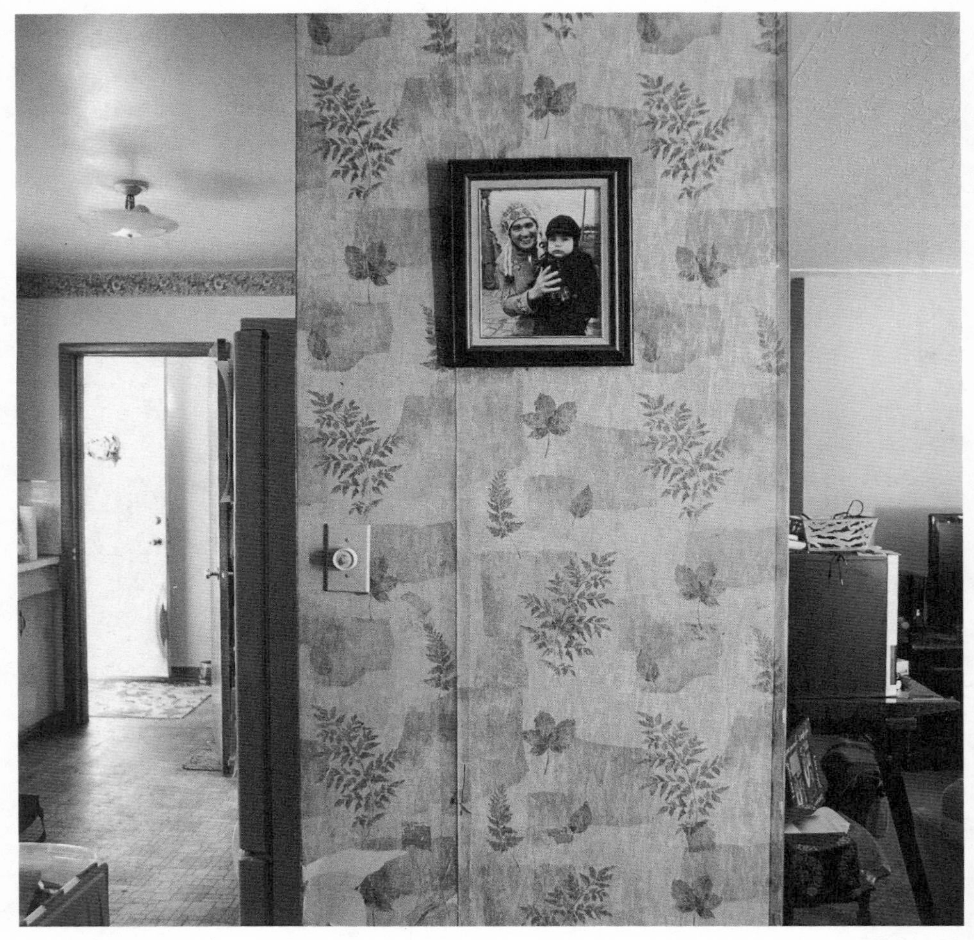

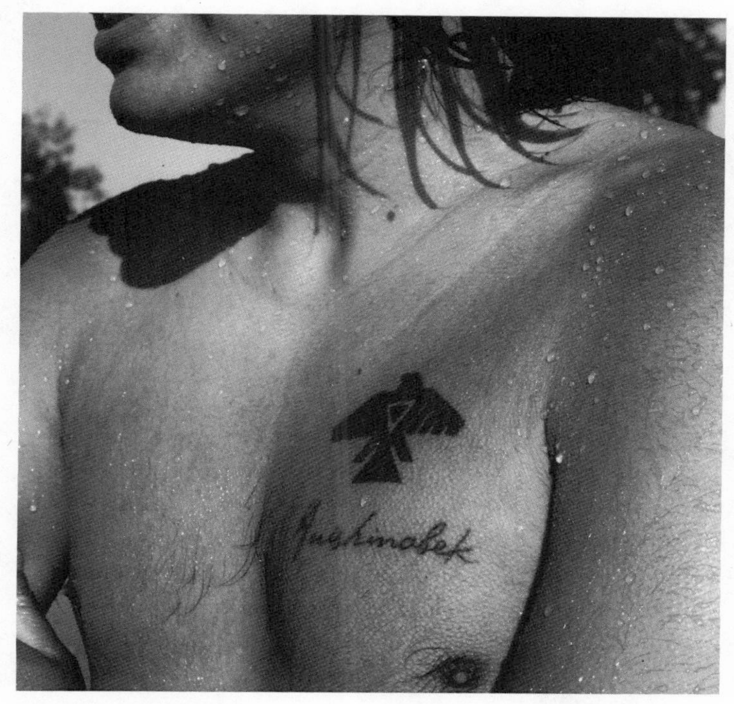

16

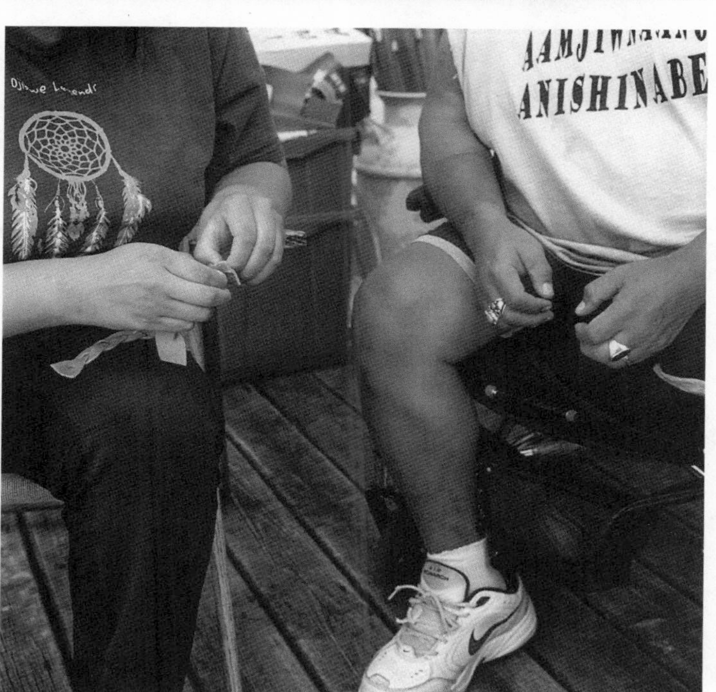

17

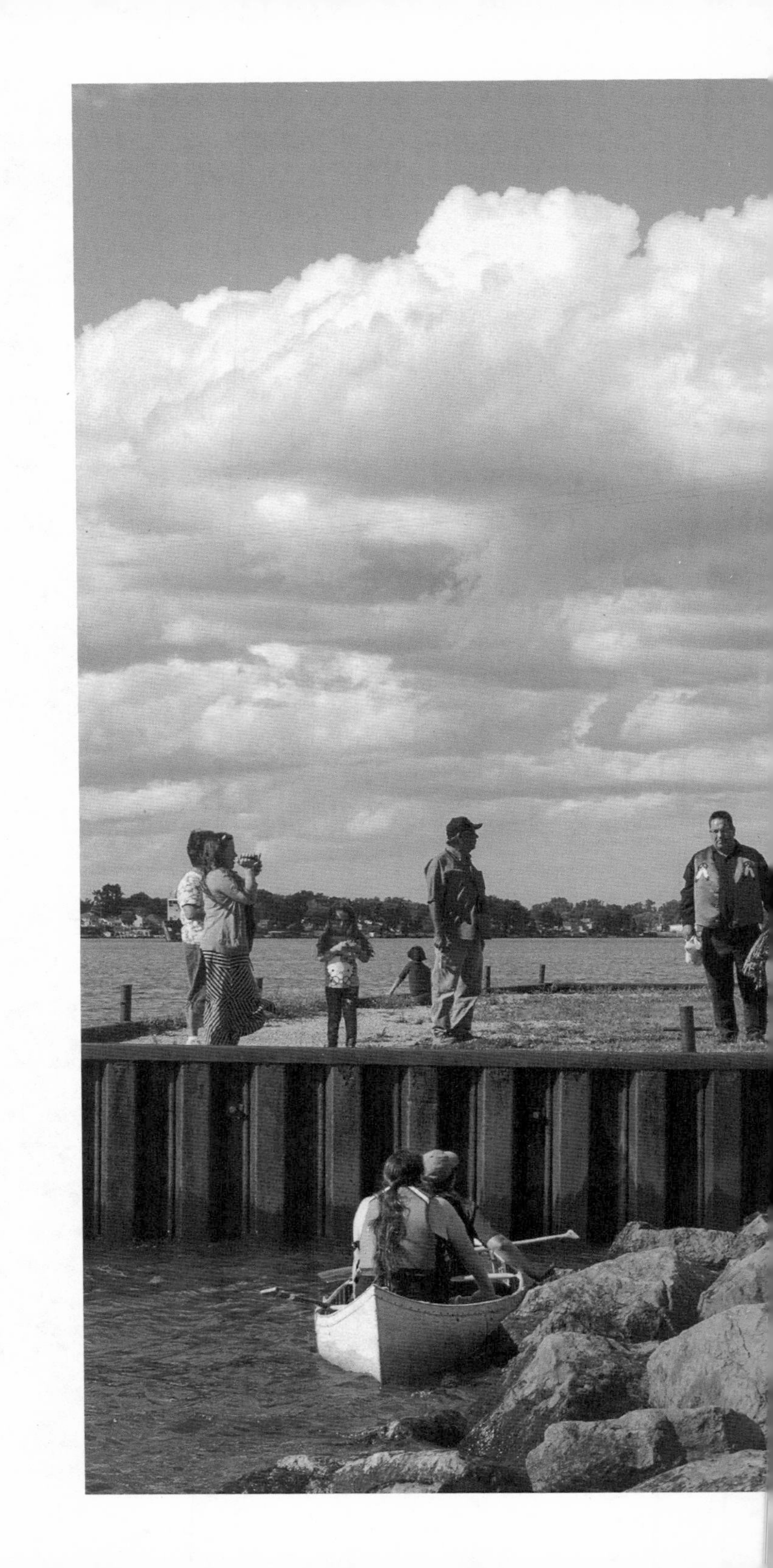

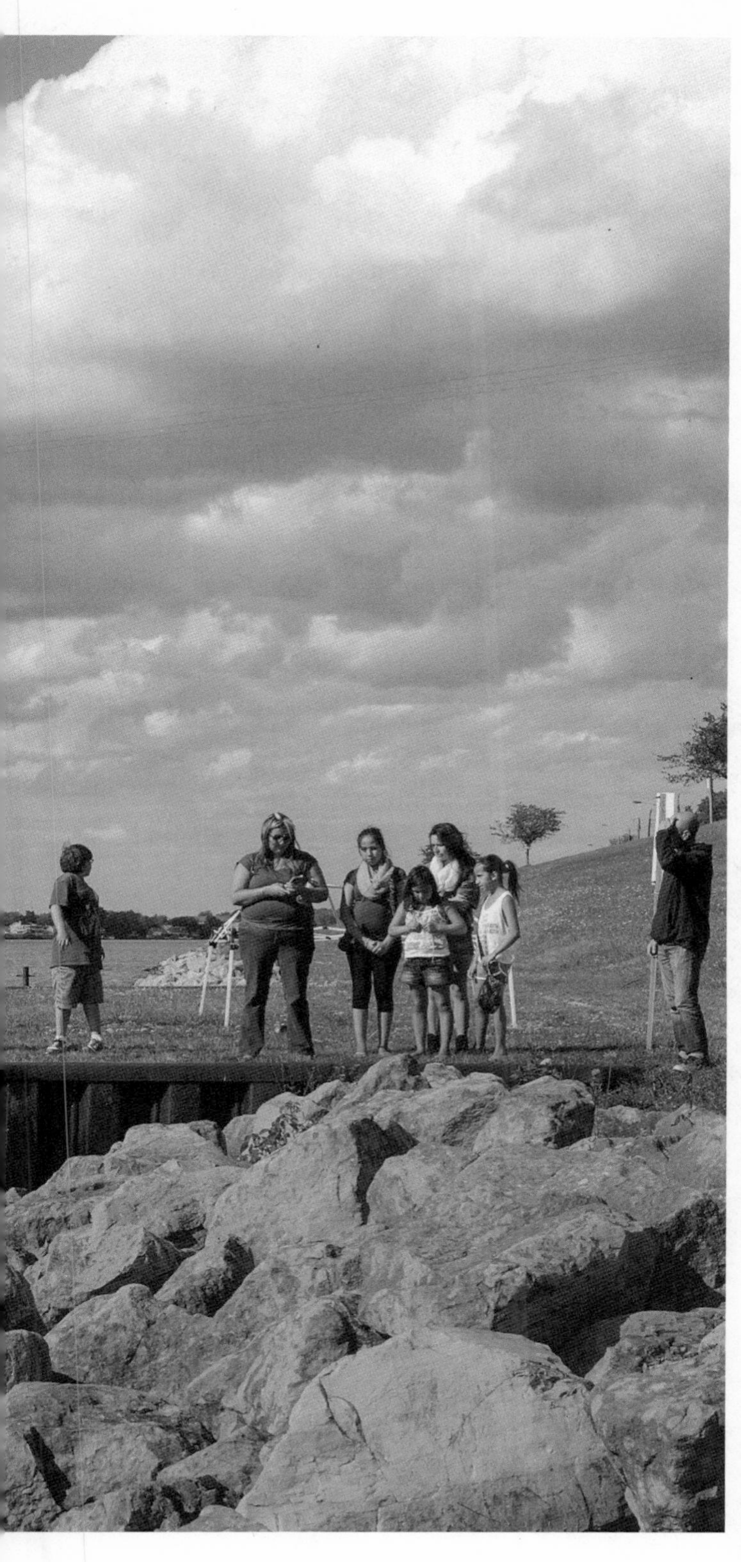

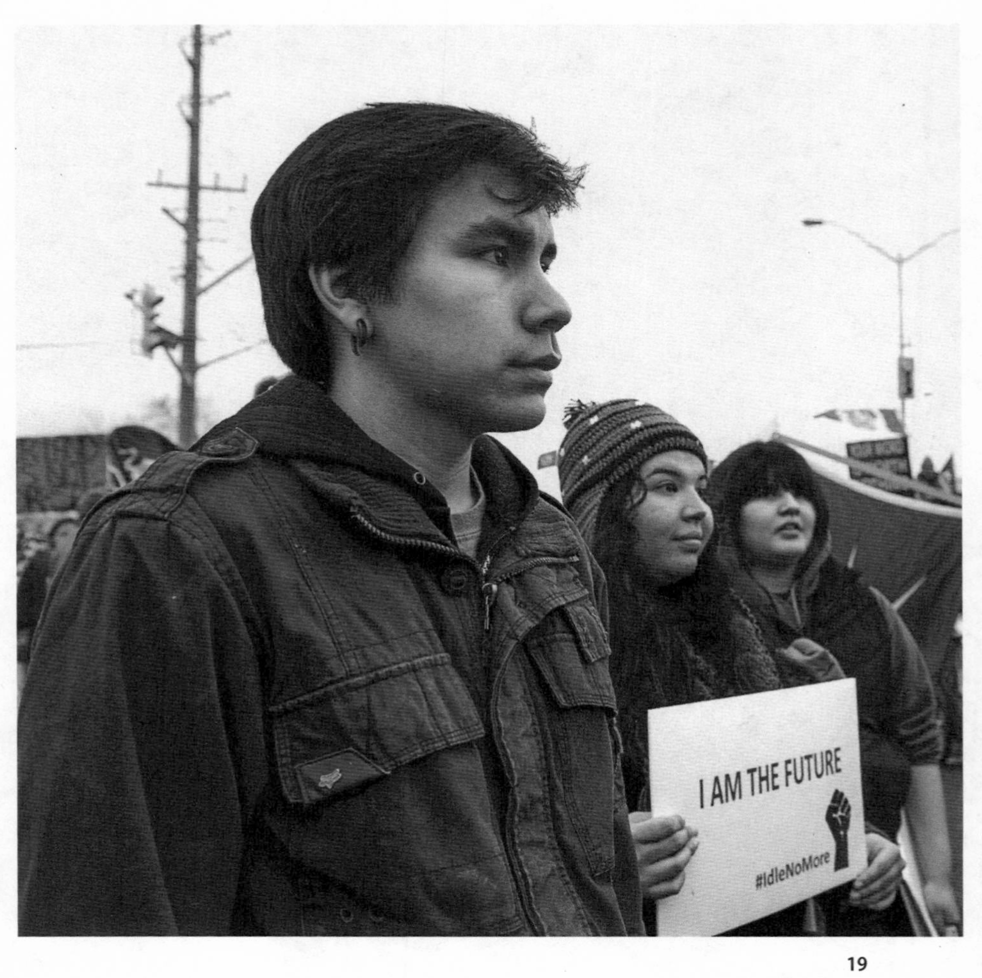
I AM THE FUTURE
#IdleNoMore

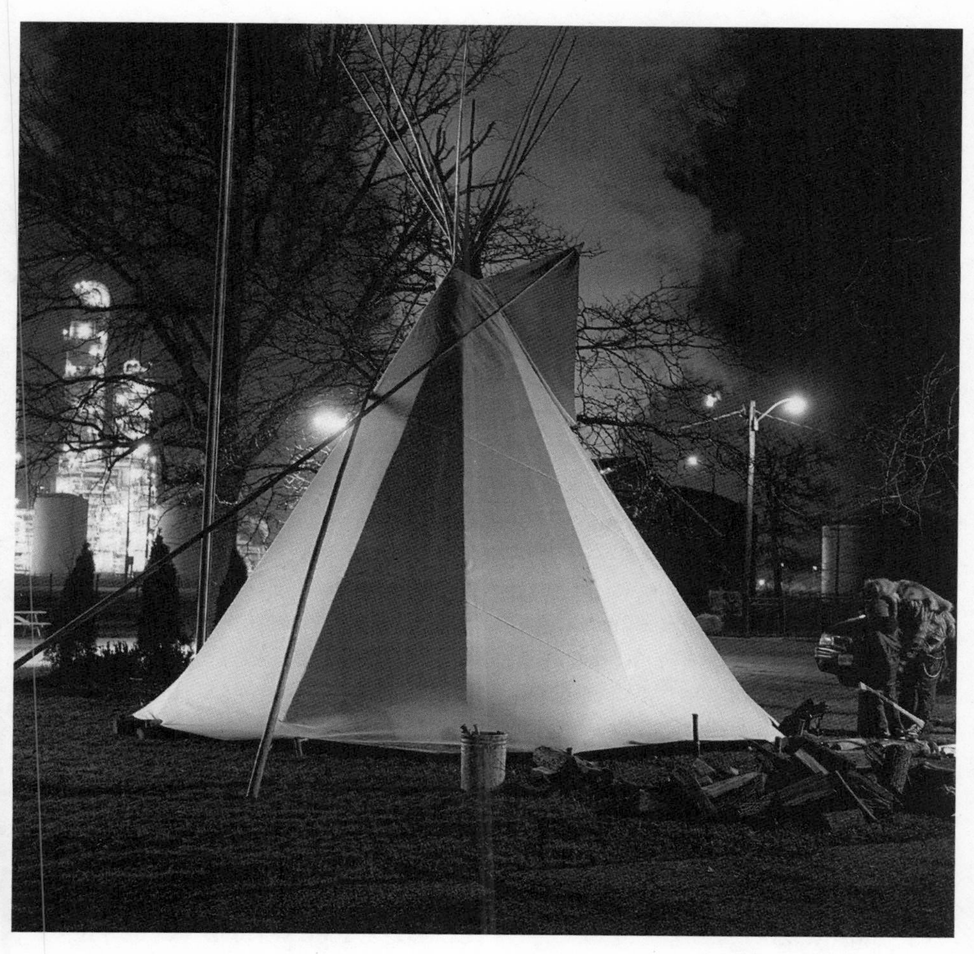

20

Resurgence

"We are not souvenirs"

Inside the teepee, where the air was thick with smoke, an earthy smell rose from a fire in the middle. About a dozen community members gathered around its warmth in humble silence. They would break it only to say "miigwetch" in thanks to Mother Earth for seeing to their needs. Gratitude also extended to their peers for being sources of strength and moral guidance. Mckay, then twenty-one years old, sat among them. He had played an instrumental role in getting everyone together.

Mckay explained that only a year prior he had remained in his basement, writing and recording rap songs, because there was nothing out there for him. But in December 2012 he came out and stood on the frontline of a campaign against new laws that would further impede his community's ability to protect itself from the impacts of the surrounding industries. For four days, he fasted. He wanted to support Chief Theresa Spence, who began a hunger strike to force Canadian Prime Minister Stephen Harper to meet with Indigenous representatives. Mckay also sought to embark on a spiritual quest in order to reconnect with his ancestors.

Across from him sat Vanessa, also in her early twenties. She had left Aamjiwnaang to go to cooking school, but after a semester, she returned, driven by the desire to bring awareness to her people's plight. Lindsey, her younger sister, was next to her. A champion of creative outlets, from traditional crafts to theatre, she uses her skills to share stories and to voice her concerns about the treatment of her community.

These young adults and their friends are torn between two ways of life: one rooted in age-old Anishinabek traditions and one ruled by consumerism; one grounded in respect for nature's gifts and the other looking to use, and abuse, them. Each day is a battle to decide which customs to keep and which to let fade away, which fights to take on and which to abandon as already lost. Every decision forces them to reconcile their pride in their heritage with the dictates of modern and Western ways. This is no easy task.

Many are driven away by the difficulty of living as they wish in a toxic environment. Some wrestle with depression and the spectre of suicide. All oscillate between moments of helplessness and moments of defiance. All, in their own way – whether through tattoos, powwows, healing walks, fasts, sweats, or public advocacy – speak up, shouting in unity that they are strong and alive, proud and spirited. They will not be reduced to museums, textbooks, or souvenirs. They will not be idle.

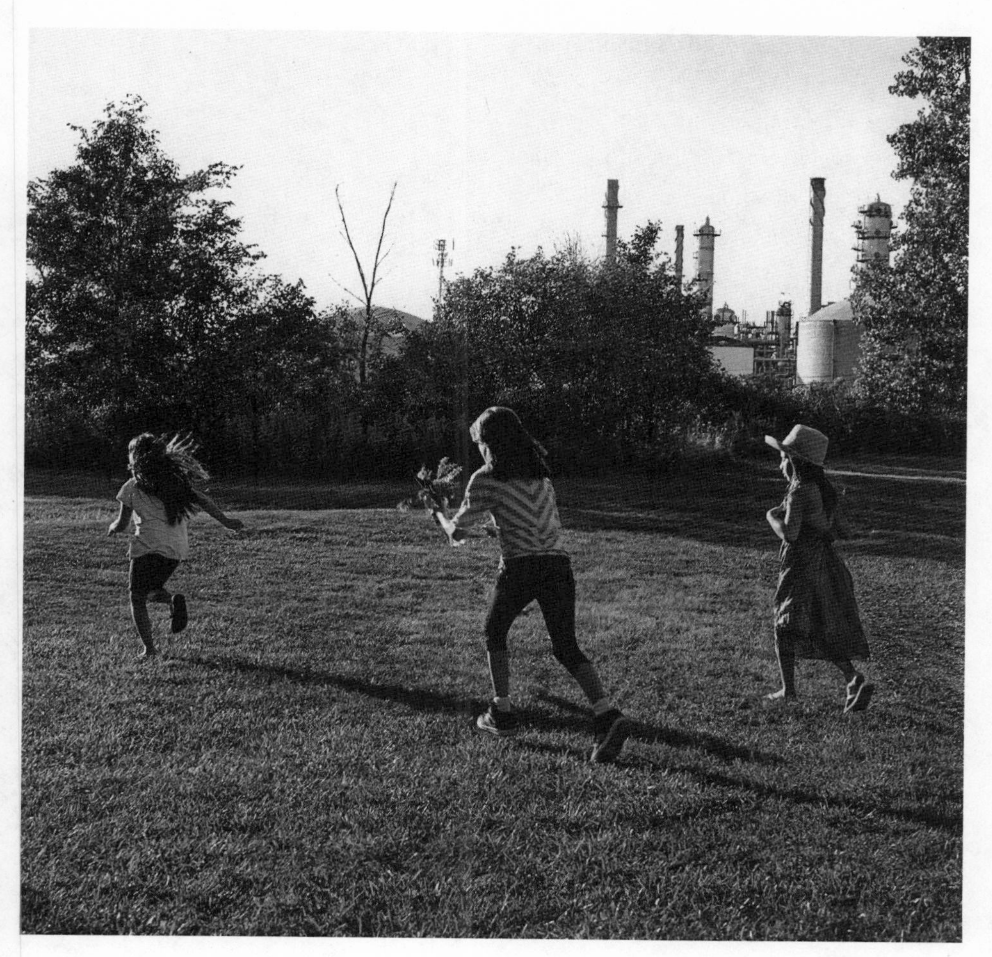

Epilogue: Life's Inspiration

I will continue to survive ...
in the midst of toxic surroundings,
that touch my being ...
I will continue to survive.

I still feel vibrant and full of life ...
with contaminations that invade my space ...
I still feel vibrant and full of life.

I am strong and still all-powerful ...

While money and greed
try to uproot my existence ...
I am strong and still all-powerful.

I stand for inspiration, pride, and determination ...
with minds bent on total destruction ...

I stand for inspiration, pride, and determination.

M'SKWAA GIIZHIG.

By Mike Plain, Aamjiwnaang First Nation,
January 2015

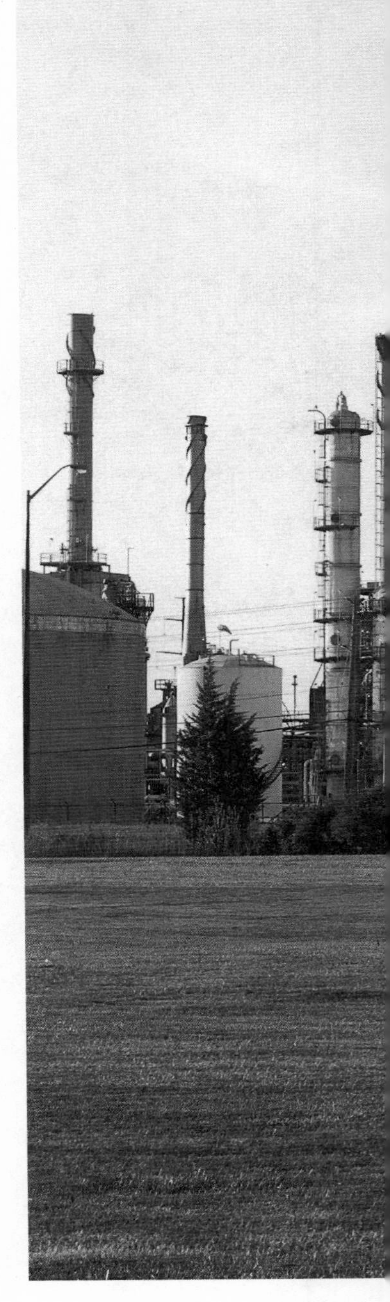

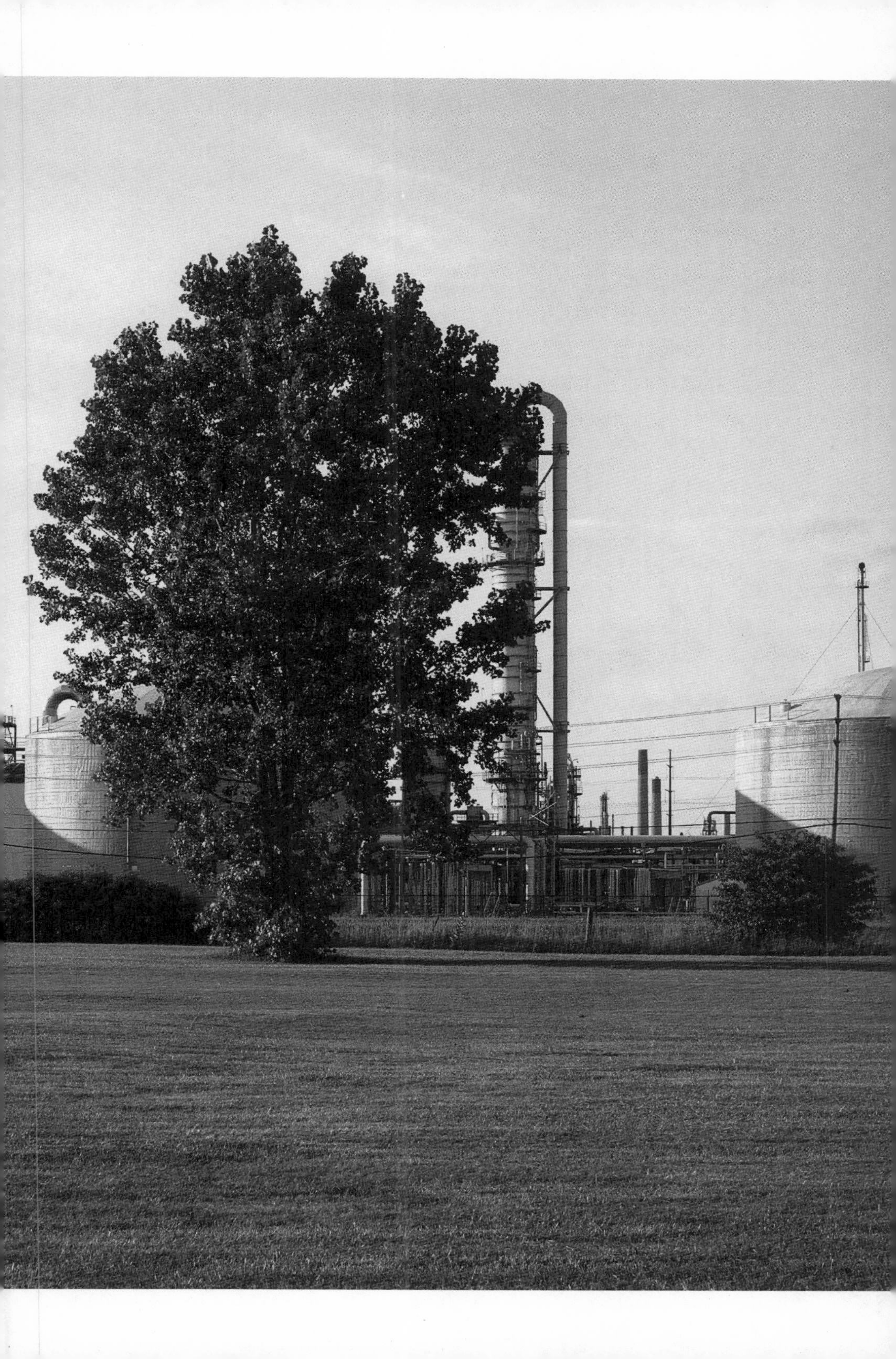

CAPTIONS

14 Clarence shows his tattoos, which honour his heritage. "Warriors," permanently inscribed on his knuckles, refers to his lineage. The diamond is a tribute to his mother and the rose to a friend who passed away. August 2013.

15 A photograph of Jake as a young child with Ovide Mercredi, then national chief, hangs in the living room. Jake went on to pursue general arts studies at nearby Lambton College in hopes of revitalizing an Ojibwe-language program in his community. August 2014.

16 Jake sports the Anishinabek emblem on his chest. Thunderbirds, the *animikii*, rule the skies. Lightning shoots from their eyes. Their cries and the flapping of their wings create the thunder. August 2014.

17 Youth leader Lindsey sits with Aamjiwnaang elder Mike Plain, who lost a leg to diabetes. Together, they make leather bracelets. Skilled artists of different generations, they exchange tips, techniques, and knowledge on how to make items such as traditional jewellery, dreamcatchers, and woven baskets. August 2012.

18 Aamjiwnaang citizens, including Chief Chris Plain (centre), welcome the paddlers taking part in a "water walk" and offer them braided sweetgrass. Three days earlier, participants left Ipperwash at the Kettle Point and Stony Point reserves by foot or canoe, sixty kilometres upstream. The journey honours Mother Earth and the water spirits. It is also a means to reconnect with traditional teachings. Women have a particular responsibility for seeing that these water teachings thrive. August 2014.

19 On a chilly December day, Jake, Vanessa, and Lindsey joined First Nations communities from across southern Ontario to take part in an Idle No More protest – a national grassroots movement defending Indigenous treaty rights. The march temporarily closed down Highway 401 near London, Ontario. December 2012.

20 At the height of the Idle No More movement, Mckay went on a four-day fast. He believed it would be a way to demonstrate support for the effort, gain spiritual strength, and bring his community together. He spent his days in a teepee raised for the occasion, welcoming peers, learning from elders, and sharing insights. December 2012.

21 Children who took part in the three-hour healing walk around Aamjiwnaang still have energy at the end to run through the field directly across from petro-chemical plants. In 2005 a study published by the journal *Environmental Health Perspectives* documented community concerns about a skewed birth ratio, known as the male "birth dearth." August 2013.

22 A large, flourishing eastern cottonwood stands tall. It faces the Lanxess polymer plant across the highway. In the midst of Chemical Valley, Aamjiwnaang and its twelve square kilometres of forest and bushes are vital green lungs. The tree is a symbol of the community's resilience, a beacon of hope, and a source of inspiration. August 2013.

Photos and text by Laurence Butet-Roch

Appendices

Appendix 1: Birth Ratio

Proportion of live male births (male live births/total live births) for Aamjiwnaang First Nation, 1984–2003

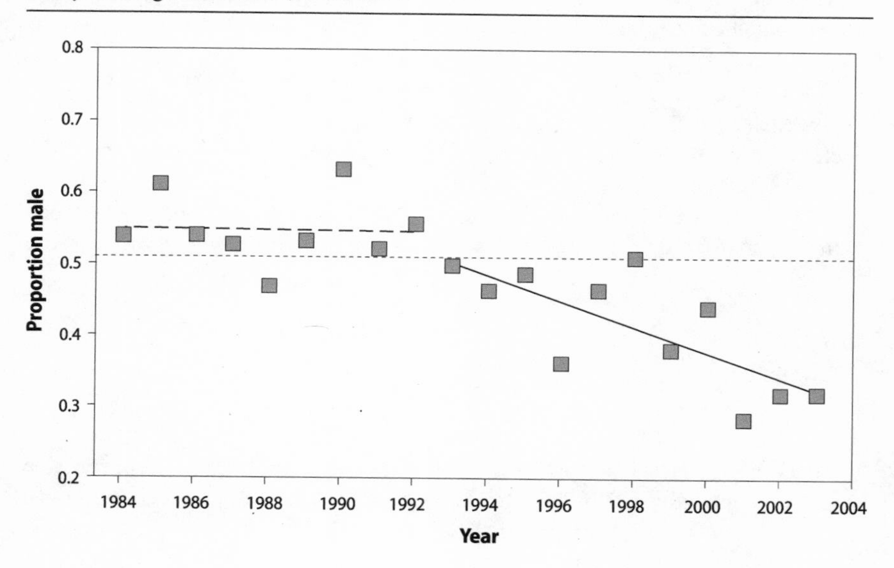

Note: The dotted line is the expected male proportion for Canada (0.512). The dashed line is the linear regression line for the period 1984–1992; $r^2 = 0.000$; slope not significantly different from zero ($p = 0.990$). The solid line is the linear regression line for the period 1993–2003; $r^2 = 0.547$; statistically significant deviation of slope from zero ($p = 0.009$).
Source: Adapted from Mackenzie, Lockridge, and Keith (2005). Reproduced with permission.

Appendix 2: Dilbit – Imperial Oil Material Safety Data Sheet, 2002[1]

4. HEALTH HAZARD INFORMATION

Nature of Hazard

Inhalation
High vapour concentrations are irritating to the eyes, nose, throat and lungs; may cause headaches and dizziness; may be anesthetic and may cause other central nervous system effects, including death.

Hydrogen sulphide gas may be released. Hydrogen sulphide may cause irritation, breathing failure, coma and death, without necessarily any warning odour being sensed. Avoid breathing vapours or mists.

Eye Contact
Irritating, but will not injure eye tissue. Hot splashes will cause eye burns and permanent eye damage.

Skin Contact
Low toxicity. Will enter the body through the skin and produce one or more toxic effects on the body. Frequent or prolonged contact may irritate the skin and cause a skin rash (dermatitis).

Exposure to hot material may cause thermal burns. Benzene may be absorbed through damaged skin and may cause blood or blood producing system disorder and/or damage.

Ingestion
Low toxicity.

Chronic
Contains polynuclear aromatic hydrocarbons (PNAs). Prolonged and/or repeated skin contact with certain PNAs has been shown to cause skin cancer. Prolonged and/or repeated exposures by inhalation of certain PNAs may also cause cancer of the lung and of other parts of the body.

Contains benzene. Human health studies (epidemiological) indicate that prolonged and/or repeated overexposures to benzene may cause damage to the blood producing system (particularly the bone marrow) and serious blood disorders including leukemia. Animal tests indicate that benzene does not cause malformations but may be toxic to the embryo/fetus. The relationship of the results to humans has not been established. Studies indicate that benzene is a known human carcinogen. Contains n–hexane. Prolonged and/or repeated exposures may cause damage to the peripheral nervous system (e.g. fingers, feet, arms etc.).

Toxicity Data
Not available for product.

Occupational Exposure Limits

Manufacturer Recommends
Although no specific hygiene standard exists, the workplace exposures to total particulates should be controlled well below a TWA value of 0.2 mg/m^3 polynuclear aromatic hydrocarbon particulates measured as benzene solubles.

ACGIH Recommends
For Hydrogen Sulphide, 10 ppm (14 mg/m3).

For Benzene, the ACGIH recommends a TLV of 0.5 ppm (1.6 mg/m3), and describes it as a confirmed human carcinogen.

For n–Hexane (skin), 50 ppm (176 mg/m3).

Local regulated limits may vary.

1 Data accessed online at http://www.msdsxchange.com/english/show_msds.cfm?paramid1=2479752 through MSDSXchange: http://www.msdsxchange.com/english/. See also Toledano (2015).

Appendix 3: List of Interview Participants

Pseudonym	Interview location	Role
Billy	Aamjiwnaang	Community member
Bob	Aamjiwnaang	Community member
Brenda	Sarnia	Policy official
Bruce	Sarnia	Policy official
Candace and Blair	Aamjiwnaang	Community members
Charlotte	Aamjiwnaang	Community member
Claire	Sarnia	Policy official
Cora	Sarnia	Policy official
Daniel	Ottawa	Policy official
Daryl	Sarnia	Policy official
Dawn	Aamjiwnaang	Community member
Denny	Aamjiwnaang	Community member
Diane	Aamjiwnaang	Community member
DJ	Aamjiwnaang	Community member
Edward	Aamjiwnaang	Community member
Edwin	Aamjiwnaang	Community member
Elle	Aamjiwnaang	Community member
Elliott	Sarnia	Policy official
Ethan	Sarnia	Policy official
Evelyn	Aamjiwnaang	Community member
Frank	Aamjiwnaang	Community member
Gerry	Toronto	Policy official
Glen	Sarnia	Policy official
Heidi	Aamjiwnaang	Community member
Henry	Sarnia	Policy official
Jake	Ottawa	Policy official
John	Sarnia	Policy official
Ken	Aamjiwnaang	Community member

Pseudonym	Interview location	Role
Kier	Sarnia	Policy official
Kimberly	Aamjiwnaang	Community member
Kirk	Aamjiwnaang	Community member
Kory and Tammy	Aamjiwnaang	Community members
Kurt	Sarnia	Policy official
Larry and Sonja	Aamjiwnaang	Community members
Lily	Aamjiwnaang	Community member
Lloyd	Sarnia	Policy official
Mike and Tracy	Aamjiwnaang	Community members
Molly	Sarnia	Policy official
Nancy and Bella	Aamjiwnaang	Community members
Nathan	Aamjiwnaang	Community member
Ned	Aamjiwnaang	Community member
Oliver	Sarnia	Policy official
Olivia	Sarnia	Policy official
Quinn	Aamjiwnaang	Community member
Sally	Sarnia	Community member
Sam	Aamjiwnaang	Community member
Sonny	Aamjiwnaang	Community member
Steve	Sarnia	Community member
Stew	Aamjiwnaang	Community member
Tanya	Aamjiwnaang	Community member
Tiffany	Aamjiwnaang	Community member
Tina	Aamjiwnaang	Policy official
Tonia	Sarnia	Community member
Wanda	Ottawa	Policy official
Walter	Aamjiwnaang	Community member
Wendy	Aamjiwnaang	Community member

Appendix 4: Additional Resources

Aamjiwnaang First Nation Health and Environment Committee News Archive. http://www.aamjiwnaangenvironment.ca/archive.html.

Anishinabek Nation. http://www.anishinabek.ca.

Auditor General of Canada. 2002. "2002 October Report of the Commissioner of the Environment and Sustainable Development." http://www.oag-bvg.gc.ca/internet/English/att_c20021002se01_e_12325.html.

Auditor General of Canada. 2009. "Chapter 6: Land Management and Environmental Protection on Reserves." In *2009 Fall Report of the Auditor General of Canada*. http://www.oag-bvg.gc.ca/internet/English/parl_oag_200911_06_e_33207.html.

Chiefs of Ontario, Environment Department. http://www.chiefs-of-ontario.org.

Coulthard, G. 2013. "Four Cycles of Indigenous Struggles for Land and Freedom: Idle No More." Presentation at the Idle? Know More! Event, January 22, Vancouver. https://www.youtube.com/watch?v=L_QruWLRDmc.

EAGLE Project. https://www.culturalsurvival.org/ourpublications/csq/article/the-eagle-project-re-mapping-canada-indigenous-perspective.

Environmental Defence. http://environmentaldefence.ca.

First Nations Environmental Health Innovation Network. http://www.fnehin.ca.

Fiske, J.-A., and A.J. Browne. 2008. *Paradoxes and Contradictions in Health Policy Reform: Implications for First Nations Women*. Vancouver: BC Centre of Excellence for Women's Health.

Honor the Earth. http://www.honorearth.org.

Idle No More. http://www.idlenomore.ca.

Indian and Northern Affairs Canada. 1966. *A Survey of the Contemporary Indians of Canada: Economic, Political, Educational Needs and Policies, Part 1 (The Hawthorn Report)*. October. http://www.collectionscanada.gc.ca/webarchives/20071120104036/http://www.ainc-inac.gc.ca/pr/pub/srvy/sci_e.html.

–. 1967. *A Survey of the Contemporary Indians of Canada: Economic, Political, Educational Needs and Policies, Part 2 (The Hawthorn Report)*. October. http://www.collectionscanada.gc.ca/webarchives/20071120103928/http://www.ainc-inac.gc.ca/pr/pub/srvy/sci3_e.html.

Indigenous Environmental Network. http://www.ienearth.org.

Institute on Governance. http://iog.ca.

Ipperwash Inquiry. 2007. *Report of the Ipperwash Inquiry.* 4 vols. http://www.attorneygeneral.jus.gov.on.ca/inquiries/ipperwash/report/.

LAC (Library and Archives Canada). 1953. "Interprovincial Pipe Line Company: Right of Way over Sarnia Indian Reserve Property." RG2, Privy Council Office, Series A-5-a, vol. 2653, access code 90, item 35978, meeting date 1953–07–06.

McDonald, Elaine, and Sarah Rang. 2007. *Exposing Canada's Chemical Valley: An Investigation of Cumulative Air Pollution Emissions in the Sarnia, Ontario Area.* http://www.ecojustice.ca/reports_publications/exposing-canadas-chemical-valley/.

Ministry of Health and Long-Term Care. 2012. "Public Health Units." http://www.health.gov.on.ca/en/common/system/services/phu.

MOE (Ministry of Environment). 1994. *Statement of Environmental Values: Ministry of Environment.* http://www.ebr.gov.on.ca/ERS-WEB-External/content/sev.jsp?pageName=sevList&subPageName=10001.

Mushkegowuk Environmental Research Centre. http://www.merc-environment.ca.

National Aboriginal Health Organization. http://www.naho.ca/.

Ontario Superior Court of Justice. 2010. "Notice of Application to Divisional Court for Judicial Review." October 9. 528/10; 2012 ONSC 2316.

Palmater, P. 2011. Interview on CBC's *8th Fire,* December. http://www.cbc.ca/8thfire/2011/12/pamela-palmater.html.

Public Health Agency of Canada. 2005. *The Pan-Canadian Healthy Living Strategy.* http://www.phac-aspc.gc.ca/hp-ps/hl-mvs/ipchls-spimmvs-eng.php.

Russell, P. 2010. "Oka to Ipperwash: The Necessity of Flashpoint Events." In *This Is an Honour Song: Twenty Years since the Blockades,* ed. L. Simpson and K. Ladner, 29–46. Winnipeg: Arbeiter Ring.

Truth and Reconciliation Commission of Canada. 2015. *Honouring the Truth, Reconciling for the Future: Summary of the Final Report of the Truth and Reconciliation Commission of Canada.* http://www.trc.ca/websites/trcinstitution/File/2015/Findings/Exec_Summary_2015_05_31_web_o.pdf.

United Nations. 2007. *Declaration on the Rights of Indigenous Peoples.* http://www.un.org/esa/socdev/unpfii/documents/DRIPS_en.pdf.

Notes

Preface

1 The Chemical Valley Emergency Coordinating Organization declares a Code 6 when full traffic control is requested in designated areas. See http://www.caer.ca/cveco/.

2 Video footage of the children's protest can be seen in *Sarnia Observer* (2013).

3 As I discuss in Chapter 7, "Idle No More" is the name of the Indigenous social movement that began in November 2012 when several Indigenous lawyers protested the Conservative government's omnibus legislation Bills C-38 and C-45, which imposed amendments to navigable waterways and reserve lands without substantive consultation. The movement, which began through social media such as Twitter and Facebook, also birthed a national day of action and a series of rallies, blockades, and flash-mobs.

4 This notion of "shelter-in-place" is considered at length by Jackson (2010, 255, 258), who discusses her own ethnographic experience as an anthropologist sheltering-in-place while residing in Sarnia and presents an analysis of the deep-rooted attachment that citizens of Aamjiwnaang have to the "sacred geography" of this place, which is "filled with memories." Jackson's text illuminates some of the ways that Aamjiwnaang has been a place of shelter for past, present, and future generations. See also http://www.caer.ca/shelter-in-place/.

Chapter 1: Skeletons in the Closet

1 The term "Anishinabek" refers to the original people and can be understood as an alternative to the word "Indian." In Ojibwe the term translates as "man made out of nothing," a "spontaneous" being on a path given by the Creator (J. Borrows 2010; Johnston 2005, 15). This term also means "the good people" and includes Odawa, Potawatomi, Ojibway, Chippewa, Mississauga, or Saulteaux (J. Borrows 2010, 241). Numerous Anishinabek communities have longstanding ties to the Great Lakes region, where their traditions and practices take place.

2 It is important to clarify my use of the term "citizenship" with respect to Anishinabek people and culture. As John Borrows (2010, 244) discusses, in any community there are multiple

perspectives on what citizenship denotes, from clan (*dodem*) member and Anishinabek to Canadian, American, and world citizen. Citizens are also part of the polities that make up watersheds, islands, valleys, countries, tribes, cities, reserves, and so on. Therefore, the term "citizen" in this book is conceptualized as site-specific while nuanced in orientation to include the multiplicity of allegiances, affinities, and attachments that embed citizens within local and global human and more-than-human communities.

3 There is an emerging group of scholars in Canada who are researching Indigenous environmental justice, such as the contributors to *Speaking for Ourselves: Environmental Justice in Canada* (Agyeman et al. 2009), in addition to numerous other authors, many of whom are cited in this book: Taiaiake Alfred, Isabel Altamirano-Jiménez, Patricia Monture Angus, John Borrows, Jeff Corntassel, Basil Johnston, Erin Marie Konsmo, Bonita Lawrence, Deborah McGregor, Val Napoleon, Pamela Palmater, Dayna Scott, Leanne Simpson, and Jessica Yee, among others. Organizations like the Native Youth Sexual Health Network in Canada and SisterSong in the United States continue to be at the forefront of scholarship on environmental reproductive justice. Globally, several others are actively contributing to this fledgling field from a radical, Indigenous, and eco-feminist orientation, including Elizabeth Hoover, Winona LaDuke, Andrea Smith, Jacinta Ruru, and Linda Tuhiwai Smith.

4 The normalization of living with catastrophe resonates with Morton's (2007, 181) discussion of "dark ecology." Although it may appear that my analysis chimes with Morton's, we depart on normative grounds. I agree that we are all implicated in a "dying world," but I disagree with his contention that we must "stay with it" (ibid., 185). His elaboration that we must not mourn for the environment as a kind of object in need of protection aligns with the view I advance in this book, as does his suggestion that "we are" the environment; however, I do not think justice is served by "preserving the dark, depressive quality of life in the shadow of ecological catastrophe" (ibid., 187). Although there is a realist bent to his eloquent and poetic formulation – indeed, we are embroiled within the "charnel ground" of all kinds of toxins and wastes – his notion is imbued with the privilege of distance (Morton 2013). Whereas he is comfortable staying put, citizens living in marginalized "sacrifice zones" contend with both dark and light ecology on a daily basis (Lerner 2010). Environmental reproductive *justice* – the motivation behind this book – requires further nuance that respects these swirling atmospheres. This contrasts with Morton's (re)production of a dualist analytical lens between "negative desire and positive fulfillment" (Morton 2007, 186). A *sensing policy* approach hones in on the charnel ground of life and death with the aim of untangling and reformulating these to create space for living otherwise.

5 The conception of "wound" advanced in this book follows Scott's (2008, 306) analysis, with reference to cultural anthropologist Sarah Jain, and highlights some of the ways that harms occur beyond a purely legalistic definition of "injury." Scott develops the argument that tort law governs accidental harms, whereas chronic, low-dose exposure to toxic chemicals is a central and inherent consequence of production itself, inextricable from a process of continuous "wounding." This understanding aligns with Nixon's (2011) concept of "slow violence."

6 For further details, see Ontario Ministry of Environment O-Reg 419/05.

7 A "bucket brigade" is a practice undertaken by the community to test air quality with individual buckets – affectionately referred to as "sniffers." The buckets are used to collect air samples in the event of a chemical spill. "Biomonitoring" refers to assessing the measurement of an individual's "body burden" and toxic chemical composition. "Body-mapping" entails gathering data about health concerns and mapping these onto large body-size posters to create a visual representation of a community's body burden.

8 About seventy kilometres away from Aamjiwnaang, this site generated attention when Indigenous protestor Dudley George was shot and killed by a member of the Ontario Provincial Police in 1995. In 2007 a provincially sanctioned inquiry completed its findings and revealed a lengthy story of state expropriation of this land base during the Second World War to build an army camp. Although some First Nations citizens now reside at the former military site on their traditional territory – in abandoned barracks – relationships among the Kettle and Stony Point First Nations continue to be in flux.

9 *Hello, I'm called Sarah. I'm from Vancouver. I am twenty-seven winters old. I am a friend of the Anishinabek.* I introduce myself in this way to illuminate the relationships I have to myself, where I was raised over the years, and recent relationships that inform the pages here. This type of introduction is commonplace in Aamjiwnaang, indicative of the importance of the embeddedness of individuals within their locales.

10 Grosz contrasts Nietzsche's emphasis on the bodily "will to power" with Foucault's focus on docility and resistance, which is to be further distinguished from Deleuze and Guattari's discussion of "becoming and transformation." Despite these variances, each theorist seeks to undermine the "pretensions of consciousness" and to critique the liberal subject's control *over* the body. Each emphasizes the capacity of the body as a generative force of social relations to counter mainstream Western philosophy's conceptual blind spot, which gives credence to a dichotomous and hierarchical ranking of the mind's superiority. I position myself in these debates somewhere between Foucault's approach and that of Deleuze and Guattari to examine the body as being bound up within power relations and simultaneously a regenerative force.

11 MacGregor (2006, 84–96) highlights three trends in contemporary approaches to ecological citizenship that are based on green theory: first, calling for sustainability and the communitarian "greening of citizenship"; second, regarding citizenship as a kind of practice of "ecological stewardship"; and third, treating individuals as "earth citizens in global society." Her feminist critique of this literature astutely highlights the subjectivity of a gender-neutral citizen embedded within this scholarship. In addition to her well-articulated criticisms, I would add that the absence of "place" in the claims making of green citizens in this literature is notable, as it heralds an atomistic yet globalized ethics for environmental citizens and emphasizes changes to "lifestyle choices" as a precondition for agency in the public sphere. A placed account of ecological citizenship accentuates the limits of this model for "active participation" in both private and public realms.

12 Laurence Butet-Roch selected each photograph as a visual representation of the accompanying text. Her documentary photography project *Our Grandfathers Were Chiefs* began in 2010, as did our collaboration. See http://www.borealcollective.com and http://www.lbrphoto.ca/. While I lived in Sarnia from January 2011 until August 2012, she continued to visit the community and to cultivate rich relationships throughout her long-term project.

Chapter 2: Sensing Policy

1 A caveat: Jenson and Papillon (2000) discuss significant challenges that the James Bay Cree posed to the Canadian political landscape and Canada's citizenship regimes, and Papillon (2008a) elaborates upon these challenges at length. Although rich and rooted in practices of political engagement, these studies remain at the macro (state) and meso (executive Aboriginal) levels, thus overlooking community-based lived experience at the micro (local) level. Their analysis scales up without scaling down, providing an incomplete account of

governmentality's effects on the ground. Kiera Ladner discusses treaty federalism at length in Ladner (2003b).

2 For a comprehensive critique of "recognition" in political thought and practice, see Coulthard (2011).

3 A chronological analysis of the Indian Act reveals some of the discursive practices that have shaped the access of Indigenous women to citizenship rights in Canada. To decode the ways that these practices inform perceptions of Indigenous women, citizenship, and nationhood, Fiske (2008) argues that the Indian Act was a sexist, patriarchal document that stripped Aboriginal women of their place in their communities. It was not until an amendment to this Act in 1985 that women who married nonstatus men could retain their Indigenous status; however, at the same time, they lost their right to collective property. The control over status itself remained, and still remains, under the authority of the federal government. As an alternative, Fiske argues for sororal citizenship, where women's reproductive roles can be conceptualized at the centre of society, and for an identity and membership grounded in relationships of mutual respect and responsibility constituted through women united by kinship and social ties. This social praxis requires reimagining citizenship from the perspective of caregivers vis-à-vis consumers. In effect, Fiske argues that we need to respect the right "to be" a citizen other than as a market consumer and producer. Language that makes citizens into "producers and consumers" is also a concern of scholars who centre their analyses on a decline of the welfare state and the formation of an increasingly hollow state.

4 My research assistance in the community for a one-year period prior to the commencement of my own research project greatly enhanced access to and relationship building with the community. I also benefited from participating in various decolonizing methodology workshops, such as the "Toward Decolonizing Methodologies" workshop, organized by the University of Ottawa's Forum for Aboriginal Studies Research, which brought academic and policy-making experts together with members of ethics boards and Indigenous communities, who made themselves available to provide guidance to graduate students interested in conducting fieldwork with Indigenous communities.

5 It is important to note that in several instances "policy makers" include community members who served on the band council or the Health and Environment Committee and those who worked at the Aamjiwnaang Environment Department. Thus it is too simple to cleanly distinguish "citizen" from "policy maker." Chapter 4 focuses on the narratives of those living on or close to the reserve, and Chapter 6 offers an account of those speaking in a more official capacity.

6 *Indian Givers* is a mixed-art documentary film produced by the Kiijig Collective (2012), based in Sarnia and Aamjiwnaang. Made collaboratively by and for Native and non-Native youth, it was shot and edited by Ian Alexander of Rocketship Productions and by Sadie Mallon, who is a student at Sarnia Collegiate Institute and Technical School. This sixty-minute film invites the audience to take a journey with the protagonists by stepping into their lives as they reveal the survival of their spiritual identities in today's world.

7 Such meaning-making practices taking shape in Aamjiwnaang are eloquently depicted by Kevin R. Smith (2008), who draws on health geography literature to discuss emergent concerns around Aamjiwnaang's "contaminated therapeutic landscape." His work addresses some of the ways that language, symbolism, ideology, and meaning affect the physical, emotional, and spiritual health of a particular place.

8 Indigenous academic Leanne Simpson takes this point further, noting how Indigenous people are all too often perceived as "resources" on lands available for exploitation rather than as people (N. Klein 2013).

9 Thinking through the reserve's social location intersects with notions of race, space, and gender. Taking a cue from intersectionality, I discuss the gendered scope of reproductive politics and struggles for reproductive justice elsewhere at length (Wiebe and Konsmo 2014).

10 The distinction between "environmental" and "ecological" is an important one for my unfolding argument. Whereas much of the literature on green governmentality and environmental citizenship emphasizes responsibilities *for* the environment, I employ the term "ecological citizenship" to refer to an ongoing, relational, and interactional approach to the more-than-human world. The term "ecological citizenship" is all too often co-opted by formal public discourse to instrumentalize citizen behaviour and to maintain a stewardship demarcation between humans and the more-than-human environment. See, for example, the discussion of "environmental citizenship" as a "personal journey" in Environment Canada (2005). This kind of greening language is also discussed at length in Darier (1996) and MacGregor and Szerszynski (2003).

11 The preamble to the Anishinabek Nation Constitution depicts these values in the Seven Grandfather Teachings: *zaagidwin* (love), *debwewin* (truth), *mnaadendmowin* (respect), *nbwaakaawin* (wisdom), *dbaadendiziwin* (humility), *gwekwaadziwin miinwa* (honesty), and *aakedhewin* (bravery). Although each of these teachings is equally important, *mnaadendmowin*/respect is considered to be a guiding principle for one's relationship with Mother Earth as a living being. See Anishinabek Nation (2015).

12 Mike is an elder from the community whose name has been used in this book with consent. The following is from a public online post by the same individual: "What is environment to you? To me, it is Bimaadziwin. Way of life. It is our life. It is all of Creation's life. It is the Seven Grandfather teachings. It is the teachings in the Medicine Wheel, circle of life. It is Human rights, Creation's rights to a comfortable and enjoyable way of living. It is maintaining, as caretakers of Mother Earth, in her entirety, sustainable beauty and flourishing entity. It is being responsible and caring. The Seven Grandfather teachings says it all. Environment is RESPECT, HONOUR, WISDOM, BRAVERY, HUMILITY, TRUTH, LOVE. IF INDUSTRY COULD ONLY UNDERSTAND THIS CONCEPT OF LIFE, AND OPERATE THIS WAY, MAYBE OUR ENVIRONMENT, OUR WAY OF LIFE, WOULD BE MORE CLEANER, MORE ENJOYABLE, MORE LIFE-LONG. We could enjoy our grandchildren, our great grandchildren, and the beauty Mother Earth gives us. MONEY – only gives us temporary satisfaction ... not a long life. It may be nice to make the money in these industries, but how long are we guaranteeing our children, our life for them. ENVIRONMENT IS BIMAADZIWIN."

Chapter 3: State Nerves

1 The concept of the "Indian" in Canadian law, policy, and discourse is charged with contested meaning. The term "Indian" is used here in direct reference to the Indian Act. This Act came into effect under Section 91(24) of the 1867 Constitution Act, which gave the federal government the exclusive authority to legislate in relation to "Indians and Land Reserved for Indians." The legislative authority over these relationships now resides with the federal minister of Aboriginal Affairs and Northern Development. Despite the explicit language in the Indian Act referring to "Indians" within Canada, this chapter uses the term "Indigenous peoples," as the concept of the "Indian" in Canada is itself a misinformed colonial creation, as discussed further by Ladner (2003a, 44). Aligned with Alfred and Corntassel (2005), I employ "Indigenous peoples" and use "Indian" only with respect to law or policy that uses this term.

2 This picture also fails to capture the vibrant life, scope, and breadth of Indigenous wellness prior to the Indian Act and prior to settler contact. As volume three of the RCAP report reveals, at the time of first contact with Europeans, Indigenous peoples for the most part enjoyed good health (RCAP 1996). As discussed by the Truth and Reconciliation Commission of Canada (2015), for over a century the Canadian government aimed to eliminate Aboriginal governments, ignored rights and treaties, outlawed venues for Aboriginal spirituality like the potlatch and the sun dance, and embarked on a program of "cultural genocide." It is now well known that Indigenous health and traditions encompass a range of culturally based healing strategies, which include sharing, healing, talking circles, sweats, ceremonies, fasts, feasts, celebrations, vision quests, and traditional medicines (Aboriginal Healing Foundation 2006; RCAP 1996). These practices and traditions predate Canadian Confederation. Creating spaces for them is crucial in the present. Doing so respects Indigenous ways of life and enables the flourishing of a vibrant and holistic approach to Indigenous self-determination for health and wellness.

3 The federal government maintains responsibility for the direct delivery of healthcare services to more than 1 million people, including status Indians living on reserves, Inuit, members of the Canadian Forces, staff of the Royal Canadian Mounted Police, eligible veterans, federal prison inmates, and refugee claimants (Picard 2011). The federal government is also responsible for public health programs and health protection measures, including food safety, regulation of pharmaceuticals and medical devices, and consumer safety. At approximately $3.3 billion a year, the federal health budget is larger than the total budget of most provinces (ibid.). Approximately one-third of the budget is allocated to health research.

4 Only Treaty 6, one of the numbered post-Confederation treaties, contained a specific "medicine chest" clause, which was awarded literal meaning by the Saskatchewan Court of Appeal in *Regina v. Johnston* (Craig 1992, 7). According to this treaty, Her Majesty agreed that a "medicine chest shall be kept at the house of each Indian Agent for the use and benefit of the Indians at the discretion of such agent" (ibid., 15). The decision in *Regina v. Johnston* found that the treaties do not give the federal government any greater legislative authority or jurisdiction than it already had. Treaties 7, 8, 10, and 11 may have made comparable provisions; consequently, some First Nations contend that they are entitled to health services as an inherent treaty right.

5 Whether this is the appropriate avenue for reconciliation remains an outstanding contentious concern (see de Costa 2009, 2013; James 2006, and Woolford 2013).

6 Ecological politics, feminism, and citizenship intersect with struggles for environmental reproductive justice. As MacGregor (2006, 6) explains, a project of "feminist ecological citizenship" considers the merits of a political approach to citizenship that engages with nonessentialist and democratic dimensions of political life. Although this book does not focus on debates within eco-feminism, in crafting an approach to *sensing policy*, it responds to MacGregor's call for us to think politically about the gendered conditions of political life itself and to reimagine relationships between the human and more-than-human worlds, both of which are required of those undertaking struggles for environmental reproductive justice.

7 According to Aboriginal Affairs and Northern Development Canada, "Health services for First Nations and Inuit are the responsibility of provincial, territorial and federal governments. The provinces/territories provide and/or pay for insured physician and hospital services. The federal government provides treatment and public health services in remote areas and public health services in non-isolated First Nation communities through the First

Nations and Inuit Health Branch of Health Canada. Services include community preventive health and health promotion programs and services and environmental health surveillance. Emergency diagnostic and treatment services are provided by the Medical Services Branch (MSB) when not available otherwise. Healthcare premiums in Alberta and British Columbia are also covered. In Yukon, Nunavut, and the Northwest Territories, the territorial governments are responsible for medical and health services." See https://www.aadnc-aandc.gc.ca/eng/1100100028564/1100100028566#hcca. Furthermore, over 50 percent of Indigenous people live off-reserve and increasingly access healthcare through provincial services and local health authorities. For details, see Browne, McDonald, and Elliott (2009).

Chapter 4: Home Is Where the Heart Is

1 Visitors to Chemical Valley will most likely experience a range of odours, from "sour" to "tarry" to "rotten egg," according to a 2002 "Imperial Oil Material Safety Data Sheet" (see Appendix 2). The data sheet continues, "High vapour concentrations are irritating to the eyes, nose, throat and lungs; may cause headaches and dizziness; may be anesthetic and may cause other central nervous system effects, including death. Hydrogen sulphide gas may be released. Hydrogen sulphide may cause irritation, breathing failure, coma and death, without necessarily any warning odour being sensed. Avoid breathing vapours or mists."
2 The sweep resulted in the issuing of thirty-two provincial offender orders (MOE 2005). Some violations were referred to MOE's Investigations and Enforcement Branch for follow-up. Concerns included fugitive emissions and steam-powered flare stacks burning multiple waste streams. MOE also identified recurring problems tracking waste-management practices and processes.
3 Since this interview took place, the Environment Department hired a full-time employee to monitor the Environmental Bill of Rights website.
4 Personal correspondence with the author, June 27, 2012.

Chapter 5: Digesting Space

1 Brownfield sites are vacant or underutilized places where past industrial or commercial activities may have left behind contamination in the form of chemical pollution. See http://www.ontario.ca/page/brownfields-redevelopment.
2 He was subsequently charged under the Criminal Code of Canada for nuisance, in addition to endangering the public (Huebl 2005).
3 For more on the issue of a regulatory gap, see Mackenzie (2013) and Moffat and Nahwegahbow (2004).
4 The primary sources for this history of the Aamjiwnaang First Nation are materials in the "Native Box," catalogued as 10(4), box 6, particularly files 10DA-D, Lambton Room, Lambton County Library, Wyoming, Ontario.
5 These sales were controversial, as they were largely enacted through the authority of federal "land agents." The Aamjiwnaang First Nation commenced legal action, declared title to unsurrendered land, and sought damages for trespass and breach of fiduciary duty. Referred to as the *Chippewas of Sarnia/Malcolm Cameron* case, this claim was rejected by the Ontario Court of Appeal in December 2000 through the court's use of "judicial discretion." According to Assembly of First Nations Resolution 31, the court ignored Section 35 of the Canadian Constitution, which recognizes and affirms Aboriginal treaty rights. Resolution 31 also

noted that the court had failed to apply Section 35, unlike in the *Sparrow, Gladstone,* and *Delgamuukw* Supreme Court cases.

6 During this time, the Sarnia Band voted to have the Kettle Point and Stony Point reserves surveyed and subdivided. Many community members resisted a survey, due to fears that it would open up the door to the sale of their land and resources. Deputy Minister of Indian Affairs Duncan Campbell Scott governed as an influential federal official who oversaw and implemented Indian policy. During his leadership, the Department of Indian Affairs sought to formally create two bands in 1919: the Sarnia Band and the Kettle and Stony Point Band.

7 Details about municipal annexations can be found in City of Sarnia (2013), which notes the relocation in 1955 of the community of Bluewater, whose former site lies just across the highway from Aamjiwnaang.

8 According to the *Sarnia Observer* (1958), the client interested in the reserve land was kept a secret by the Crown Trust Company.

9 New England Industries, an American development, mining, pulp, chemical, shipping, and investment corporation, provided a plan to purchase all of the Indian reserve lands in Sarnia for general industrial development. The company stated that it was not buying this land as a "wildcat speculator," and it pledged to align itself with industries already in Sarnia as well as other cooperating industries. Its intent was to develop the area as an "industrial park" through direct site resale or by building on a lend-lease basis. On March 22, 1957, the band council agreed to a land surrender in exchange for close to $9 million and the company's promise that it would build a "model riverfront village for all Indians families involved." Half of the purchase price was to be distributed among the 457 band members, and the remainder was to be placed "in trust" with the federal government on behalf of the Indian citizens. See Nicholson (1959).

10 According to Indigenous and Northern Affairs Canada (2013), the term "locatee" refers to band members with the right to occupy and to lease out land, often made official by a certificate of possession.

11 In 1958 negotiations took place between realtors D.B. White and Sons and representatives of the Toronto-based Crown Trust Company. It is not clear what role band members themselves played in these high-level, high-stakes deliberations. It was also suggested during this time that "locatees" would be forced to move their homes to the proposed 361-acre "Indian Village." Immediately following the land surrender, payments would go to the receiver general, subject to terms approved by the Crown.

12 In addition to this dealing, two other negotiations remained underway yet in the background. One was with the city regarding a sewage treatment plant, which on December 9 saw the band council vote in favour of selling five acres of reserve land to the city for $29,000 for the city's new multimillion-dollar sewage disposal unit. Another was with the Ontario Hydro-Electric Power Commission for a new transformer station. Thus industrial encroachment has perpetually pinched the geopolitical landscape of this community from all angles. For details, see Government of Canada (1959) and Government of Ontario (1960).

13 Archival notes reveal that the land was independently appraised at $5.5 million, and Veterans' Lands Act officials appraised buildings and other improvements at $250,000. See LAC (1959a).

14 For details on Cabinet conclusions, see LAC (1959a, 1959b, 1959c).

15 See also Government of Canada (1960, 1963).

16 In June 1978 the Ontario Superior Court of Justice dismissed the Chippewas' land claims for "fairly legal and complicated reasons." Specifically, because the Crown has the right to

grant title to Indian reserve land, there was no claim against the lands by the Indians under the Registry Act, and there existed "no prior knowledge" that Indians "owned" the land (*Sarnia Observer* 1978). Members of the Jacobs family had received land from the band council upon enfranchisement, and since this land was no longer registered under the Indian Land Act, it did not require a government proclamation to be mortgaged or sold. It could be treated like any other private property. In September of that year, the band was refused the right to appeal the decision.

17 As stated in the *Sarnia Observer*, local member of Parliament and minister of employment and immigration Bud Cullen had been informed about the situation (Stevenson 1978). It was the second time that the band had requested ministerial intervention regarding a disputed land claim that summer.

Chapter 6: Seeking Reproductive Justice

1 Worldwide, the sex ratio of human live births is remarkably constant, ranging between 102 and 108 male to 100 female live births; in Canada, the sex ratio is generally reported to be 105 males to 100 females (m = 0.512) (Mackenzie, Lockridge, and Keith 2005). In Aamjiwnaang an analysis of the most recent interval period (1999-2003) revealed that nearly two females were being born for each male (m = 0.348) (ibid.).

2 The study's coauthors used linear regression to model the relationship between a scalar y variable and one or more explanatory x variables. The use of one explanatory variable is commonly referred to as "simple regression," whereas more than one explanatory variable is known as "multiple regression."

3 The y variable, which is endogenous (i.e., regressed, responsive, and measured), is the dependent variable, whereas the x variable, which is exogenous (i.e., the regressor or predictor, explanatory, and covariate), is the independent variable. According to the study's "design matrix," x must have a full p value to hold; the p value holds when a "null hypothesis" is rejected as statistically significant. It correlates to the probability of obtaining a test statistic, which can be performed by a chi-square test, to assess the probability distribution. In this study, a Pearson's chi-square test was used to look at the "control group" of a Chippewa First Nation.

4 For example, as cited in Wiebe and Konsmo (2014), historically, many Indigenous communities and First Nations had places for community members whose gender represented both masculine and feminine roles. Whenever gender is discussed in relation to Indigenous peoples, it should be understood that "in Native North America, there were and still are cultures in which more than two gender categories are marked" (Jacobs, Thomas, and Lang 1997, 2).

5 Andrea Smith (2005) observes that examining reproductive justice in an Indigenous context requires recognition of colonialism's ongoing persistence.

6 Weisskopf and colleagues (2003) found that mothers who had consumed large amounts of PCB-contaminated fish from the Great Lakes were more likely to have girls. It is difficult to say how exactly the effects of endocrine disruptors impact the general population; however, there is little doubt that endocrine-disrupting pollutants affect the sexual development of wildlife near Aamjiwnaang.

7 Because hormones are so important to the development and healthy performance of the body's organs, endocrine disruptors have a wide range of potential effects, from damage to the brain and sex organs to decreased sperm production and immune suppression in

adults (De Guerre 2008). They may also be responsible for rising cancer rates, reproductive abnormalities, and declining sperm counts.

8 Whereas this scientific language tends to construct gender changes in animals caused by environmental change as abnormal or simply defective, I seek to challenge this notion and its dominance in environmental discourse. As discussed in Wiebe and Konsmo (2014), Indigenous communities have multifaceted ideas about gender and identity, whereas scientific Western research may tend to fall back upon binaristic gendered concepts. Although providing a comprehensive, gendered, historical account of colonization is beyond the scope of this book, I reiterate here that it is significant to acknowledge the ways that discourse and deliberative processes are "gendering." Perceptions pertaining to the relationship between gender changes and environmental degradation often perpetuate narratives that fail to account for more nuanced and/or Indigenous views of gender.

9 For example, email correspondence between federal policy makers in November 2005 contains the following subject heading: "WHO THE FRIG IS THE LEAD." Obtained through an "access to information and privacy request" under the Access to Information Act.

10 Government documents gathered pertaining to this request were copied to relevant federal authorities, including the Ministry of Health, Ministry of Indian Affairs, and Office of the Auditor General of Canada, as well as to the provincial Ministry of Environment and Ministry of Health and Long Term Care. The request followed a four-hour meeting with representatives of Aamjiwnaang, the Cities of Sarnia, St. Clair, and Point Edward, Occupational Health Clinics for Ontario Workers Incorporated, Health Canada, the Sarnia Community Round Table, the Sarnia-Lambton Environmental Association, Connecting Environmental Professionals of Canada, and the Ontario Ministry of Environment. Correspondence reveals that the core outcome of this meeting was the determination that funding for a health study should come from responsible federal and provincial authorities. It was also noted that funding for the health of the Aamjiwnaang First Nation is a federal, not a local, responsibility.

11 In February 2013 LCHS chair Anne Marie Gillis announced that the board would develop a Sustainability Action Plan to ensure completion of the health study (LCHS 2013).

12 How to work respectfully and effectively with the federal government to conduct ethical health research is a recurring concern, as *regulatory gaps* in Canada affect communities faced with contamination (see Mackenzie 2013; and Moffat and Nahwegahbow 2004). Aamjiwnaang officials noted that Health Canada did provide funding for a feasibility study in 2007-08, which sought to determine the scope of Aamjiwnaang's environmental health concerns, but since that time there has been limited federal involvement with respect to environmental health. According to a report of the First Nations Environmental Health Innovation Network (2008, 5), community members raised the issue of data ownership and analysis, drawing upon their experience with the EAGLE Project, where the First Nations and the government could not reach an agreement on who would conduct the analysis of the raw data, which led to the project's funding being pulled. For more on the EAGLE Project, see http://www.chiefs-of-ontario.org/node/115.

13 Random numbers were assigned to this interview in order to maintain privacy and ensure confidentiality. The original numbers have been removed and randomly selected numbers used in their place.

14 The term "Indian" is used here with reference to the Indian Act, which is a federal act that continues to govern Indigenous peoples across the country today.

15 For the purposes of consultation, "health" is not specifically included under Section 35 of the Constitution, which protects Aboriginal rights. This has caused some officials to note that there are gaps in Canada's constitutional design for policy making regarding on-reserve environmental health.
16 Information on the protocols of the duty to consult and accommodate is available at Indigenous and Northern Affairs Canada (2011). Most government decisions that trigger adherence to these protocols occur at the provincial level. On the role of the Ontario Ministry of Aboriginal Affairs in the consultation process, see https://www.ontario.ca/page/duty-consult-aboriginal-peoples-ontario. For more on the Province of Ontario's Environmental Bill of Rights, see MOE (1994).
17 While conducting participant observation, I attended a series of Regulation 419 meetings in Toronto with members of the Aamjiwnaang Health and Environment Committee, members of the Ministry of Environment, and other environment and public health stakeholders in the province. I also received ongoing email updates. At my first meeting, it was apparent that in the days prior, as part of the Open for Business initiative, the premier had met with industry representatives, whose concerns were consequently given precedence over the interests of environmental stakeholders respecting amendments to the existing regulations. Whereas industry members met directly with the premier, stakeholders present at the meetings met with midlevel public servants. The granting of access to one set of interests over another was striking. Information on this initiative is available in MOE (2012b).

Chapter 7: Shelter-in-Place?

1 Murray Sinclair, introductory *Big Thinking* lecture, Congress of the Humanities and Social Sciences, Ottawa, May 30, 2015, http://congress2015.ca/program/videos.
2 See http://www.huffingtonpost.ca/news/attawapiskat/3.
3 Leanne Simpson (2013) highlights the significance of fish broth as symbolic of hardship and sacrifice.
4 Details about Canada's Truth and Reconciliation Commission are available at http://www.trc.ca/websites/trcinstitution/index.php?p=830. The commission built upon the mandate set out in the 1998 "Statement of Reconciliation" by advocating an ongoing individual and collective process to achieve reconciliation between all those affected by the legacy of Canada's residential schools. In this process, all Canadians are called upon to witness our shared dark past in pursuit of moving toward a brighter future.
5 For the court injunction's impacts on Ron Plain, see Aboriginal Peoples Television Network (2013) and Scott (2013).
6 As an experiential approach to policy making, this framework aligns with the contention of the Canadian Political Science Association's past president Jill Vickers that the discipline must respect gendered ways of knowing and feminist scholarship in theory, method, and practice. Jill Vickers, presidential address, Congress of the Humanities and Social Sciences, Ottawa, June 2, 2015.
7 See Chapter 2's discussion of Tully's (1995, 24–25) conception of "multilogue." Mouffe (2005a, 17, 61) finds her bearings in Tully's work to critique an imperial and monological form of reasoning, oriented toward a postimperial philosophy and practice of constitutionalism.
8 Concerned with political scientist David Held's notion of "cosmopolitan citizenship" and with law professor Richard Falk's notion of "citizen pilgrims," both of which involve shifting

loyalties to an "invisible political community of their hopes and dreams," Mouffe (2005a, 37) gestures toward a new kind of citizenship unhitched to this seeming boundlessness.

9 For more on the compelling significance of witnessing Canada's colonial history, as well as an example of a project that thrusts this history into view, see Indigenous artist Carey Newman's *Witness Blanket,* a large-scale art installation that documents the legacy of Canada's residential schools: http://witnessblanket.ca/.

10 This comment was made by an audience member regarding research, ethics, and filmmaking during a fireside chat with documentary filmmaker Alanis Obomsawin at the University of British Columbia, March 7, 2012. This kind of intersubjective approach draws inspiration from French curator and art critic Nicolas Bourriaud's notion of "relational aesthetics," popularized by art and culture critic Hennessy Youngman (a.k.a. Jayson Musson) in his video clip "Art Thoughtz: Relational Aesthetics": https://www.youtube.com/watch?v=7yea4qSJMx4&feature=related. In this respect, "art" takes shape as a shared and interactive practice. The "audience" is considered to be community, challenging the formation of a strict viewer-object binary. Thus the meanings of these artistic practices are formed collectively, which gestures toward an aesthetics that is more democratic than the aesthetics of a "spectacle" produced only for consumption. In addition to participating in community events and creative endeavours like photography and filmmaking, I also shared resources with community members on an iterative basis. Some of these resources are included in Appendix 4.

References

Aboriginal Affairs and Northern Development Canada. 2014. *Acts*. https://www.aadnc-aandc.gc.ca/eng/1100100032317/1100100032318.

Aboriginal Healing Foundation. 2006. *Final Report of the Aboriginal Healing Foundation*. Vol. 1, *A Healing Journey: Reclaiming Wellness*. http://www.ahf.ca/downloads/final-report-vol-1.pdf.

Aboriginal Peoples Television Network. 2013. "Idle No More Activist Faced Death Threats, Fighting 'Goliath' in Court." March 14. http://aptn.ca/news/2013/03/14/idle-no-more-activist-faced-death-threats-fighting-goliath-in-court/.

Acres Research and Planning Ltd. 1965. *The Sarnia Reserve Industrial Society*. Sarnia, ON: Acres Research and Planning Ltd.

Adkin, L. 2009. *Environmental Conflict and Democracy in Canada*. Vancouver: UBC Press.

Agyeman, J., P. Cole, R. Haluza-DeLay, and P. O'Riley. 2009. *Speaking for Ourselves: Environmental Justice in Canada*. Vancouver: UBC Press.

Alfred, T. 2005. *Wasáse: Indigenous Pathways of Action and Freedom*. Peterborough, ON: Broadview.

–. 2009. *Peace, Power, Righteousness: An Indigenous Manifesto*. Oxford: Oxford University Press.

Alfred, T., and J. Corntassel. 2005. "Being Indigenous: Resurgences against Contemporary Colonialism." *Government and Opposition* 40 (4): 597–614. http://dx.doi.org/10.1111/j.1477-7053.2005.00166.x.

Anderson, B. 2014. *Encountering Affect: Capacities, Apparatuses, Conditions*. Surrey, BC: Ashgate.

Anishinabek Nation. 2015. *Restoration of Jurisdiction*. http://www.anishinabek.ca/roj/anishinaabe-chi-naaknigewin.asp#.

Aristotle. 1962. *Politics*. London: Penguin Classics.

Asch, M. 2014. *On Being Here to Stay: Treaties and Aboriginal Rights in Canada*. Toronto: University of Toronto Press.

Auditor General of Canada. 2009. "Chapter 6: Land Management and Environmental Protection on Reserves." In *2009 Fall Report of the Auditor General of Canada*. http://www.oag-bvg.gc.ca/internet/English/parl_oag_200911_06_e_33207.html.

Auditor General of Canada. 2011. *2011 June Status Report of the Auditor General of Canada*. Ottawa: Government of Canada.

Bargu, B. 2011. "Forging Life into a Weapon." *Social Text*, May 21. http://socialtextjournal.org/periscope_article/the_weaponization_of_life_-_banu_bargu/.

Barry, J. 1999. *Rethinking Green Politics: Nature, Virtue and Progress*. London: Sage.

–. 2002. "Vulnerability and Virtue: Democracy, Dependency and Ecological Stewardship." In *Democracy and the Claims of Nature*, ed. B. Minteer and B.P. Taylor, 133–52. Lanham, MD: Rowman and Littlefield.

Bellamy, M. 2007. *Profiting the Crown: Canada's Polymer Corporation, 1942–1990*. Montreal and Kingston: McGill-Queen's University Press.

Bertram, L. 2011. "Resurfacing Landscapes of Trauma: Multiculturalism, Cemeteries and the Migrant Body, 1875 Onwards." In *Home and Native Land: Unsettling Multiculturalism in Canada*, ed. M. Chazan, L. Helps, A. Stanley, and S. Thakkar, 157–74. Toronto: Between the Lines.

Borrows, J. 2002. *Recovering Canada: The Resurgence of Indigenous Law*. Toronto: University of Toronto Press.

–. 2010. *Canada's Indigenous Constitution*. Toronto: University of Toronto Press.

–. 2013. "*Maajitaadaa:* Nanaboozhoo and the Flood, Part 2." In *Centering Anishinaabeg Studies: Understanding the World through Stories*, ed. J. Doerfler, N.J. Sinclair, and H. Stark, ix–xiv. Winnipeg: University of Manitoba Press.

Borrows, L. n.d. "Otter's Journeys: Indigenous Language and Legal Revitalization." Unpublished manuscript.

Bowen, N. 1994. "Lack of Communication Caused Evacuation Problems." *Sarnia Observer*, January 26.

–. 2004a. "Battle over Barrels Continues." *Sarnia Observer*, November 3.

–. 2004b. "Cleanup Orders Issued; Ministry of Environment Acts on Chemicals Found at Site on Scott Road." *Sarnia Observer*, May 22.

Boyer, Y. 2004. "First Nations, Metis, and Inuit Health Care: The Crown's Fiduciary Obligation." *NAHO Discussion Paper Series in Aboriginal Health: Legal Issues* (2): 1–55.

Brady, M. 2011. "Researching Governmentalities through Ethnography: The Case of Australian Welfare Reforms and Programs for Single Parents." *Critical Policy Studies* 5 (3): 264–82. http://dx.doi.org/10.1080/19460171.2011.606300.

Braun, B. 2007. "Biopolitics and the Molecularization of Life." *Cultural Geographies* 14 (1): 6–28. http://dx.doi.org/10.1177/1474474007072817.

Brown, W. 1988. *Manhood and Politics: A Feminist Reading in Political Theory*. Totowa, NJ: Rowman and Littlefield.

–. 1995. *States of Injury: Power and Freedom in Late Modernity*. Princeton, NJ: Princeton University Press.

Browne, A.J., H. McDonald, and D. Elliott. 2009. *First Nations Urban Aboriginal Health Research Discussion Paper: A Report for the First Nations Centre, National Aboriginal Health Organization*. Ottawa: National Aboriginal Health Organization. http://www.naho.ca/documents/fnc/english/UrbanFirstNationsHealthResearchDiscussionPaper.pdf.

Bryan, B. 2000. "Property as Ontology: On Aboriginal and English Conceptions of Ownership." *Canadian Journal of Law and Jurisprudence* 13 (1): 3–31.
Bryant, B. 1995. *Environmental Justice: Issues, Policies, Solutions*. Washington, DC: Island University Press.
Bullard, R. 1993. *Confronting Environmental Racism: Voices from the Grassroots*. Boston: South End.
Burnham, P., K. Gilland Lutz, W. Grant, and Z. Layton-Henry. 2008. *Research Methods in Politics*. New York: Palgrave Macmillan.
Butler, J. 1993. *Bodies That Matter: On the Discursive Limits of Sex*. New York: Routledge.
–. 2004. *Precarious Life: The Powers of Mourning and Violence*. London: Verso.
Cairns, A. 2000. *Citizens Plus: Aboriginal Peoples and the Canadian State*. Vancouver: UBC Press.
Campbell, D. 2007. "Geopolitics and Visuality: Sighting the Darfur Conflict." *Political Geography* 26 (4): 357–82. http://dx.doi.org/10.1016/j.polgeo.2006.11.005.
Carruthers, D. 2010. "Plain to Lead Aamjiwnaang First Nation." *Sarnia Observer*, July 12.
CBC. 2008a. "A History of Residential Schools in Canada." http://www.cbc.ca/news/canada/a-history-of-residential-schools-in-canada-1.702280.
–. 2008b. "Stephen Harper's Statement of Apology." June 11. http://www.cbc.ca/news/canada/prime-minister-stephen-harper-s-statement-of-apology-1.734250.
City of Sarnia. 2013. *History of the City Planning Department*. http://www.sarnia.ca/planning.
Clarke, L., and J. Agyeman. 2011. "Shifting the Balance in Environmental Governance: Ethnicity, Environmental Citizenship and Discourses of Responsibility." *Antipode* 43 (5): 1773–800. http://dx.doi.org/10.1111/j.1467-8330.2010.00832.x.
Code, L. 2006. *Ecological Thinking: The Politics of Epistemic Location*. Oxford: Oxford University Press. http://dx.doi.org/10.1093/0195159438.001.0001.
Coulthard, G. 2011. "Subjects of Empire: Indigenous Peoples and the Politics of Recognition in Canada." In *Home and Native Land: Unsettling Multiculturalism in Canada*, ed. M. Chazan, L. Helps, A. Stanley, and S. Thakkar, 31–50. Toronto: Between the Lines.
–. 2014. *Red Skin, White Masks: Rejecting the Colonial Politics of Recognition*. Minneapolis: University of Minnesota Press. http://dx.doi.org/10.5749/minnesota/9780816679645.001.0001.
Craig, B. 1992. "Jurisdiction for Aboriginal Health in Canada." LLM thesis, University of Ottawa.
Cresswell, T. 2004. *Place: A Short Introduction*. Oxford: Blackwell.
Cruikshank, B. 1999. *The Will to Empower: Democratic Citizens and Other Subjects*. Ithaca, NY: Cornell University Press.
Curry, B. 2011. "Cost of Residential School Redress Rising." *Globe and Mail*, November 19.
CVECO (Chemical Valley Emergency Coordinating Organization). 2011. Accessed April 19, 2011. http://www.caer.ca/cveco.html.
Darier, E. 1996. "Environmental Governmentality: The Case of Canada's Green Plan." *Environmental Politics* 5 (4): 585–606. http://dx.doi.org/10.1080/09644019608414294.
Dean, M. 2010. *Governmentality: Power and Rule in Modern Society*. London: Sage.
Debassige, L., and S. Pyne. 2011. "Devilotion/Devolution: Profits from the Wilderness." In *Anishinaabewin NIIZH: Culture Movements, Critical Moments*, ed. A. Corbiere and D.M. Migwans. M'Chigeeng, ON: Ojibwe Cultural Foundation.

de Costa, R. 2009. "Apologia Pro Vita Sua: Truth and Reconciliation in Canada." Paper presented at the Critical Race Conference "Compassion, Complicity and Conciliation: The Politics, Cultures and Economics of 'Doing Good,'" June 5–7, Montreal.

–. 2013. "Indigenous Peoples and Democratic Politics." Paper presented at the Centre for the Study of Democratic Institutions, University of British Columbia, March 1, Vancouver.

De Guerre, M. 2008. *The Disappearing Male*. Documentary. Canadian Broadcasting Corporation.

Deleuze, G., and F. Guattari. 1987. *A Thousand Plateaus: Schizophrenia and Capitalism*. Minneapolis: University of Minnesota Press.

Dixon, D. 2014. "The Way of the Flesh: Life, Geopolitics and the Weight of the Future." *Gender, Place and Culture* 21 (2): 136–51. http://dx.doi.org/10.1080/0966369X.2013.879110.

Dixon, D., and S. Marston. 2011. "Introduction: Feminist Engagements with Geopolitics." *Gender, Place and Culture* 18 (4): 445–53. http://dx.doi.org/10.1080/0966369X.2011.583401.

Dobson, A. 2003. *Citizenship and the Environment*. Oxford: Oxford University Press. http://dx.doi.org/10.1093/0199258449.001.0001.

Dobson, C. 2006a. "Public Health Study Wanted: Industry Aims to Put End to Speculation." *Sarnia Observer*, April 19.

–. 2006b. "Thousands to Be Checked for Chemicals." *Sarnia Observer*, May 31.

–. 2010. "City Firm Mopping Up at Gulf Oil Spill." *Sarnia Observer*, September 9.

Doerfler, J., N.J. Sinclair, and H.K. Stark, eds. 2013. *Centering Anishinaabeg Studies: Understanding the World through Stories*. Winnipeg: University of Manitoba Press.

Dowler, L., and J. Sharp. 2001. "A Feminist Geopolitics?" *Space and Polity* 5 (3): 165–76. http://dx.doi.org/10.1080/13562570120104382.

Dryzek, J. 2000. *Deliberative Democracy and Beyond: Liberals, Critics, Contestations*. Oxford: Oxford University Press.

Ecojustice. 2007a. *Exposing Canada's Chemical Valley: An Investigation of Cumulative Air Pollution Emissions in the Sarnia, Ontario Area*. http://www.med.uottawa.ca/sim/data/Images/Env_Health_Sarnia_air_pollution_report.pdf.

–. 2007b. "Spills to First Nation Lands: A Legal Memo to the Environmental Commissioner of Ontario." September 27.

–. 2010. "Chemical Valley Faces Canada's Charter." Press release, November 1.

Elford, J.T. 1982. *Canada West's Last Frontier: A History of Lambton*. Sarnia, ON: Lambton County Historical Society.

Environment Canada. 2005. *From the Mountains to the Sea: A Journey in Environmental Citizenship*. http://infohouse.p2ric.org/ref/14/13416.pdf.

–. 2012. *St. Clair River Area of Concern*. https://www.ec.gc.ca/raps-pas/default.asp?lang=En&n=FB15DE20-1.

Environmental Protection Agency (EPA). 2011. "Environmental Justice." http://www3.epa.gov/environmentaljustice/.

Epstein, S. 1996. *Impure Science: AIDS, Activism, and the Politics of Knowledge*. Los Angeles: University of California Press.

First Nations Environmental Health Innovation Network. 2008. *Summary Report of Contaminants and Environmental Health: A Discussion Group for First Nations in Ontario*.

August 5. http://www.chiefs-of-ontario.org/sites/default/files/files/NAHO-COO-FNEHIN%20workshop%20draft%20report.pdf.

Fischer, F. 2003. *Reframing Public Policy: Discursive Politics and Deliberative Practices.* Oxford: Oxford University Press. http://dx.doi.org/10.1093/019924264X.001.0001.

–. 2007. "Deliberative Policy Analysis as Practical Reason: Integrating Empirical and Normative Arguments." In *Handbook of Public Policy Analysis: Theory, Politics, and Methods,* ed. F. Fischer, G.J. Miller, and M.S. Sidney, 223–36. Boca Raton, FL: CRC Press.

–. 2009. *Democracy and Expertise: Reorienting Policy Inquiry*. Oxford: Oxford University Press. http://dx.doi.org/10.1093/acprof:oso/9780199282838.001.0001.

Fischer, F., and J. Forester. 1993. *The Argumentative Turn in Policy Analysis and Planning.* Durham, NC: Duke University Press. http://dx.doi.org/10.1215/9780822381815.

Fischer, F., and M.A. Hajer. 1999. *Living with Nature: Environmental Politics as Cultural Discourse*. Oxford: Oxford University Press. http://dx.doi.org/10.1093/019829509X.001.0001.

Fiske, J. 2008. "Constitutionalizing the Space to Be Aboriginal Women: The Indian Act and the Struggle for First Nations Citizenship." In *Aboriginal Self-Government in Canada: Current Trends and Issues,* 3rd ed., ed. Y. Belanger, 309–31. Saskatoon: Purich.

Flanagan, T. 2000. *First Nations, Second Thoughts*. Montreal and Kingston: McGill-Queen's University Press.

Flicker, S., J.Y. Danforth, C. Wilson, V. Oliver, J. Larkin, J.-P. Restoule, C. Mitchell, E. Konsmo, R. Jackson, and T. Prentice. 2014. "'Because we have really unique art': Decolonizing Research with Indigenous Youth Using the Arts." *International Journal of Indigenous Health* 10 (1): 16–34. http://www.mmduvic.ca/index.php/ijih/article/viewFile/13271/pdf_3.

Flicker, S., B. Savan, B. Kolenda, and M. Mildenberger. 2008. "A Snapshot of Community-Based Research in Canada: Who? What? Why? How?" *Health Education Research* 23 (1): 106–14. http://dx.doi.org/10.1093/her/cym007. Medline:17322572

Foucault, M. 1977. *Power/Knowledge: Selected Interviews and Other Writings*. New York: Pantheon.

–. 1994a. "Governmentality." In *The Essential Foucault: Selections from the Essential Works of Foucault, 1954–1984,* ed. P. Rabinow and N. Rose, 229–45. New York: New Press.

–. 1994b. "Nietzsche, Genealogy, History." In *The Essential Foucault: Selections from the Essential Works of Foucault, 1954-1984,* ed. P. Rabinow and N. Rose, 351–69. New York: New Press.

Fridkin, A. 2012. "Decolonizing Policy Processes: An Intersectionality-Based Policy Analysis of Policy Processes Surrounding the Kelowna Accord." In *An Intersectionality-Based Policy Analysis Framework,* ed. O. Hankivsky, 115–31. Vancouver: Institute for Intersectionality Research and Policy, Simon Fraser University.

Fung, K.Y., I. Luginaah, K.M. Gorey, and G. Webster. 2005. "Air Pollution and Daily Hospitalization Rates for Cardiovascular and Respiratory Diseases in London, Ontario." *International Journal of Environmental Studies* 62 (6): 677–85.

Gabrielson, T., and K. Parady. 2010. "Corporeal Citizenship: Rethinking Green Citizenship through the Body." *Environmental Politics* 19 (3): 374–91. http://dx.doi.org/10.1080/09644011003690799.

Garrick, R. 2015. "Sisters Host 'Toxic Tours' of Their Home in Canada's Chemical Valley." *Anishinabek News,* January 7. http://anishinabeknews.ca/2015/01/07/sisters-host-toxic-tours-of-their-home-in-canadas-chemical-valley/

Giese, R. 2008. "How to Fix a Toxic Town." *Chatelaine*, June, 237–48. http://www.chatelaine.com/health/canadas-toxic-town/.

Government of Canada. 1959. *House of Commons Debates*. 24th Parliament, 2nd Session, vol. 4.

–. 1960. *House of Commons Debates*. 24th Parliament, 3rd Session, vol. 5.

–. 1963. *House of Commons Debates*. 25th Parliament, 1st Session, vol. 1.

–. 1969. *Statement of the Government of Canada on Indian Policy, 1969*. http://www.aadnc-aandc.gc.ca/DAM/DAM-INTER-HQ/STAGING/texte-text/cp1969_1100100010190_eng.pdf.

–. 1978. *The Historical Development of the Indian Act*. 2nd ed. Ottawa: Treaties and Historical Research Centre, Indian and Northern Affairs Canada.

–. 1985. *Indian Act*. http://laws.justice.gc.ca/eng/acts/I-5/FullText.html.

–. 1991. "Aboriginal People: History of Discriminatory Laws." November. http://publications.gc.ca/collections/Collection-R/LoPBdP/BP/bp175-e.htm.

Government of Ontario. 1960. *Report of the Royal Commission Appointed to Investigate Charges Relating to the Purchase of Lands in the City of Sarnia by the Hydro-Electric Power Commission of Ontario from Dimensional Investments Limited*.

–. 1993. *Environmental Bill of Rights*. http://www.ontario.ca/laws/statute/93e28.

Grosz, E. 1994. *Volatile Bodies: Toward a Corporeal Feminism*. Bloomington: Indiana University Press.

Gunnarsson, S. 2010. *Force of Nature*. Documentary. National Film Board of Canada.

Hall, B., E. Jackson, R. Tandon, and N. Lall, eds. 2013. *Knowledge, Democracy and Action: Community-University Research Partnerships in Global Perspectives*. Manchester, UK: University of Manchester Press.

Haluza-DeLay, R. 2007. "Environmental Justice in Canada." *Local Government* 12 (6): 557–63.

Hankivsky, O., ed. 2012. *An Intersectionality-Based Policy Analysis Framework*. Vancouver: Institute for Intersectionality Research and Policy, Simon Fraser University.

Hankivsky, O., and A. Christoffersen. 2008. "Intersectionality and the Determinants of Health: A Canadian Perspective." *Critical Public Health* 18 (3): 271–83. http://dx.doi.org/10.1080/09581590802294296.

Hankivsky, O., and R. Dhamoon. 2013. "Which Genocide Matters the Most? An Intersectionality Analysis of the Canadian Museum of Human Rights." *Canadian Journal of Political Science* 46 (4): 899–920. http://dx.doi.org/10.1017/S000842391300111X.

Haraway, D. 1991. *Simians, Cyborgs, and Women: The Reinvention of Nature*. New York: Routledge.

Health Canada. 1979. "Indian Health Policy 1979." http://www.hc-sc.gc.ca/ahc-asc/branch-dirgen/fnihb-dgspni/poli_1979-eng.php.

–. 2003. "A Statistical Profile on the Health of First Nations in Canada: Determinants of Health, 1999 to 2003." http://www.hc-sc.gc.ca/fniah-spnia/pubs/aborig-autoch/2009-stats-profil/index-eng.php#high-sail.

–. 2010. "Your Health at Home – Radio Public Service Announcements." http://www.hc-sc.gc.ca/fniah-spnia/promotion/public-publique/home-maison/radio-eng.php.

–. 2011a. "First Nations and Inuit Health." http://www.hc-sc.gc.ca/fniah-spnia/pubs/finance/_agree-accord/2004_trans_handbook-guide_1/index-eng.php.

–. 2011b. "History of Providing Health Services to First Nations People and Inuit." http://www.hc-sc.gc.ca/ahc-asc/branch-dirgen/fnihb-dgspni/services-eng.php.

Hindess, B. 2002. "Neo-liberal Citizenship." *Citizenship Studies* 6 (2): 127–43. http://dx.doi.org/10.1080/13621020220142932.
–. 2004. "Citizenship for All." *Citizenship Studies* 8 (3): 305–15. http://dx.doi.org/10.1080/1362102042000257023.
Hobson, K. 2013. "On the Making of the Environmental Citizen." *Environmental Politics* 22 (1): 56–72. http://dx.doi.org/10.1080/09644016.2013.755388.
Hoover, E., K. Cook, R. Plain, K. Sanchez, V. Waghiyi, P. Miller, R. Dufault, C. Sislin, and D.O. Carpenter. 2012. "Indigenous Peoples of North America: Environmental Exposures and Reproductive Justice." *Environmental Health Perspectives* 120 (12): 1645–49. http://dx.doi.org/10.1289/ehp.1205422. Medline:22899635
Huebl, S. 2005a. "Chemical Barrels Case Will Go to Trial." *Sarnia Observer,* November 26.
–. 2005b. "Leaky Barrels Case to Be Heard: Local Man Charged for Improper Storage." *Sarnia Observer,* November 23.
Indigenous and Northern Affairs Canada. 2011. "Aboriginal Consultation and Accommodation." http://www.aadnc-aandc.gc.ca/eng/1100100014664/1100100014675.
–. 2013. "Locatee Lease Policy and Directive." https://www.aadnc-aandc.gc.ca/eng/1374091139187/1374091182369.
Ignatieff, M. 2009. *True Patriot Love: Four Generations in Search of Canada.* Toronto: Penguin.
Ingold, T. 2000. *The Perception of the Environment: Essays on Livelihood, Dwelling and Skill.* London: Routledge. http://dx.doi.org/10.4324/9780203466025.
–. 2011. *Being Alive: Essays on Movement, Knowledge and Description.* London: Routledge.
Irlbacher-Fox, S. 2009. *Finding Dahshaa: Self-Government, Social Suffering, and Aboriginal Policy in Canada.* Vancouver: UBC Press.
Isin, E. 1997. "Who Is the New Citizen? Towards a Genealogy." *Citizenship Studies* 1 (1): 115–32. http://dx.doi.org/10.1080/13621029708420650.
–. 2002. *Being Political: Genealogies of Citizenship.* Minneapolis: Minnesota University Press.
–. 2004. "The Neurotic Citizen." *Citizenship Studies* 8 (3): 217–35. http://dx.doi.org/10.1080/1362102042000256970.
Israel, B.A., A.J. Schulz, E.A. Parker, A.B. Becker, and Community-Campus Partnerships for Health. 2001. "Community-Based Participatory Research: Policy Recommendations for Promoting a Partnership Approach in Health Research." *Education for Health* 14 (2): 182–97.
Jackson, D.D. 2010. "Shelter in Place: A First Nation Community in Canada's Chemical Valley." *Interdisciplinary Environmental Review* 11 (4): 249–62. http://dx.doi.org/10.1504/IER.2010.038080.
Jacobs, S.E., W. Thomas, and S. Lang. 1997. "Introduction." *Two-Spirit People: Native American Gender Identity, Sexuality, and Spirituality,* 1–18. Urbana and Chicago: University of Illinois Press.
Jain, S. 2006. *Injury: The Politics of Product Design and Safety Law in the United States.* Princeton, NJ: Princeton University Press.
James, M. 2006. "Do Campaigns for Historical Redress Erode the Canadian Welfare State?" In *Multiculturalism and the Welfare State: Recognition and Redistribution in Contemporary Democracies,* ed. K. Banting and W. Kymlicka, 222–46. Oxford: Oxford University Press. http://dx.doi.org/10.1093/acprof:oso/9780199289172.003.0008.
Jeffords, S. 2010. "Lawsuit Targets Local Industry, Ministry." *Sarnia Observer.* 1 November.
Jeffrey, T. 2011. "Sarnia's Air Canada's Worst." *Sarnia Observer,* 27 September. http://www.theobserver.ca/2011/09/26/sarnias-air-canadas-worst.

Jenson, J., and M. Papillon. 2000. "Challenging the Citizenship Regime: The James Bay Cree and Transnational Action." *Politics and Society* 28 (2): 245–64. http://dx.doi.org/10.1177/0032329200028002005.

Johnston, B. 2005. *Ojibwe Heritage*. Toronto: McClelland and Stewart.

Kavanagh, R.J., G.C. Balch, Y. Kiparissis, A.J. Niimi, J. Sherry, C. Tinson, and C.D. Metcalfe. 2004. "Endocrine Disruption and Altered Gonadal Development in White Perch *(Morone americana)* from the Lower Great Lakes Region." *Environmental Health Perspectives* 112 (8): 898–902.

Keefer, T. 2014. "A Short Introduction to the Two Row Wampum." *Briarpatch*, March 10. https://briarpatchmagazine.com/articles/view/a-short-introduction-to-the-two-row-wampum.

Kelm, M.-E. 1998. *Colonizing Bodies: Aboriginal Health and Healing in British Columbia, 1900–1950*. Vancouver: UBC Press.

Kiijig Collective. 2012. *Indian Givers*. Documentary. https://www.youtube.com/watch?v=pot411GJzdM.

Kinew, W. 2012. "Idle No More Is Not Just an 'Indian Thing.'" *Huffington Post*, December 17. http://www.huffingtonpost.ca/wab-kinew/idle-no-more-canada_b_2316098.html.

Klein, A. 2013. "The Genius of Spence." *NOW*, January 31. https://www.nowtoronto.com/news/story.cfm?content=191010.

Klein, N. 2013. "Dancing the World into Being: A Conversation with Idle No More's Leanne Simpson." *Yes! Magazine*, March 5. http://www.yesmagazine.org/peace-justice/dancing-the-world-into-being-a-conversation-with-idle-no-more-leanne-simpson.

–. 2014. "Missing and Murdered Indigenous Women: No One Saw Anything." *Globe and Mail*, December 20.

Kovach, M. 2009. *Indigenous Methodologies: Characteristics, Conversations, and Contexts*. Toronto: University of Toronto Press.

Kreuter, M.W., C. De Rosa, E.H. Howze, and G.T. Baldwin. 2004. "Understanding Wicked Problems: A Key to Advancing Environmental Health Promotion." *Health Education and Behavior* 31 (4): 441–54. http://dx.doi.org/10.1177/1090198104265597. Medline: 15296628

Kubik, J. 2009. "Ethnography of Politics: Foundations, Applications, Prospects." In *Political Ethnography: What Immersion Contributes to the Study of Power*, ed. E. Schatz, 25–52. Chicago: University of Chicago Press.

Kymlicka, W. 1989. *Liberalism, Community and Culture*. Oxford: Clarendon.

–. 1995. *Multicultural Citizenship: A Liberal Theory of Minority Rights*. Oxford: Clarendon.

–. 2001. *Politics in the Vernacular: Nationalism, Multiculturalism and Citizenship*. Oxford: Oxford University Press. http://dx.doi.org/10.1093/0199240981.001.0001.

–. 2004. *Finding Our Way: Rethinking Ethnocultural Relations in Canada*. Toronto: Oxford University Press.

LAC (Library and Archives Canada). 1959a. "Sale of Portion of Sarnia Indian Reserve Lands to Dimensional Investments Limited." RG2, Privy Council Office, Series A-5-a, vol. 2744, access code 90, item 18112, meeting date 1959–03–07. http://www.bac-lac.gc.ca/eng/discover/politics-government/cabinet-conclusions/Pages/list.aspx?k=Sarnia&.

–. 1959b. "Sale of Portion of Sarnia Indian Reserve Lands to Dimensional Investments Limited." RG2, Privy Council Office, Series A-5-a, vol. 2744, access code 90, item 18129, meeting date 1959–03–14. http://www.bac-lac.gc.ca/eng/discover/politics-government/cabinet-conclusions/Pages/list.aspx?k=Sarnia&.

–. 1959c. "Sale of Sarnia Indian Reserve lands." RG2, Privy Council Office, Series A-5-a, vol. 2744, access code 90, item 18401, meeting date 1959–05–19. http://www.bac-lac.gc.ca/eng/discover/politics-government/cabinet-conclusions/Pages/list.aspx?k=Sarnia&.
Lack, K. 1958a. "New Indian Land Offer Seen: 2nd Meeting Slated Nov. 19." *Sarnia Observer*, November 13.
–. 1958b. "$6,500,000 Sale: 3,000 Acres Purchased by Crown Trust." *Sarnia Observer*, December 20.
Laclau, E., and C. Mouffe. 2014. *Hegemony and Socialist Strategy: Towards a Radical Democratic Politics*. London: Verso.
Ladner, K. 2003a. "Rethinking Aboriginal Governance." In *Reinventing Canada: Politics of the 21st Century*, ed. J. Brodie and L. Trimble, 43–60. Toronto: Prentice Hall.
–. 2003b. "Treaty Federalism: An Indigenous Vision of Canadian Federalisms." In *New Trends in Canadian Federalism*, 2nd ed., ed. F. Rocher and M. Smith, 167–96. Peterborough, ON: Broadview.
LaDuke, W. 1994a. *All Our Relations: Struggles for Land and Life*. Cambridge, MA: South End Press.
–. 1994b. "A Society Based on Conquest Cannot Be Sustained." In *The New Resource Wars: Native and Environmental Struggles against Multinational Corporations*, ed. A. Gedicks, ix–xv. Boston: South End.
–. 1994c. "Traditional Ecological Knowledge and Environmental Futures." *Colorado Journal of International Environmental Law and Policy* 5 (1): 127–48.
–. 1997. "Voices from White Earth." In *People, Land and Community: Collected E.F. Schumacher Society Lectures*, ed. H. Hannum, 22–37. Great Barrington, MA: E.F. Schumacher Society.
Lalonde, M. 1974. *A New Perspective on the Health of Canadians*. Ottawa: Health and Welfare Canada.
Latour, B. 1999. "On Recalling ANT." In *Actor Network and After*, ed. J. Law and J. Hassard, 15–25. Oxford: Blackwell.
LCHS (Lambton Community Health Study). 2007. "Reproductive Health." *Lambton Community 2007 Health Status Report*. Community Health Services Department. Point Edward, ON.
–. 2011. http://www.lambtonhealthstudy.ca/Pages/default.aspx.
–. 2013. "Health Study Board to Create Sustainability Action Plan." February 28. http://www.lambtonhealthstudy.ca/News/Pages/default.aspx.
–. 2014. "Lambton Community Health Study Requests Federal Funding." November 18. http://www.lambtonhealthstudy.ca/News/Pages/default.asp.
–. 2015. "Community Health Study Group Announces Academic Partnership." May 26.
Leadley, T., and G. Haffner. 1996. *The Chippewas of Sarnia Environmental Assessment*. Windsor, ON: Great Lakes Institute for Environmental Research, University of Windsor.
Lerner, S. 2010. *Sacrifice Zones: The Front Lines of Toxic Chemical Exposure in the United States*. Cambridge, MA: MIT Press.
Leslie, John F. 2002. "The Indian Act: An Historical Perspective." *Parliamentary Review* 25 (2): 23–27. http://www.revparl.ca/english/issue.asp?art=255¶m=83.
Loppie, C., and N. Marsden. 2014. "Welcome to the International Journal of Indigenous Health." *International Journal of Indigenous Health* 10 (1): 1–2.
Luginaah, I., K. Smith, and A. Lockridge. 2010. "Surrounded by Chemical Valley and 'Living in a Bubble': The Case of the Aamjiwnaang First Nation, Ontario." *Journal of Environ-*

mental Planning and Management 53 (3): 353–70. http://dx.doi.org/10.1080/0964056 1003613104.

Lynes, K. 2013. *Prismatic Media, Transnational Circuits: Feminism in a Globalized Present.* Global Cinema Series. New York: Palgrave Macmillan.

MacGregor, S. 2006. *Beyond Mothering Earth: Ecological Citizenship and the Politics of Care.* Vancouver: UBC Press.

MacGregor, S., and B. Szerszynski. 2003. "Environmental Citizenship and the Administration of Life." Paper presented at the Citizenship and Environment Workshop, Newcastle University, Newcastle upon Tyne, September 4–6.

Mackenzie, C.A., A. Lockridge, and M. Keith. 2005. "Declining Sex Ratio in a First Nation Community." *Environmental Health Perspectives* 113 (10): 1295–98. http://dx.doi.org/10.1289/ehp.8479. Medline:16203237

Mackenzie, J. 2013. "Environmental Laws on First Nations Reserves: Bridging the Regulatory Gap." In *Site Remediation in B.C.: From Policy to Practice,* 1–29. Vancouver: BC Ministry of Environment and Aboriginal Law Section, Department of Justice Canada.

Madison, S. 2005. *Critical Ethnography: Method, Ethics and Performance.* Thousand Oaks, CA: Sage.

Martineau, J. 2014. "Fires of Resistance." *New Inquiry,* December 12. http://thenewinquiry.com/essays/fires-of-resistance/.

Massaro, V., and J. Williams. 2013. "Feminist Geopolitics." *Geography Compass* 7 (8): 567–77. http://dx.doi.org/10.1111/gec3.12054.

Massey, D. 1994. *Space, Place and Gender.* Minneapolis: University of Minnesota Press.

–. 2005. *For Space.* London: Sage.

Mathewson, G. 1992. "Chippewas of Sarnia Upset by Benzene Leak Evacuation." *Sarnia Observer,* July 14.

–. 2004a. "Guarding the Environment." *Sarnia Observer,* March 31.

–. 2004b. "On the Front Line." *Sarnia Observer,* April 13.

–. 2004c. "Suncor Spill Report Late." *Sarnia Observer,* May 1.

McCaffery, D. 1993. "Communications Problems Mar Evacuation of Reserve: Critics." *Sarnia Observer,* December 16.

McGregor, D. 2009. "Honouring Our Relations: An Anishnaabe Perspective on Environmental Justice." In *Speaking for Ourselves: Environmental Justice in Canada,* ed. J. Agyeman, P. Cole, R. Haluza-DeLay, and P. O'Riley, 27–41. Vancouver: UBC Press.

McGregor, D., and S. Plain. 2013. "Anishinaabe Research Theory and Practice: Place-Based Research." In *Anishinaabewin NIIWIN: Four Rising Winds,* ed. A.O. Corbiere, 93–114. M'Chigeeng, ON: Ojibwe Cultural Foundation.

McKee, L. 2009. "Post-Foucauldian Governmentality: What Does It Offer Critical Social Policy Analysis?" *Critical Social Policy* 29 (3): 465–86. http://dx.doi.org/10.1177/0261018309105180.

Miner, J. 2005. "Drop in Male Births Raises Serious Fears." *London Free Press,* August 19.

Mittelstaedt, M. 2004. "Where the Boys Aren't." *Globe and Mail,* July 31.

–. 2005. "Pollution Debate Born of Chemical Valley's Girl-Baby Boom." *Globe and Mail,* November 15.

MOE (Ministry of Environment). 1990. *Environmental Protection Act.* https://www.ontario.ca/laws/statute/90e19.

–. 1994. *Statement of Environmental Values: Ministry of Environment.* http://www.ebr.gov.on.ca/ERS-WEB-External/content/sev.jsp?pageName=sevList&subPageName=10001.

–. 2005. *Environmental Compliance in the Petrochemical Industry in the Sarnia Area.* http://booksnow1.scholarsportal.info/ebooks/oca10/7/8844.ome/8844.pdf.
–. 2012a. *Environmental Registry.* http://www.ebr.gov.on.ca/ERS-WEB-External/content/about.jsp?f0=aboutTheRegistry.info&menuIndex=0_1.
–. 2012b. *Summary of Standards and Guidelines to Support Ontario Regulation 419: Air Pollution — Local Air Quality (Includes Schedule 6 of Reg. 419 on Upper Risk Thresholds).* https://dr6j45jk9xcmk.cloudfront.net/documents/1426/3-7-5-chemical-abstracts-service-en.pdf.
Moffat, J., and D. Nahwegahbow. 2004. "Roundtable on Environmental Management and the On-Reserve 'Regulatory Gap.'" http://iog.ca/publications/roundtable-on-environmental-management-and-the-on-reserve-regulatory-gap/.
Morden, Paul. 2010. "Health Study Inching Along." *Sarnia Observer,* September 16.
Morton, T. 2007. *Ecology without Nature: Rethinking Environmental Aesthetics.* Cambridge, MA: Harvard University Press.
–. 2013. "Thinking the Charnel Ground (The Charnel Ground Thinking): Auto-Commentary and Death in Esoteric Buddhism." *Glossator* 7: 73–94. https://scholarship.rice.edu/handle/1911/71540.
Mouffe, C. 2005a. *The Democratic Paradox.* London: Verso.
–. 2005b. *On the Political.* New York: Routledge.
Murray, K. 2004. "Do Not Disturb: 'Vulnerable Populations' in Federal Government Policy Discourses and Practices." *Canadian Journal of Urban Research* 13 (1): 50–69.
–. 2007. "Governmentality and the Shifting Winds of Policy Studies." In *Critical Policy Studies,* ed. M. Orsini and M. Smith, 161–84. Vancouver: UBC Press.
Native Women's Association of Canada. 2009. *Sisters in Spirit Research Strategy: Reflecting on Method and Process.* Ottawa: NWAC-SIS Initiative.
NEB (National Energy Board). 2014. "Hearing Order OH-001-2014." In *Trans Mountain Pipeline ULC: Trans Mountain Expansion.* http://www.neb-one.gc.ca/pplctnflng/mjrpp/trnsmntnxpnsn/index-eng.html.
Nicholson, P. 1959. "Cabinet at Ottawa Pass $6,500,000 Deal." *Sarnia Observer,* March 14.
Nixon, R. 2011. *Slow Violence and the Environmentalism of the Poor.* Cambridge, MA: Harvard University Press. http://dx.doi.org/10.4159/harvard.9780674061194.
Ochocka, J., and R. Janzen. 2014. "Breathing Life into Theory: Illustrations of Community-Based Research, Hallmarks, Functions and Phases." *Gateways: International Journal of Community Research and Engagement* 7 (1): 18–33. http://dx.doi.org/10.5130/ijcre.v7i1.3486.
Office of the Environmental Commissioner of Ontario. 2006. "Minutes of the Aamjiwnaang First Nation Transjurisdictional Meeting, January 24, 2006."
Orsini, M. 2007. "Discourses in Distress: From 'Health Promotion' to 'Population Health' to 'You Are Responsible for Your Own Health.'" In *Critical Policy Studies,* ed. M. Orsini and M. Smith, 347–64. Vancouver: UBC Press.
Orsini, M., and M. Smith. 2010. "Social Movements, Knowledge and Public Policy: The Case of Autism Activism in Canada and the US." *Critical Policy Studies* 4 (1): 38–57. http://dx.doi.org/10.1080/19460171003714989.
–, eds. 2007. *Critical Policy Studies.* Vancouver: UBC Press.
Papillon, M. 2008a. *Federalism from Below? The Emergence of Aboriginal Multilevel Governance in Canada: A Comparison of the James Bay Crees and Kahnawá:ke Mohawks.* Toronto: University of Toronto Press.

–. 2008b. “Is the Secret to Have a Good Dentist? Canadian Contributions to the Study of Federalism.” In *The Comparative Turn in Canadian Political Science,* ed. L.A. White, R. Simeon, R. Vipond, and J. Wallner, 123–39. Vancouver: UBC Press.

–. 2009. “Towards Post-colonial Federalism? The Challenges of Aboriginal Self-Determination in the Canadian Context.” In *Contemporary Canadian Federalism: Foundations, Traditions, Institutions,* ed. A.-G. Gagnon, 405–27. Toronto: University of Toronto Press.

Parr, J. 2010. *Sensing Changes: Technologies, Environments and the Everyday*. Vancouver: UBC Press.

Pattenaude, D. 1978. “Chippewas Battle over Ownership of 200 Acres.” *Sarnia Observer,* June 5.

Petersen, M. 2009. “The Lost Boys of Aamjiwnaang.” *Men's Health Magazine*. 5 November. http://www.menshealth.com/health/industrial-pollution-health-hazards.

Petryna, A. 2002. *Life Exposed: Biological Citizens after Chernobyl*. Princeton, NJ: Princeton University Press.

Picard, A. 2011. “Don't Let Leaders Duck Health Issues This Election.” *Globe and Mail,* March 31.

Plain, D. 2007. *The Plains of Aamjiwnaang: Our History*. Victoria, BC: Trafford.

Poirier, J. 2004a. “MOE Wants a Cleanup: Barrels Must Be Cleared by August 3.” *Sarnia Observer,* July 23.

–. 2004b. “Spills Anger First Nation.” *Sarnia Observer,* February 27.

–. 2004c. “‘We've had enough’: Chief Maness Declares Emergency over Barrels.” *Sarnia Observer,* May 20.

–. 2005a. “Gender-Bending Issue Featured in Prestigious Journal.” *Sarnia Observer,* August 18.

–. 2005b. “Natives Need Better Protection.” *Sarnia Observer,* August 18.

Rabinow, P., and N. Rose, eds. 1994. *The Essential Foucault: Selections from the Essential Works of Foucault, 1954-1984*. New York: New Press.

Rancière, J. 2004. “Who Is the Subject of the Rights of Man?” *South Atlantic Quarterly* 103 (2–3): 297–310. http://dx.doi.org/10.1215/00382876-103-2-3-297.

Razack, S. 2002. *Race, Space and the Law: Unmapping a White Settler Society*. Toronto: Between the Lines.

RCAP (Royal Commission on Aboriginal Peoples). 1996. *People to People, Nation to Nation: Highlights from the Report of the Royal Commission on Aboriginal Peoples*. http://www.aadnc-aandc.gc.ca/eng/1100100014597/1100100014637.

Rose, N. 2007. *The Politics of Life Itself: Biomedicine, Power, and Subjectivity in the Twenty-First Century*. Princeton, NJ: Princeton University Press. http://dx.doi.org/10.1515/9781400827503.

Rutherford, S. 2007. “Green Governmentality: Insights and Opportunities in the Study of Nature's Rule.” *Progress in Human Geography* 31 (3): 291–307. http://dx.doi.org/10.1177/0309132507077080.

–. 2011. *Governing the Wild: Ecotours of Power*. Minneapolis: University of Minnesota Press. http://dx.doi.org/10.5749/minnesota/9780816674404.001.0001.

Sarnia Free Press. 1963. “Indian Band to Get $600,000.” September 14.

Sarnia Observer. 1958. “Indians OK Talks for Sale of Land.” August 29.

–. 1977. “Polysar Seeks Right-of-Way from Indians.” June 27.

–. 1978. “Supreme Court Dismisses Chippewas' Land Claims.” June 30.

–. 2011. "Small Fire at Nova." April 11.
–. 2013. "PROTEST: Demonstrators March Near Refinery." January 16. http://www.theobserver.ca/2013/01/16/protest-demonstrators-march-near-refinery.
Schatz, E. 2009. *Political Ethnography: What Immersion Contributes to the Study of Power*. Chicago: University of Chicago Press. http://dx.doi.org/10.7208/chicago/9780226736785.001.0001.
Schlosberg, D. 2013. "Theorising Environmental Justice: The Expanding Sphere of a Discourse." *Environmental Politics* 22 (1): 37–55. http://dx.doi.org/10.1080/09644016.2013.755387.
Schwartz-Shea, P., and D. Yanow. 2012. *Interpretive Research Design: Concepts and Processes*. New York: Routledge.
Scott, D.N. 2005. "Shifting the Burden of Proof: The Precautionary Principle and Its Potential for the Democratization of Risk." In *Law and Risk*, ed. Law Commission of Canada, 50–85. Vancouver: UBC Press.
–. 2008. "Confronting Chronic Pollution: A Socio-legal Analysis of Risk and Precaution." *Osgoode Hall Law Journal* 46 (2): 293–343.
–. 2009. "'Gender-Benders': Sex and Law in the Constitution of Polluted Bodies." *Feminist Legal Studies* 17 (3): 241–65. http://dx.doi.org/10.1007/s10691-009-9127-4.
–. 2013. "The Forces that Conspire to Keep Us 'Idle.'" *Canadian Journal of Law and Society* 28 (3): 425–28. http://dx.doi.org/10.1017/cls.2013.48.
Scott, D.N., and A. Smith. 2012. "The Green Teens of Aamjiwnaang Make the Connection." *Canadian Dimension* 46 (1): 20–21.
Sharp, J. 2011. "Subaltern Geopolitics: Introduction." *Geoforum* 42 (3): 271–73. http://dx.doi.org/10.1016/j.geoforum.2011.04.006.
Shaw, K. 2008. *Indigeneity and Political Theory: Sovereignty and the Limits of the Political*. London: Routledge.
Simeon, R. 2004. *Political Science and Federalism: Seven Decades of Scholarly Engagement*. Kingston, ON: Institute of Intergovernmental Relations, Queen's University.
Simpson, A. 2003. "To the Reserve and Back Again: Kahnawake Mohawk Narratives of Self, Home and Nation." PhD diss., McGill University, Montreal.
Simpson, L. 2011. *Dancing on Our Turtle's Back: Stories of Nishnaabeg Re-Creation, Resurgence, and a New Emergence*. Winnipeg: Arbeiter Ring.
–. 2012. "Aambe! Maajaadaa! (What #IdleNoMore Means to Me)." Blogpost. *Decolonization: Indigeneity, Education and Society*, December 21. https://decolonization.wordpress.com/2012/12/21/aambe-maajaadaa-what-idlenomore-means-to-me/.
–. 2013. "Fish Broth & Fasting." Blogpost. *Divided No More*, January 16. http://dividednomore.ca/2013/01/16/fish-broth-fasting/.
SisterSong. 2013. "What Is Reproductive Justice?" http://sistersong.net/reproductive-justice/.
SLEP (Sarnia Lambton Economic Partnership). 2011. "Key Benefits." http://www.sarnialambton.on.ca/main/ns/20/doc/291/lang/EN.
Smith, A. 2005. *Conquest: Sexual Violence and the American Indian Genocide*. Boston: South End.
Smith, K.R. 2008. "Contaminated Therapeutic Landscape: Perceptions in Aamjiwnaang First Nation." MA thesis, University of Western Ontario.
Smith, L.K., and G. Smith. 1976. *Historical Reference to Sarnia Indian Reserve: Sarnia Indian Reserve Series #4*. Bright's Grove, ON: George Smith.

Smith, L.T. 1999. *Decolonizing Methodologies: Research and Indigenous Peoples.* London: Zed Books.

Soja, E. 1996. *Thirdspace: Journeys to Los Angeles and Other Real-and-Imagined Places.* Cambridge, UK: Blackwell.

–. 2010. *Seeking Spatial Justice.* Minneapolis: University of Minnesota Press. http://dx.doi.org/10.5749/minnesota/9780816666676.001.0001.

Sontag, S. 1997. *On Photography.* New York: Picador.

Spears, T. 2005. "Doctors Fear Pollution Is Skewing Birth Rates." *Ottawa Citizen,* September 8.

Statistics Canada. 2006. "Lambton Community Profile." In *2006 Community Profiles.* http://www12.statcan.ca/census-recensement/2006/dp-pd/prof/92-591/details/Page.cfm?Lang=E&Geo1=CD&Code1=3538&Geo2=PR&Code2=35&Data=Count&SearchText=Lambton&SearchType=Begins&SearchPR=01&B1=All&Custom=.

Stein, M. 2006. "Your Place or Mine: The Geography of Social Research." In *The Sage Handbook of Fieldwork,* ed. D. Hobbs and R. Wright, 59–75. London: Sage.

Stevenson, K. 1978. "Chippewas Lay Claim to Land." *Sarnia Observer,* September 29.

Suleman, Z. 2011. *Vancouver Dialogues: First Nations, Urban Aboriginal and Immigrant Communities.* Vancouver: Social Policy, City of Vancouver.

Taussig, M. 1987. *Shamanism, Colonialism and the Wild Man: A Study in Terror and Healing.* Chicago: University of Chicago Press. http://dx.doi.org/10.7208/chicago/9780226790114.001.0001.

Taylor, C. 1994. "The Politics of Recognition." In *Multiculturalism and the Politics of Recognition,* ed. A. Gutman, 25–74. Princeton, NJ: Princeton University Press.

Thornton, G. 2008. *Being and Place among the Tlingit.* Seattle: University of Washington Press.

Titley, B.E. 1986. *A Narrow Vision: Duncan Campbell Scott and the Administration of Indian Affairs in Canada.* Vancouver: UBC Press.

Toledano, M. 2015. "Enbridge Bailed on Its Own Open House in Aamjiwnaang." *VICE Magazine,* January 27. http://www.vice.com/en_ca/read/enbridge-bailed-on-their-own-open-house-in-aamjiwnaang-911.

Tourism Sarnia-Lambton. 2011. "Discover Bluewater Country." Accessed November 22, 2011. http://www.tourismsarnialambton.com/.

Truth and Reconciliation Commission of Canada (TRC). 2015. *Honouring the Truth, Reconciling for the Future: Summary of the Final Report of the Truth and Reconciliation Commission of Canada.* http://www.trc.ca/websites/trcinstitution/File/2015/Findings/Exec_Summary_2015_05_31_web_o.pdf.

Tuan, Y.-F. 1975. "Place: An Experiential Perspective." *Geographical Review* 65 (2): 151–65. http://dx.doi.org/10.2307/213970.

Tully, J. 1995. *Strange Multiplicity: Constitutionalism in an Age of Diversity.* Oxford: Oxford University Press. http://dx.doi.org/10.1017/CBO9781139170888.

–. 2008a. *Public Philosophy in a New Key.* Vol. 1, *Democracy and Civic Freedom.* Cambridge, UK: Cambridge University Press.

–. 2008b. *Public Philosophy in a New Key.* Vol. 2, *Imperialism and Civic Freedom.* Cambridge, UK: Cambridge University Press.

UBC (University of British Columbia). 2015. *Indigenous Foundations.* http://indigenousfoundations.arts.ubc.ca/home/government-policy/the-indian-act.html.

Waldram, J.B., D.A. Herring, and T.K. Young. 2004. *Aboriginal Health in Canada: Historical, Cultural and Epidemiological Perspectives.* Toronto: University of Toronto Press.

Weir, L. 2006. *Pregnancy, Risk and Biopolitics: On the Threshold of the Living Subject*. New York: Routledge.

Weisskopf, M.G., H.A. Anderson, L.P. Hanrahan, and Great Lakes Consortium. 2003. "Decreased Sex Ratio Following Maternal Exposure to Polychlorinated Biphenyls from Contaminated Great Lakes Sport-Caught Fish: A Retrospective Cohort Study." *Environmental Health* 2: 2–15. http://www.ncbi.nlm.nih.gov/pmc/articles/PMC153540/

Wiebe, S.M. 2010. Review of Linda C. McClain and Joanna L. Grossman, "Gender Equality: Dimensions of Women's Equal Citizenship." *Canadian Journal of Political Science* 43 (4): 1044-45.

–. 2012. "Bodies on the Line: The In/Security of Everyday Life in Aamjiwnaang." In *Natural Resources and Social Conflict: Towards Critical Environmental Security,* ed. M.A. Schnurr and L.A. Swatuk, 215–36. New York: Palgrave Macmillan.

–. 2013. "Affective Terrain: Approaching the Field in Aamjiwnaang." In *Research Methods in Critical Security Studies,* ed. M. Salter and C. Mutlu, 158–61. New York: Routledge.

Wiebe, S.M., and E.M. Konsmo. 2014. "Indigenous Body as Contaminated Site? Examining Reproductive Justice in Aamjiwnaang." In *Fertile Ground: Reproduction in Canada,* ed. F. Scala and S. Paterson, 325–58. Montreal and Kingston: McGill-Queen's University Press.

Wiebe, S.M., and M. Taylor. 2014. "Pursuing Excellence in Collaborative Community-Campus Research." Paper presented at the 2014 CCCR National Summit, Waterloo, November.

Woolford, A. 2013. "Indigenous Peoples and Democratic Politics." Paper presented at the Truth, Reconciliation and Apology Panel, Centre for the Study of Democratic Institutions, March 1, Vancouver.

Wright, H. 2013. "Idle on the Tracks." *Maclean's,* January 21, 36.

Yanow, D. 1998. "Space Stories: Studying Museum Buildings as Organizational Spaces While Reflecting on Interpretive Methods and Their Narration." *Journal of Management Inquiry* 7 (3): 215–39. http://dx.doi.org/10.1177/105649269873004.

–. 2003. "Assessing Local Knowledge." In *Deliberative Policy Analysis: Understanding Governance in the Network Society,* ed. M. Hajer and H. Wagenar, 228–46. Cambridge, UK: Cambridge University Press. http://dx.doi.org/10.1017/CBO9780511490934.010.

Young, I.M. 1989. "Polity and Group Difference: A Critique of the Ideal of Universal Citizenship." *Ethics* 99 (2): 250–74. http://dx.doi.org/10.1086/293065.

Index

Note: "(f)" following a number indicates a figure; "(t)" following a number indicates a table